MW00795271

EMILY'S FRESH KITCHEN

COOK YOUR WAY TO BETTER HEALTH

BY EMILY MAXSON

PHOTOGRAPHS BY BELÉN FLEMING

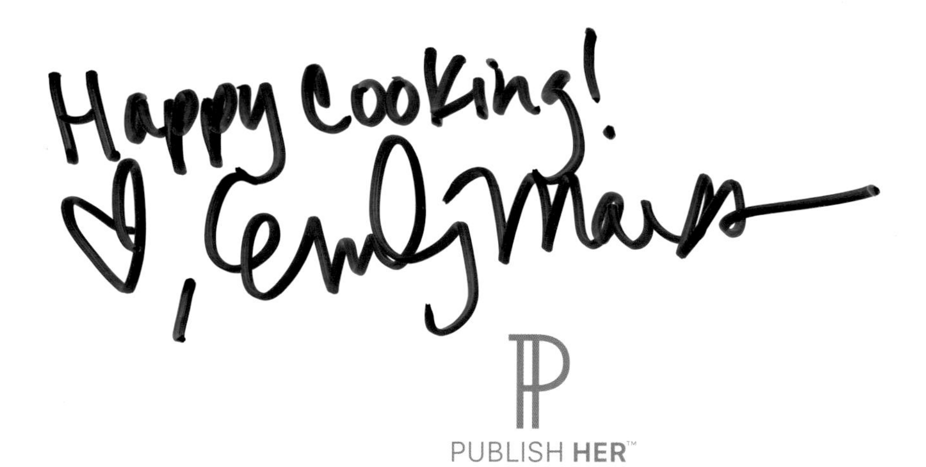

ABOUT THE AUTHOR

After a Crohn's disease diagnosis at age 28 and more than a decade of unsuccessful traditional treatment, Emily Maxson discovered the positive effects of the Specific Carbohydrate Diet and the transformative power of food to improve health. A trained chef, she poured her heart into creating delectable dishes that met the diet's rigorous guidelines. She soon felt better physically, mentally and emotionally. This way of eating, coupled with her faith in God, gave Emily newfound hope for the future. Emily believes preparing food at home is one of the best ways to impact your health and that good food doesn't have to be complicated. With more than 100 delicious recipes that are approachable and adaptable, "Emily's Fresh Kitchen" cookbook is a great starting point for cooking your way to better health.

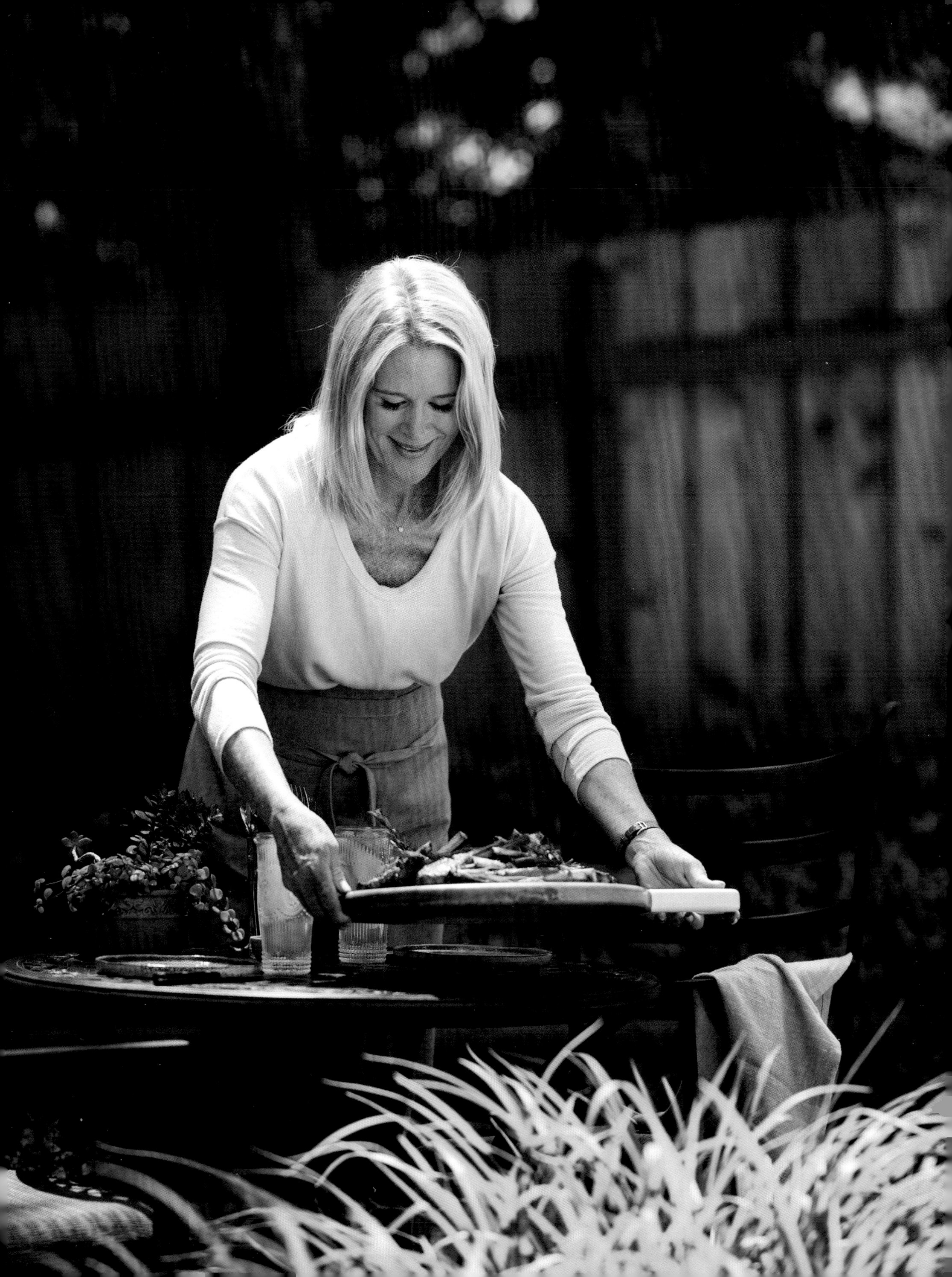

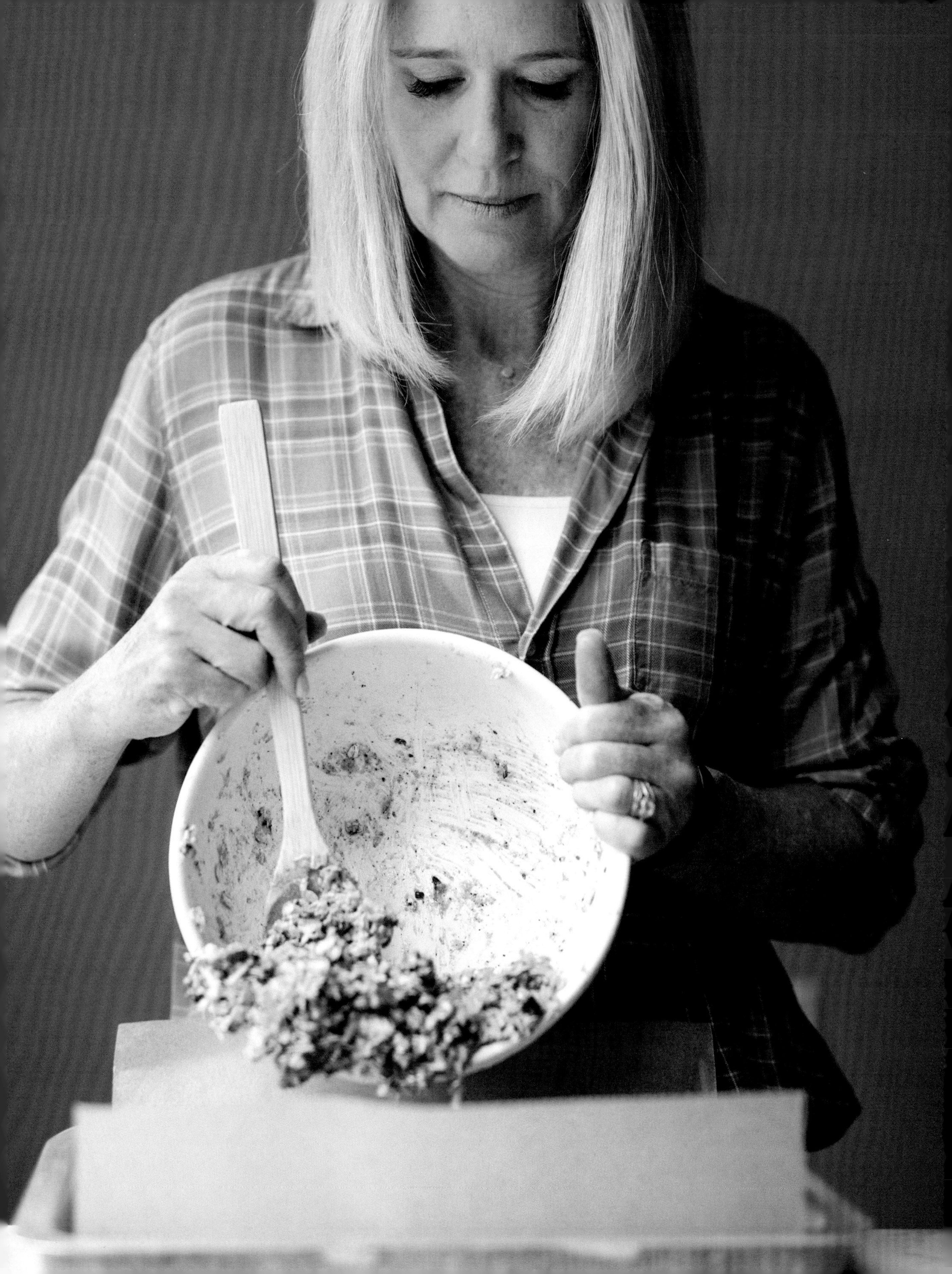

ADVANCE PRAISE

"Emily Maxson understands firsthand the power that food has to help and heal. The recipes in 'Emily's Fresh Kitchen' cookbook are ideal for anyone with food sensitivities or anyone who wants to cook healthier meals. The recipes are easy to follow and delicious, and the photography brings food to life in a stunning way!"

—Chris Freytag, author, speaker and founder of Get Healthy U TV

"'Emily's Fresh Kitchen' cookbook is a testament to the immense impact that the Specific Carbohydrate Diet can have in the healing and recovery of people suffering from inflammatory bowel disease. Leveraging the insights she gleaned from her journey, along with the skills she mastered at culinary school, Emily explored new 'treatments' in her kitchen. Her cookbook delivers the results through thoughtfully developed and delicious recipes presented in vivid photographs. It's an inspiring gift and resource for anyone looking to restore health and well-being with fresh and flavorful food."

—Bernhard J. Hering, MD, director of University of Minnesota Schulze Diabetes Institute

"'Emily's Fresh Kitchen' cookbook is full of colorful, exceptionally flavorful and easy recipes, which fit into many different dietary lifestyles. The meals, snacks and beverages are fun and inspirational, and you'll want to make them over and over again. If eating great food, cooking with seasonal ingredients, and not feeling deprived are your goals, this collection of recipes is a must for your kitchen!"

—Patricia Wall, owner of The Market at Malcolm Yards

"Emily Maxson bringing 'Emily's Fresh Kitchen' cookbook to life is exactly what we all need. Her personal experience pushed her to challenge herself in many ways. The result is more than 100 healthy and approachable recipes that every cook will want to create. She has done all the work and research so we don't have to."

—Chef Michael Shaughnessy, executive chef and owner of Advellum Vegetable Eatery

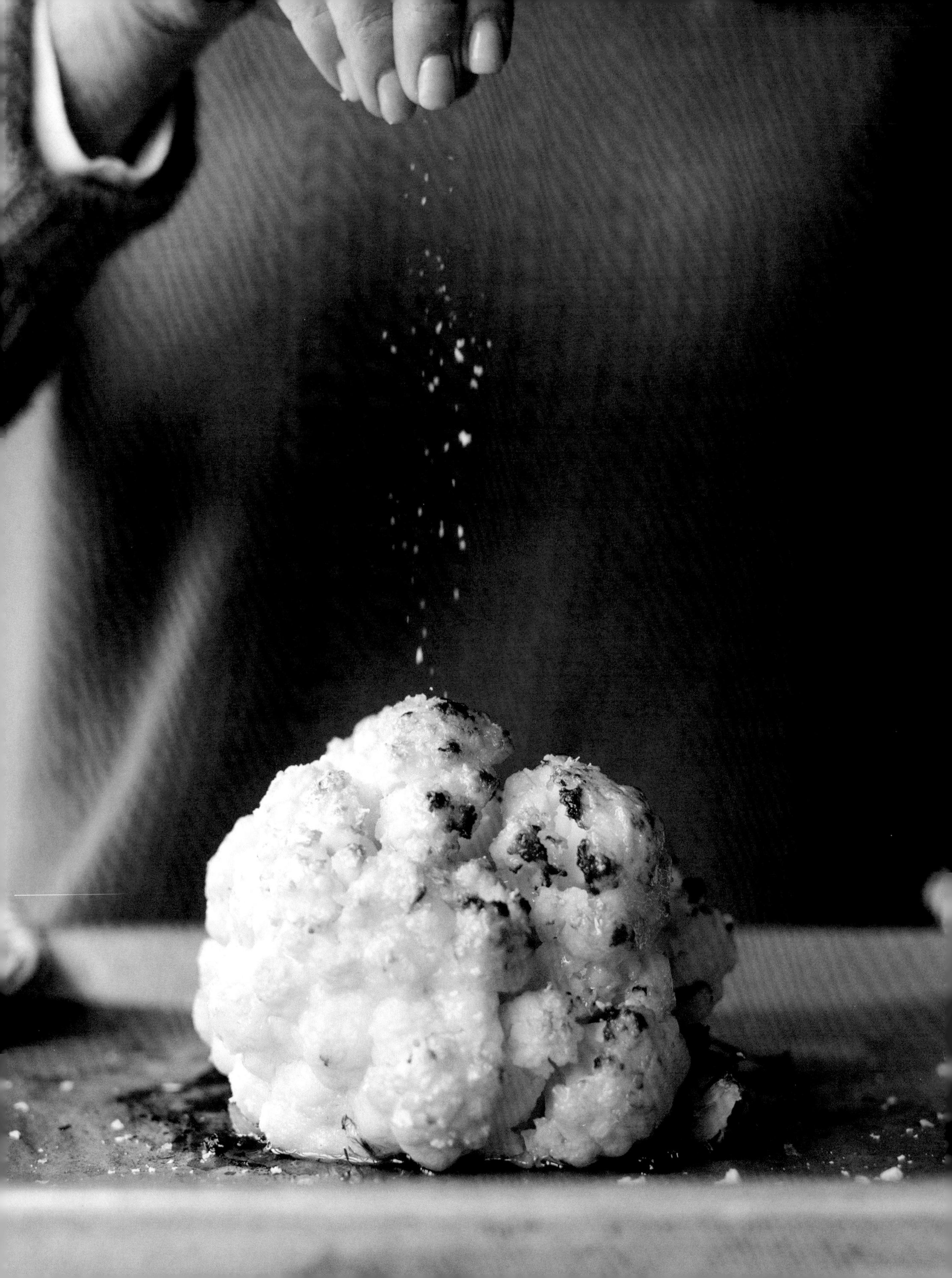

CONTENTS

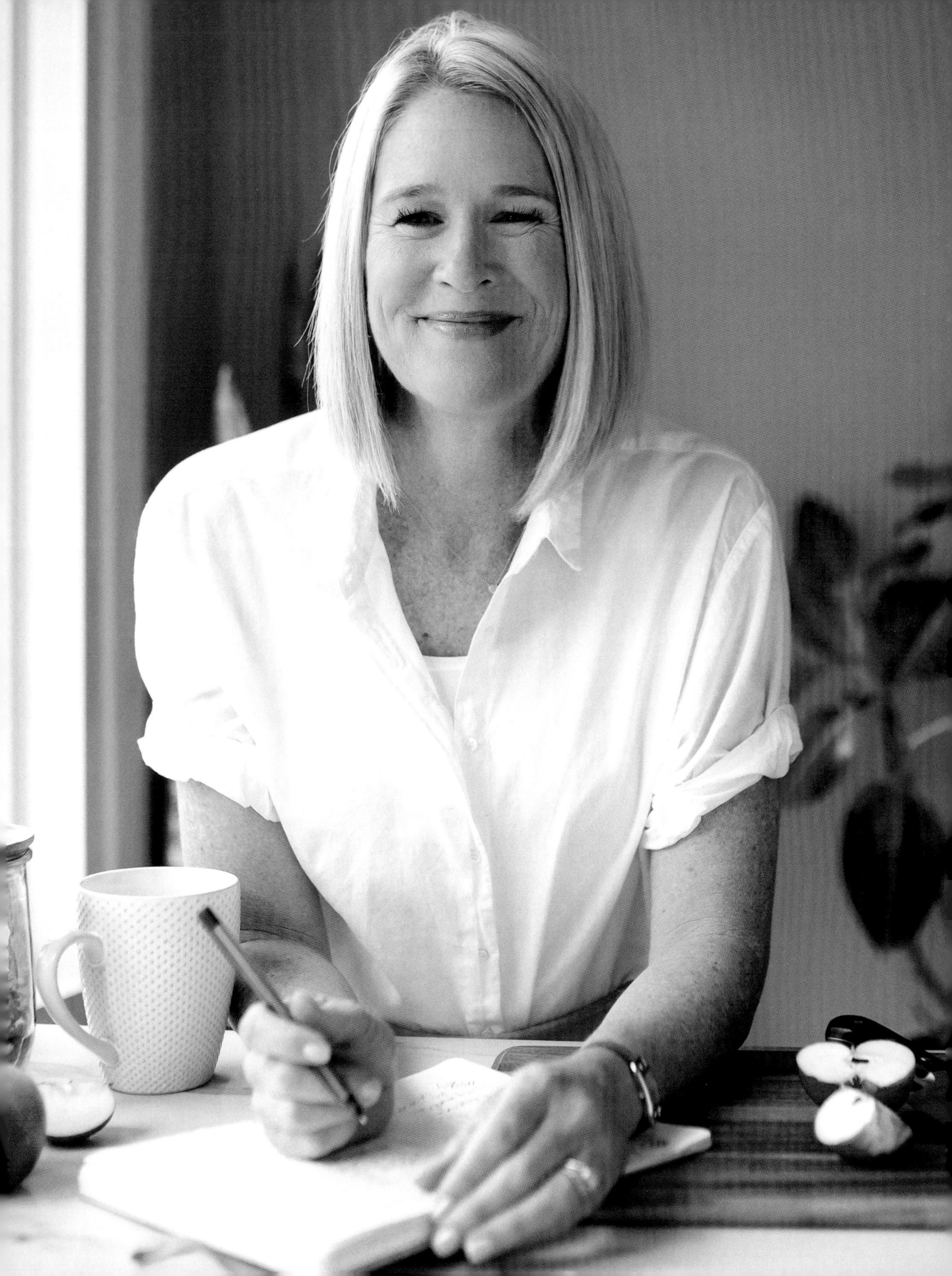

MY HEALTH STRUGGLES

THE DAY EVERYTHING CHANGED

It was a beautiful morning during the summer of 1998. With a quick kiss goodbye, my husband left for work and I hopped in the shower. I got ready for the day, sat down to write a menu for an event I was catering later that week, and was drinking my first cup of coffee. Suddenly I felt a sharp pain pierce my abdomen. Ouch! What was that? I thought.

Before I could set my cup down, another pain hit. It was sharper than the first one. I took some deep breaths and slid down my chair onto the kitchen floor. It felt like I was being stabbed in the stomach. I curled into the fetal position hoping to soften the pain; instead it became excruciating. I could barely move.

With tears streaming down my face, I crawled across the floor and reached up for the telephone. I frantically pushed the buttons of my mother's phone number. When she answered I blurted out, "I am in so much pain that I can barely move!"

"You need to go to the hospital," she said. "I will be right there." About 15 minutes later my mom was in my kitchen helping me off the floor and into her car. At 28 years old, I felt like a child unable to take care of myself and scared about what was happening to me.

My mom sped to the closest hospital and brought me into the emergency room. I was visibly in extreme pain so they quickly rushed me through the intake process and got me into a room. The nurses gave me an IV with medication to help the pain. After some tests, they determined I must have appendicitis. They couldn't find my appendix with an ultrasound, but they were confident it had burst and needed to be removed. My husband met us in the emergency room. We talked it over with the surgeon and decided to go ahead with the 45-minute surgery they recommended. I was prepped and rolled back to the operating room.

IT WAS NOT APPENDICITIS

During the procedure, Chris and my parents were sitting in the hospital waiting room. They were told someone would speak with them when the surgery was done to report how it went. After two hours passed without hearing anything, they asked about me at the information desk. The attendant called the operating room for an update, and a nurse told her that part of my small intestine had been removed and they were starting to remove a portion of my large intestine. My family was shocked and confused. Small and large intestines? Not an appendectomy?

Concerned, Chris and my parents returned to the waiting area and prayed. They anxiously waited for me to come out of a surgery that had turned into something bigger than anyone had originally thought. After a few more hours, the surgeon told them I was in the recovery room and would be moved up to a hospital room once I was stable. He explained that after they had opened me up to remove my appendix, they saw my intestines were damaged with disease. He removed the damaged sections and sent samples to pathology to determine the cause. It would be a few days before we would get the results, he explained, adding that I would need to stay in the hospital to recover.

When I began to wake up from my deep anesthetized sleep, I felt lost. It took me a few minutes to remember the pain from earlier in the day in my kitchen and that I was at the hospital. My body hurt, especially my abdomen. As my memory was being jogged, I heard a toilet flush. I looked toward the sound, and a bald woman emerged from a door wiping her mouth. She looked at me with deep sympathy, shook her head and said, "You poor thing," then pulled the privacy curtain closed as she collapsed in the bed on the other side of the room.

She called me poor thing? A woman who I deduced was throwing up from chemotherapy or some other awful treatment was feeling sorry for me? If she had pity for me, what did I look like? A nurse abruptly walked into the room and brusquely told me I needed to get up and walk. I was barely awake and in pain. The last thing I wanted to do was walk. I stared at her blankly, not understanding the reason for her command. "You need to get your body moving," she said, "so you can get your intestines working again."

I was confused. What was she talking about? I told the nurse I wasn't ready to walk yet, that I'd had an appendectomy and needed time to wake up. She measured my vital signs and informed me I had also undergone a bowel resection. She said the doctor would be in shortly to talk to me about it.

As I tried making sense of her words, Chris came into the room, rushed to my bedside and hugged me. We held each other tightly and cried. "What happened?" I asked between sobs. He told me the surgeon found disease on my intestines, ended up having to remove part of them, and the surgery had taken more than four hours. Chris glanced at the curtain that divided the room and apologized. He said he asked the hospital to move me into a private room when I got out of surgery. They didn't have one available until later that day, and I would be moved as soon as possible. I smiled softly. Leave it to Chris to think about my needs and advocate on my behalf to make sure those needs were met. I was so blessed to have him by my side during this journey.

LEARNING ABOUT CROHN'S DISEASE

After I was moved into my own room, a doctor from the gastroenterology department came in to speak to me, Chris and my mom. We learned that when the surgeon went in to perform the appendectomy, he discovered part of my intestines were covered in sores and lesions, which indicated disease. He removed the damaged sections and sent samples of the tissue to the pathology department. The gastroenterologist said that I likely had Crohn's disease and they were waiting for the pathology report to confirm their findings. He explained that Crohn's was a disease that can affect the entire digestive tract, starting at the mouth and ending at the anus. It is a chronic disease that I would have for the rest of my life, and it would require management with medication and possibly future surgeries. He said my appendix was fine but that they removed it so they could rule out appendicitis in the event of another bout of severe abdominal pain in the future. The doctor told us the internet had a lot of information about the disease and suggested we look online to learn more about it. He seemed rushed to get to his next patient and said another doctor would be back tomorrow to check on me.

We were stunned. None of us had heard about Crohn's before that. It was 1998, so the hospital didn't have Wi-Fi and we didn't have smartphones. I couldn't Google "Crohn's disease" from my hospital bed to start learning about this newly discovered part of me or quickly find other people's stories complete with happy endings. It was a lot to process for all of us, and we had no idea how we would manage the changes that Crohn's would require.

Fortunately, Chris was able to get some information online when he returned home that evening. He also had a family friend who was a doctor and answered a lot of our questions. The doctor explained to Chris that during my type of procedure the surgeon takes the intestines out of the body to work on them. Once the surgery is complete the intestines are placed back in the body. Because the surgery began as an appendectomy, the incision was quite small where the intestines were pushed back into my abdomen. My intestines were most likely twisted and needed to get resettled in their right place. This can cause pain and cramping in addition to the anticipated pain experienced during recovery from any surgery. There would also be air bubbles trapped in my bowels that would cause pain as they tried to escape. He prepared Chris with the expectation that my recovery could take weeks.

SLOW RECOVERY

My days in the hospital were difficult and long. In order for me to be well enough to be released, I needed to have a bowel movement and I needed to eat solid food. The narcotics prescribed slowed down my digestive system. I was in a lot of pain and had to find a balance between pain relief and pushing through it without medication to expedite my recovery. I was extremely uncomfortable and it was hard to sleep. Nurses woke me up several times throughout the night to check my vital signs. I threw up frequently and moaned in pain. I prayed constantly for comfort and relief. As that first nurse originally told me, I would need to walk to help get things moving. Determined to get better and go home, I clung to my IV pole, walking as often as I could muster the strength. I couldn't even tolerate clear liquids so I wasn't eating. A nasogastric tube was inserted up my nose and down into my stomach to drain the bile that had accumulated in hopes of giving my stomach some relief and to stop the vomiting.

After a week, I had lost a tremendous amount of weight. My skin was ashen and my eyes were sunken and hollow. I looked like a shell of my former self. My mother implored the nurse to do something about my weight loss. I was grateful to have her advocating for me. Because of my mom's persistence, the nurse got an order to have a peripherally inserted central catheter (PICC) line inserted in my neck for liquid nutrition. Over the next few days, I started gaining some strength and color back. Eventually I stopped throwing up and they were able to remove the nasogastric tube. I increased the frequency of my walks, venturing down and back all four of the hallways that stemmed off of the nurses station. After two weeks, I was able to tolerate a small amount of food and complete a bowel movement. My prayers had been answered and my hard work and determination had paid off. I was finally released.

Riding home from the hospital was surreal. It was wonderful to feel the fresh air blowing across my face in the sunshine. I had not been outside of the hospital once during my recovery. Looking out the car window, I watched people walking and crossing the streets who appeared to have places to go and things to do. Their lives had gone on while mine stopped for more than two weeks. It was strange to feel like I had been plucked from daily life for a period of time and was now being dropped back in. As happy as I was to go home, I was also afraid. I had a new sense of vulnerability not knowing what my life would be like now that I would be living with this disease. I was both physically and emotionally fragile.

After my surgery and hospital stay, I followed up with a gastroenterologist. The pathology report confirmed I had Crohn's disease. He prescribed medications to manage the disease and told me that due to the type of surgery I had undergone it would be difficult for me to have children. I was heartbroken. My husband and I had been married for less than a year, and having children was something we both really wanted. My dream of having a family was crushed. I could handle living with a disease for life, but not having children was difficult for me to accept.

I made an appointment with a naturopath named Sunny who I had seen off and on since I was a teenager. Sunny explained that the part of my intestines that had been removed absorbed certain vitamins and minerals. Because that part of my body was gone, I would need to take extra supplements to make up for it. She shared that many of those nutrients are essential to support carrying a baby, and she was confident that if I took these vitamins and minerals, I would be able to get pregnant and carry a baby to term. I was filled with a new sense of hope and gratitude.

Within the next two and a half years, Chris and I were blessed with two beautiful daughters, and I was able to carry them both full term. They were (and still are) the greatest joy of our lives.

THE PHARMACEUTICAL LADDER

Over the next 10 years that joy was mixed with hard times. The medication and supplements I was taking would manage the disease for a while, but then they would stop working. I experienced bouts of extreme pain and nausea. I was fatigued. Sometimes I required short hospitalizations and weeks of steroids to get better. I would start a new medication, get my energy back and feel great, only to get sick again. I climbed what is referred to as the "pharmaceutical ladder." A drug would manage the Crohn's disease and then my body would get used to it and the drug would prove ineffective. I would then climb the next rung of the ladder to a new drug. I was experiencing this while raising two young girls. My husband, who traveled for work, was often not home. Each day I pushed through the malaise while playing school and Polly Pockets, walking to the park, and cutting finger sandwiches and bite-sized fruits and vegetables. I used all of my energy to be the best mother I could during the day and then collapsed as soon as they were asleep.

FIRST INTRODUCTION TO THE SPECIFIC CARBOHYDRATE DIET

Throughout this period of time, I was actively researching dietary theories and natural wellness. I read book after book and experimented with different ways of eating to help manage my symptoms. I continued seeing my naturopath and started making lifestyle changes. I was near the top of the pharmaceutical ladder, traveling to the Mayo Clinic every eight weeks for intravenous therapy, when my naturopath recommended the Specific Carbohydrate Diet (SCD). She encouraged me to read the book "Breaking the Vicious Cycle" by Elaine Gottschall, a biochemist whose daughter was gravely ill with severe ulcerative colitis. The girl's doctor wanted to remove all of her intestines, but Elaine was desperate to prevent that from happening. In her quest to help her daughter, she discovered the SCD. After implementing the diet, her daughter had a miraculous recovery and didn't have the surgery. Elaine went on to write the book and share this dietary theory with the world.

I was grateful for the new resource and picked up a copy. It sounded promising. I read through the book and did more research online. The SCD is based on the chemical structure of carbohydrates. The allowed carbohydrates on the diet are monosaccharides and have a single molecule structure that is easily absorbed by the intestines. Complex carbohydrates that are disaccharides (double molecules) and polysaccharides (chain molecules) are more difficult to absorb and are not allowed because the complex carbohydrates not assimilated are left behind and become food for bad bacteria in the digestive tract. These bad bacteria overgrow, causing damage and inflammation in the intestines. The goal of the diet is to starve these bad bacteria by taking away their food source and restoring bacterial balance in the gut.

The science behind the SCD made a lot of sense, but it was very restrictive. The foods not allowed on the diet include grains, starches and starchy vegetables, most dairy and sugars, and processed, refined, and packaged foods. Following it would require a tremendous amount of home cooking. Simple everyday ingredients like ketchup, mayonnaise and salad dressings would need to be made from scratch. I was busy raising my young family and didn't think I could make the time to prepare special food just for me. I also loved to eat good food. Before starting my family, I went to culinary school and became a chef. I wasn't ready to give up eating all of the ingredients that weren't allowed or give up trying new dishes at restaurants. In order to have success with the program, the diet had to be followed perfectly for one to two years to allow enough time for the intestines to heal. The limitations and time involved were overwhelming to think about. At the time, my medication managed the disease fairly well. I mentally filed the information away and moved on.

GIVING THE SPECIFIC CARBOHYDRATE DIET A REAL CHANCE

Not long after reading "Breaking the Vicious Cycle" I got sick and found myself on a new medication. Once again, I had reached the top of the ladder. The new drug worked well to manage the disease, but I was concerned that once it stopped working, as all the others had, I would have nothing new to try. I was on the last rung. I also started worrying about some of the long-term side effects associated with the medications I had been on, including the one I was currently taking. My chances of getting certain cancers and other diseases had increased. The future of my health was looking ominous. I began to pray and ask God what I should do.

Shortly after I started to pray about it, my mother shared that a former neighbor had suffered from Crohn's disease and started following the SCD. She was having great results. A few weeks later, I heard about another person who had ulcerative colitis and was on the diet. That person no longer needed medication and was managing symptoms by strictly following the SCD. Sunny and I had not spoken about the diet for quite some time, but at my next appointment she brought it up again. She told me she had many patients who were having great success following the diet and really encouraged me to try it. After not hearing anything about the SCD since reading the book, I was suddenly bombarded with testimonies about it. God was clearly giving me the answer to my prayers. It was time for me to try it.

THE THREE-MONTH EXPERIMENT

I decided I would commit to following the SCD for three months. I thought this would be enough time to see if I noticed a difference in how I felt and whether or not I had the self-discipline to stick to it. Being on a strict diet got me back into the kitchen doing a lot of scratch cooking. Because the SCD is so restrictive, I was stretched creatively. I used ingredients I had never worked with before and found new ways to make favorite recipes. My family was eating mostly the same things as I ate. It was easier than I anticipated. I felt great. I had energy and didn't get fatigued by the end of the day. My whole family was feeling good with the healthier meals I was preparing. At the end of the three months, I was convinced I could keep it going.

A LEAP OF FAITH

I met with my gastroenterologist at the Mayo Clinic and told him I was following the SCD and wanted to stop taking my medications. He reminded me that my insurance company and I paid him a lot of money to tell me what he knows. He shared that the likelihood of me relapsing after discontinuing the drugs was very high. He also explained that if I needed to go back on my medication the chances of it working again were very slim. Once the drugs were out of my system, if reintroduced, my body might not respond to them. There were currently no new medications for me to try if that happened. But he also understood my reasons for not wanting to manage the Crohn's with drugs any longer and said he would support whatever I decided.

The idea that there might not be a medication that would help me if the diet didn't work was scary. Chris and I talked and prayed about it. We both agreed that I would discontinue the drugs and continue with the SCD. It was a leap of faith.

Over the next 15 months, I followed the Specific Carbohydrate Diet to a T. I felt great and didn't experience any Crohn's symptoms. After a total of 18 months of

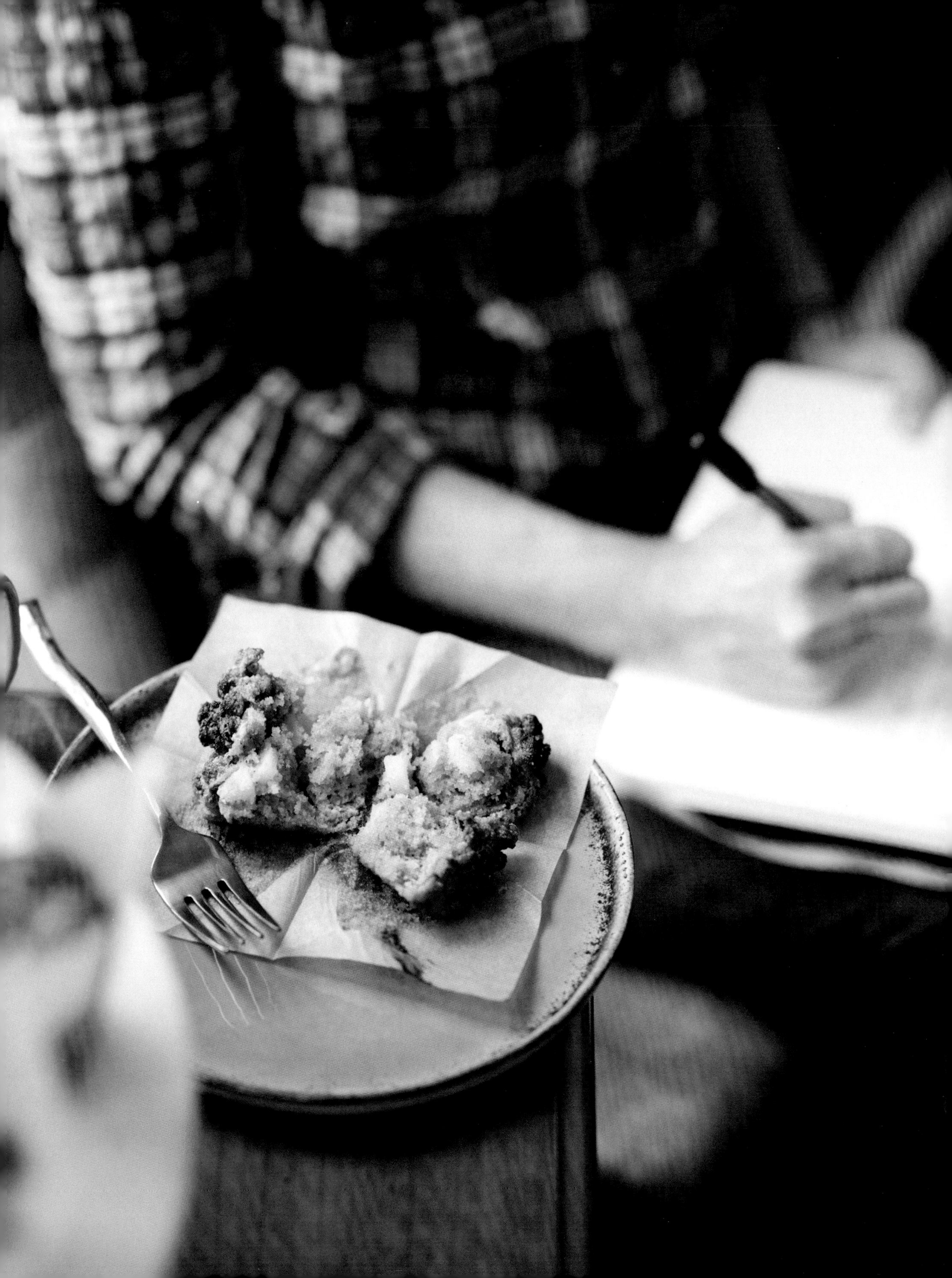

being on the SCD and completely symptom-free, I went back to the Mayo Clinic. My team ran a few tests and the results showed no active disease. They remarked that after my last visit they were sure I would be back in three months with symptoms. They were happy to see that they were wrong and glad they had a testimony to share with patients who were interested in alternate treatments.

HOW I EAT TODAY

Following the Specific Carbohydrate Diet, I cooked myself out of disease and into good health. While the diet was strict, the results were miraculous. It was such a blessing to not have to take medications or spend time in hospitals. My gut was healthy again and I was able to start introducing foods that were not allowed while following the diet. I added things one by one and waited to see how my body reacted. I was able to tolerate most foods but enjoyed them sparingly at first. Over time I was able to find balance with a regular diet focusing on fresh whole foods while allowing for some indulgences.

Today, I strive for my diet to be 80 percent plant-based. I focus on fiber and try to get a variety of different plant foods in my diet daily, including some gluten-free whole grains. That is what is currently working for me and keeps my microbiome balanced. After following a strict diet for so long, I now enjoy what I like to call food freedom. I am not as rigorous but still careful about what I eat. While I believe that what we eat has a direct impact on our overall health, we are all created differently and each do better eating different foods. What works for one person may not necessarily work for the next. If you are having digestive issues and are interested in trying the SCD, I recommend first reading the book "Breaking the Vicious Cycle" and talking with your nutritionist or health practitioner. There are also many resources online.

This cookbook is the culmination of my journey. In it you will find recipes that follow the SCD guidelines and some that don't. The majority are adaptable to different dietary needs. Most recipes are gluten-, grain- and dairy-free, but some recipes have more standard ingredients. There is something in this book for everyone. The spotlight is on clean, real-ingredient food used in simple recipes. Cooking our own food is one of the best things we can do for our overall health. My goal is to offer thoughtfully developed recipes that are nutrient-dense and easy to make. Food doesn't need to be complicated to be good.

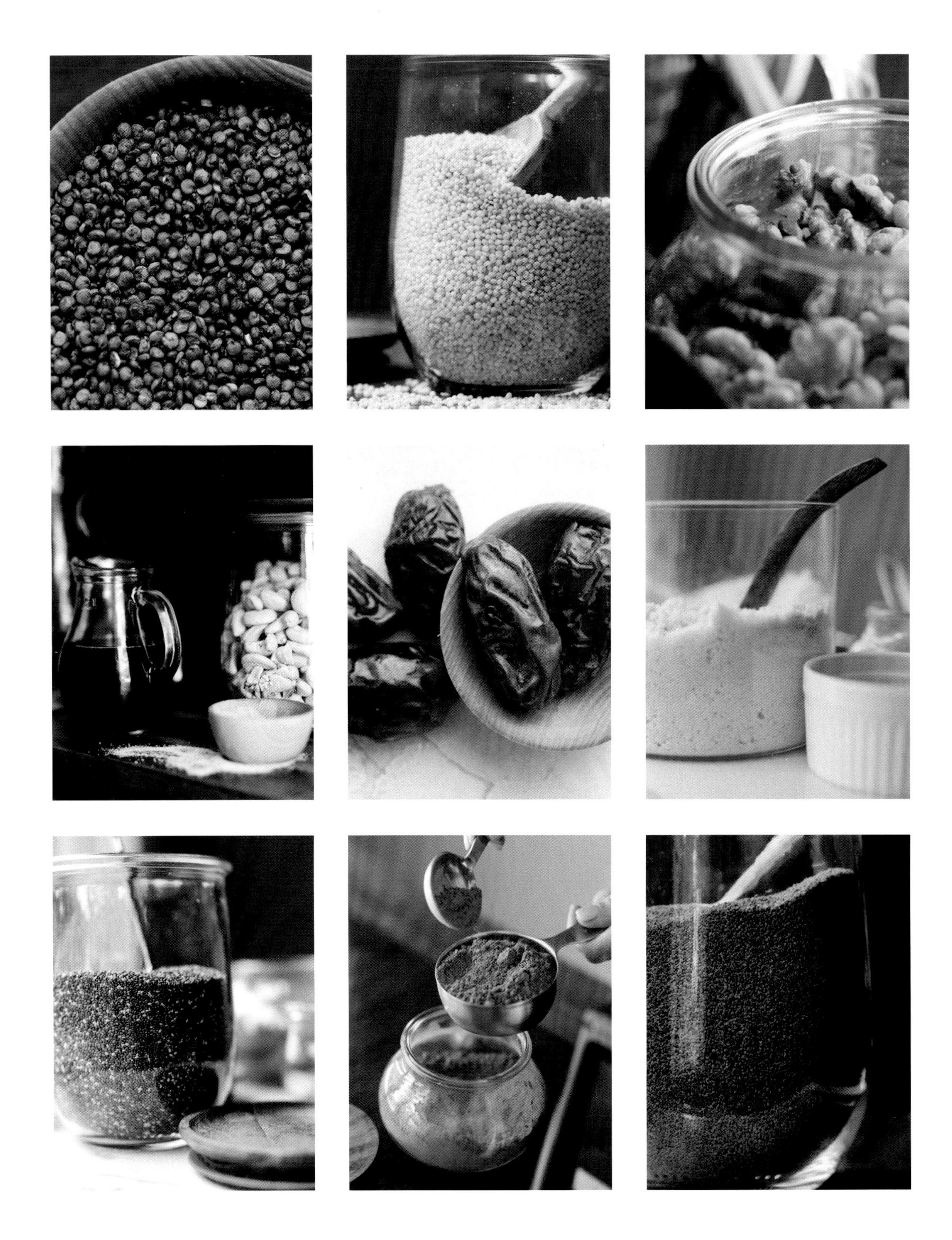

WHAT'S IN MY PANTRY

When I changed my way of eating, my kitchen pantry got a makeover. The Specific Carbohydrate Diet doesn't allow for grains, starches, sugars (other than those occurring naturally in fruit and honey), processed foods and most dairy. I had to replace a lot of the ingredients I had been using with new ones. I have since been able to add back some ingredients that were not allowed on the diet. I created a list of the staples that I keep in my kitchen today and are used in the recipes in this book.

BAKING AND DRY GOODS

Almond flour
Arrowroot powder
Baking soda
Coconut flour
Grain-free baking powder
Maca powder
Maldon sea salt flakes
Matcha
Palm shortening
Pink Himalayan sea salt or Redmond Real Salt
Puffed quinoa*
Raw cacao nibs
Raw cacao powder
Unsweetened coconut flakes
Unsweetened shredded coconut

**This is one of my favorite ingredients to work with. It is crunchy like Rice Krispies but made from quinoa. I order it from nuts.com.*

NUTS AND SEEDS

Almonds
Cashews
Chia seeds
Hazelnuts
Hemp seeds
Macadamia nuts
Peanuts
Pecans
Pepitas
Pine nuts
Sesame seeds
Sunflower seeds
Walnuts

OILS AND FATS

Avocado oil
Coconut oil
Extra virgin olive oil
Ghee
Grass-fed butter
Hazelnut oil
Macadamia nut oil
Toasted sesame oil
Walnut oil

CANNED AND SHELF-STABLE GOODS

Black beans
Cannellini beans
Chicken broth
Full-fat coconut milk
Garbanzo beans
Great Northern beans
Kidney beans
Pumpkin
Tomatoes from Italy
Vegetable broth

GRAINS AND LENTILS

Brown basmati rice
Brown lentils
Gluten-free oats
Green lentils
Millet
Red lentils
Red quinoa
Sushi rice
Tricolor quinoa
White quinoa
Wild rice

SWEETENERS

Coconut sugar
Dark chocolate
Dates
Local raw honey
Pure maple syrup
Unsweetened applesauce

SPICES

Black peppercorns
Black pepper, ground
Cayenne pepper
Chili powder
Cinnamon
Cloves, ground
Coriander
Crushed red pepper flakes
Cumin
Curry powder
Dill
Dried onion
Fennel seeds
Ginger
Granulated garlic
Mustard powder
Nutmeg
Oregano
Smoked paprika
Turmeric
Vanilla extract
White pepper

CONDIMENTS

Apple cider vinegar
Avocado oil mayonnaise
Balsamic vinegar
Chili garlic sauce
Coconut aminos
Dijon mustard
Horseradish
Natural almond butter
Natural cashew butter
Natural peanut butter
Tahini
Tamari (gluten-free soy sauce)
White balsamic vinegar

REFRIGERATED AND FROZEN FOODS

Fresh and frozen organic fruits and vegetables
Frozen fresh coconut purée
Frozen riced cauliflower
Frozen unsweetened açaí purée
Grass-fed and pasture-raised meats and poultry
Nut milks
Pasture-raised eggs, size large
Some organic and grass-fed cheeses
Wild-caught fish and shrimp

BRANDS I LIKE

Butcher Box brand meat, poultry and seafood
Eden Foods brand beans
Hain brand baking soda
Hu brand chocolate and crackers
Kerrygold brand butter from grass-fed cows
Malk brand nut milk
Native Forest brand simple coconut milk
Primal Kitchen brand condiments
Siete brand tortillas, taco shells and chips
Simple Mills brand crackers and baking mixes
Sir Kensington's brand mayonnaise and condiments
Three Trees brand nut milk
Yai's Thai brand sauces

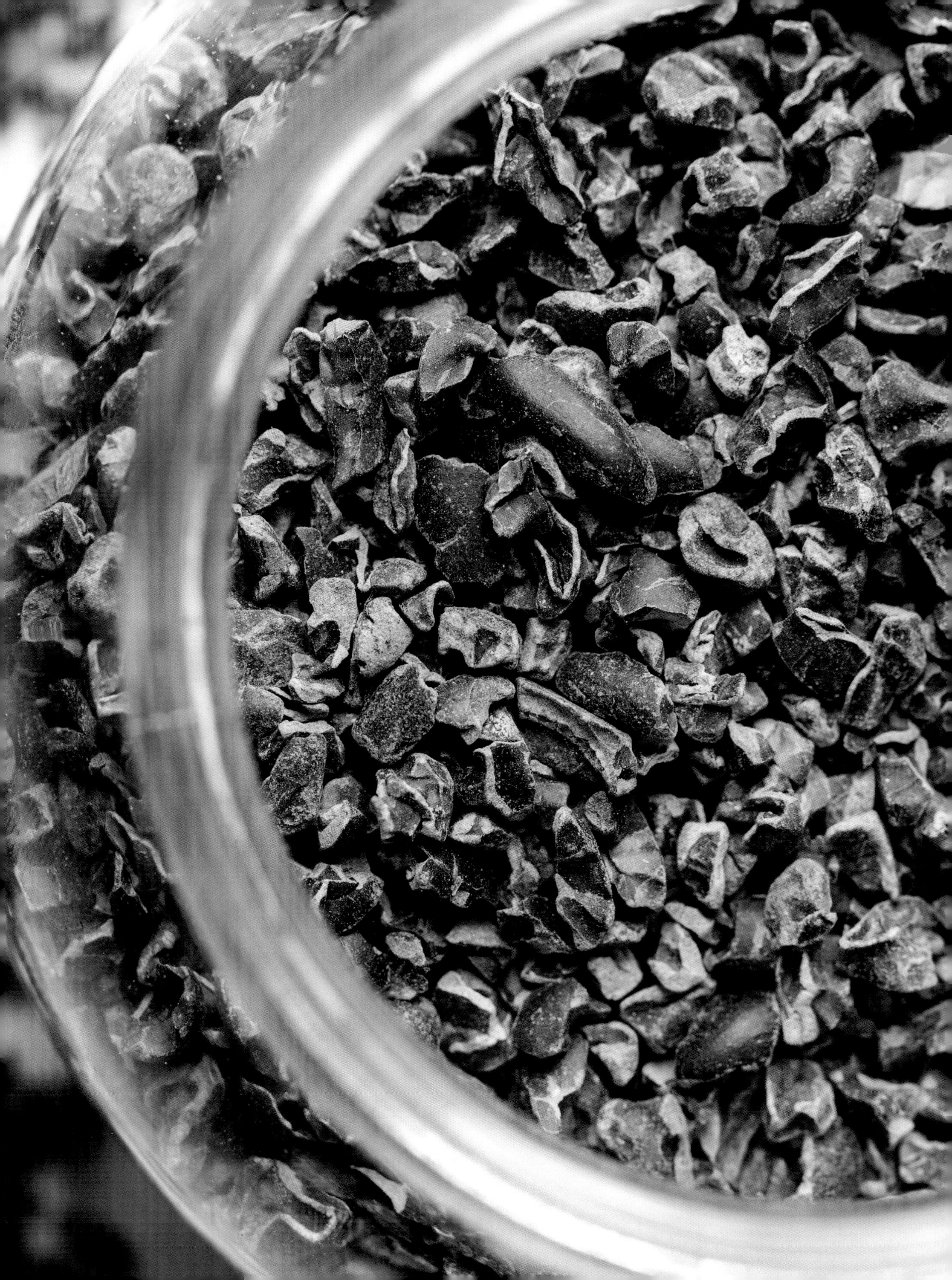

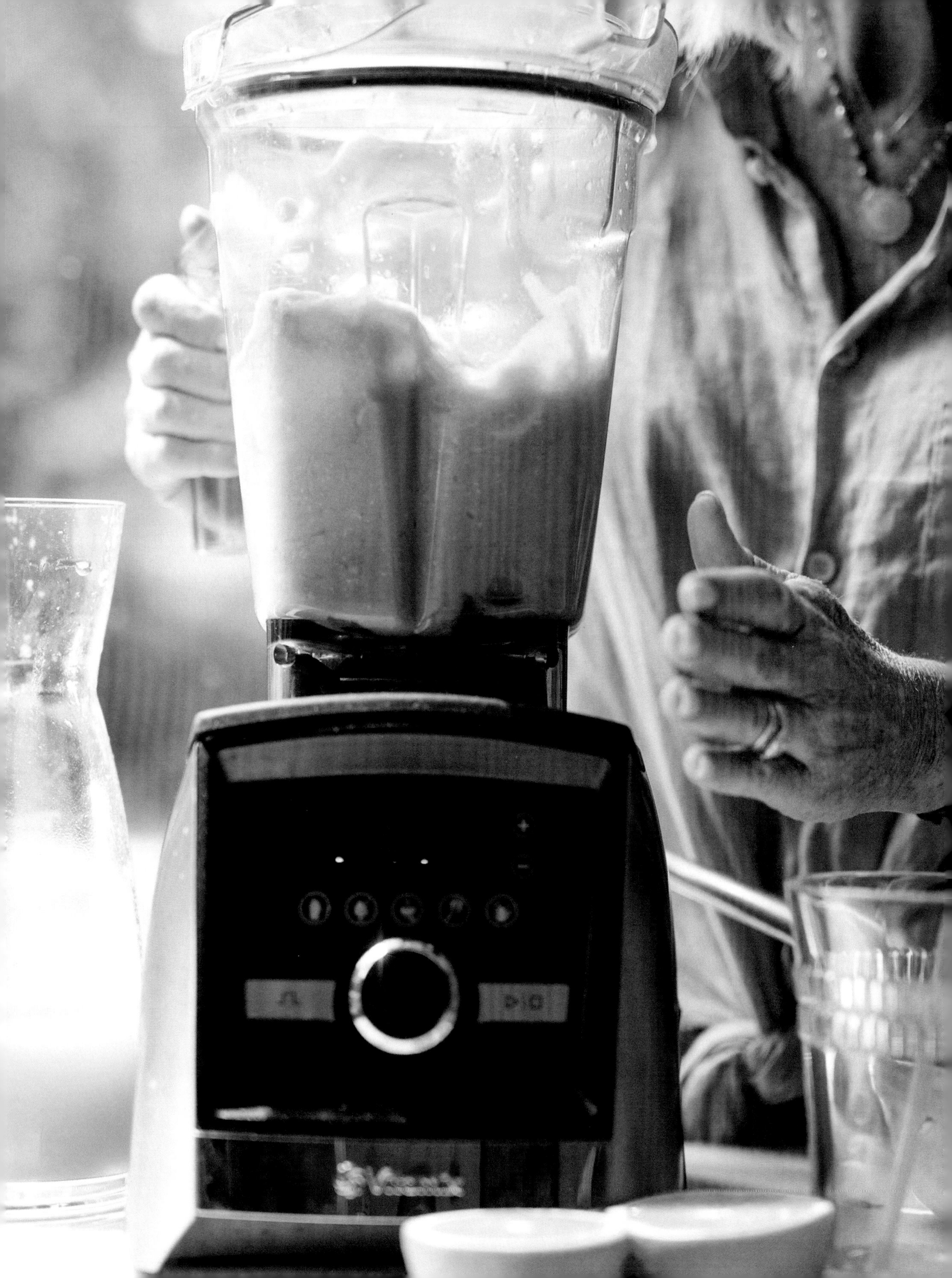

MY FAVORITE KITCHEN TOOLS

HIGH-POWER BLENDER

The Vitamix is expensive, but it is the most used appliance in my kitchen. I use it for smoothies, soups, sauces, vegetable purées, ice cream and more. The Ninja is a more affordable brand.

MINI AND STANDARD FOOD PROCESSOR

I use my mini food processor all of the time. It's great for chopping garlic and nuts and making dips and sauces. The standard size works well for larger batches of ingredients as well as shredding cheese and chopping vegetables.

IMMERSION BLENDER

This tool is perfect for blending soups and other items without having to transfer to a blender or food processor. I like to use it when I want the dish to have some texture and not be completely smooth.

DUTCH OVEN

Dutch ovens are great for making soups and stews, browning, searing, roasting and frying. They are very versatile and can be used on the stovetop as well as in the oven. They come in a variety of colors and sizes. I use the 5 1/2-quart and 7-quart sizes most often.

SLOW COOKER

I love the convenience of a slow cooker. It makes it easy to prepare meals ahead of time. It's also great for making stocks and broths.

STAND-UP OR HAND MIXER

I use either a stand-up or hand mixer for making batters and doughs for baking.

SPIRALIZER

A spiralizer is an inexpensive tool that can turn almost any vegetable into noodles.

MICROPLANE GRATER

This tool is great for zesting lemons and grating ginger and garlic.

MANDOLINE SLICER

I use a mandoline for quickly slicing and cutting foods uniformly. It's a great time-saver and keeps the sizing consistent.

ELECTRIC CITRUS JUICER

I use a lot of fresh citrus juice in my recipes so I have a Breville electric juicer. You can get a less expensive one from Amazon or Target.

ICE CREAM MAKER

Ice cream makers are great for making dairy-free frozen desserts like my cashew chocolate ice cream.

ALMOND COW

I finally splurged on an Almond Cow plant-based milk maker, and I love it. Making nut milk and cleaning up afterward has never been easier.

MORTAR AND PESTLE

A mortar and pestle is a sturdy bowl and heavy rod used to grind spices, pound garlic, crush nuts, and make pastes and thick sauces.

PARCHMENT PAPER

Lining pans with parchment paper keeps things from sticking and makes cleaning up significantly easier.

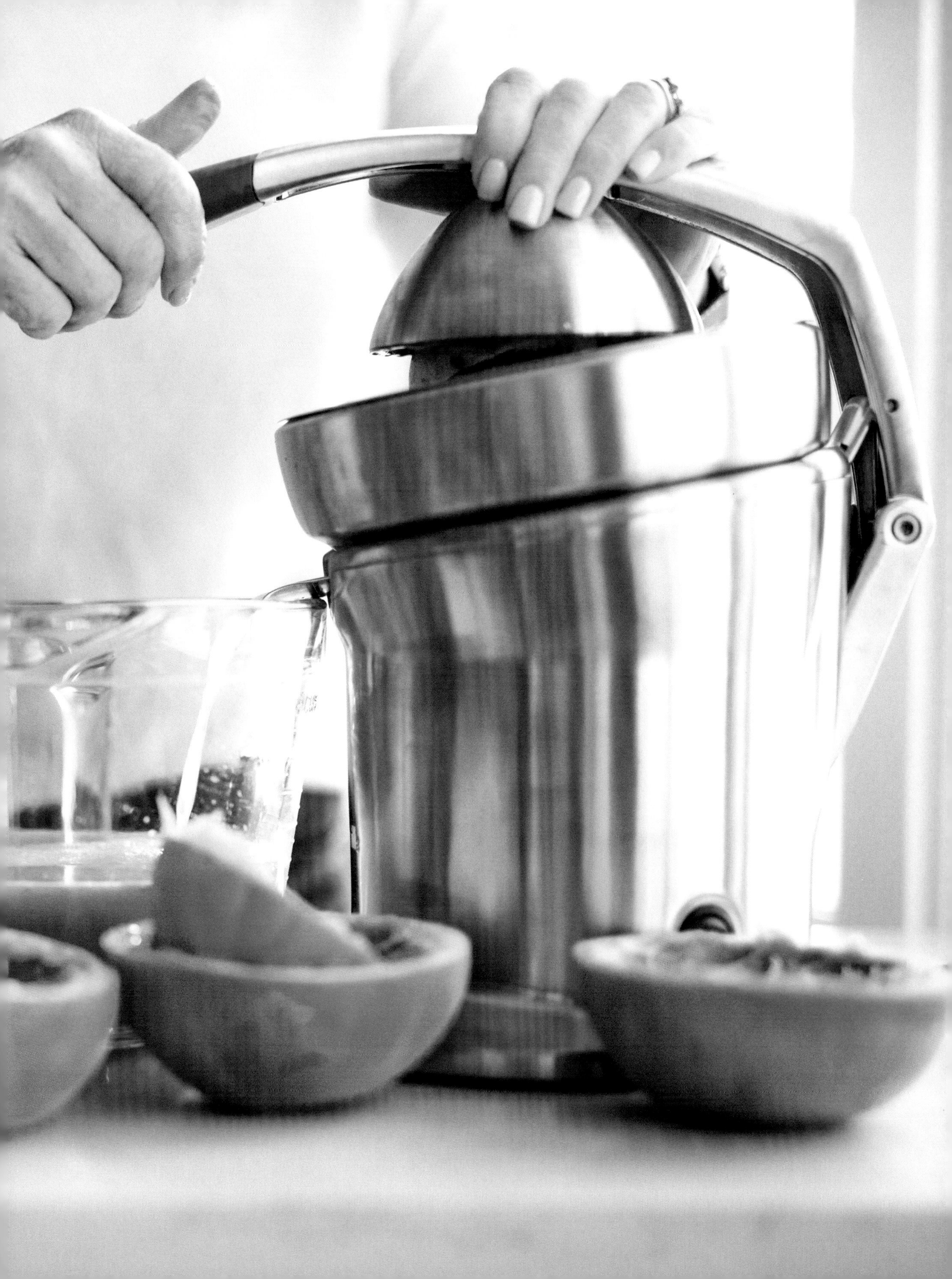

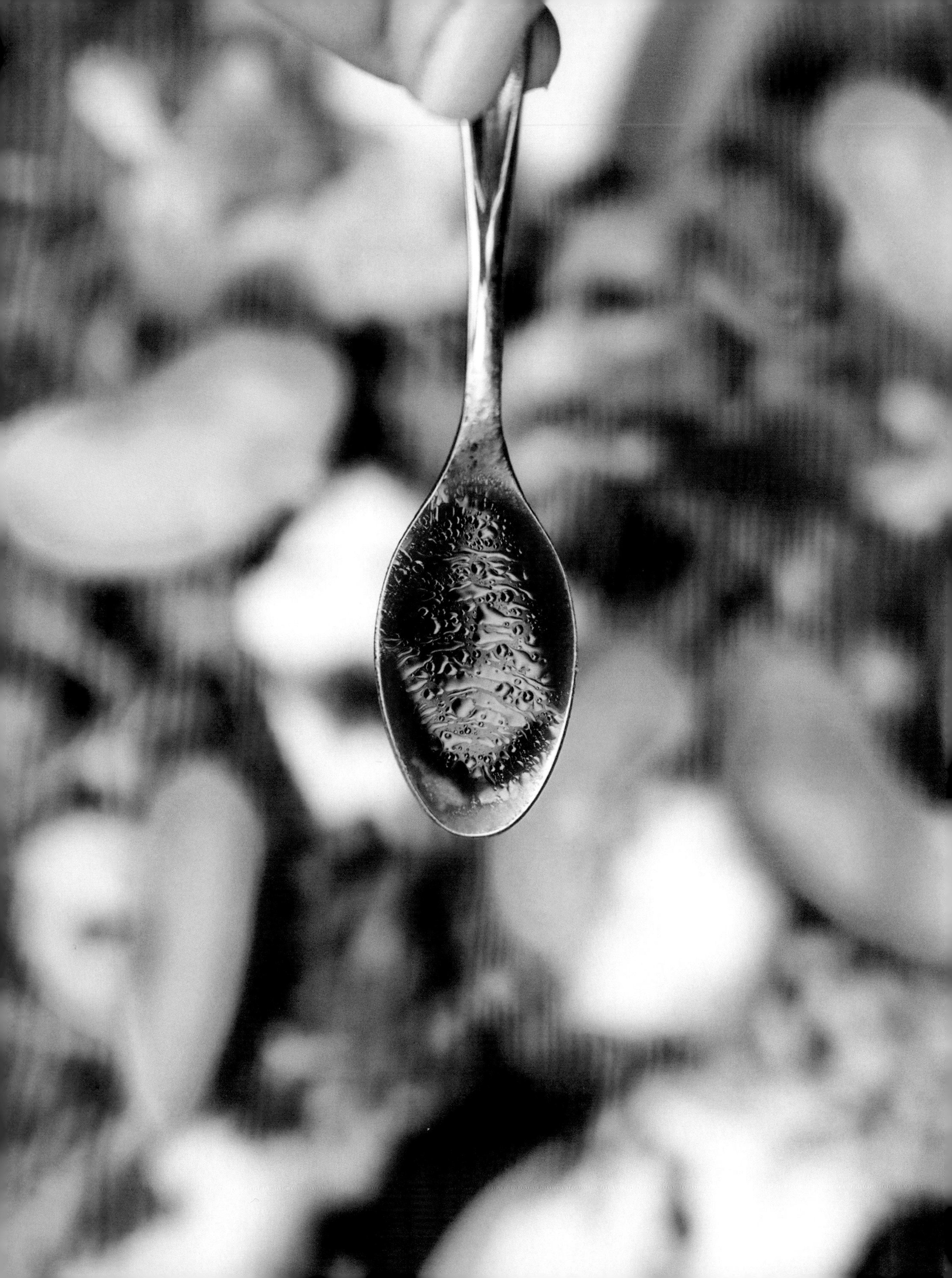

SALADS

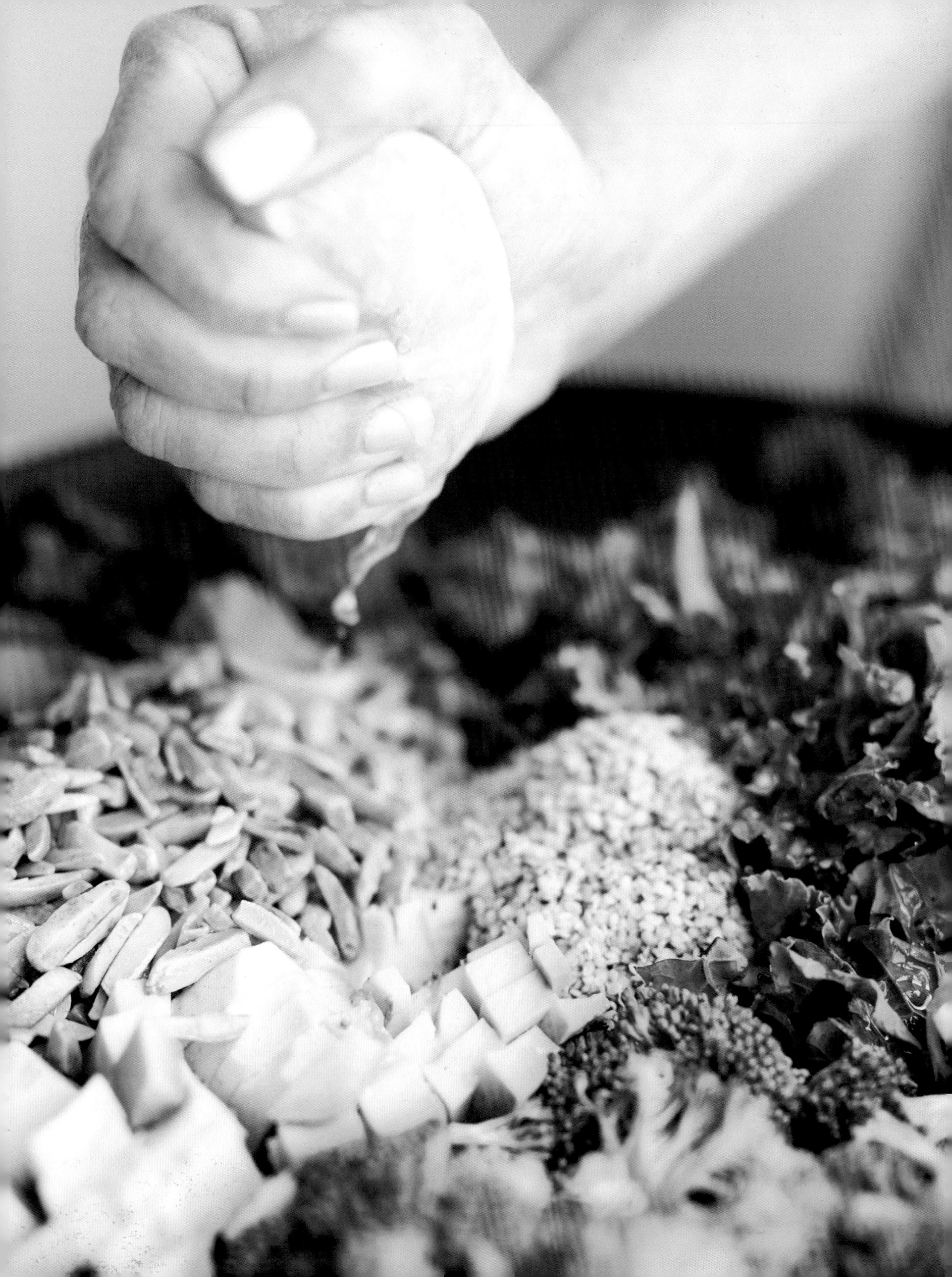

CHOPPED GREEN SALAD

Dairy-Free, Gluten-Free, Grain-Free, Paleo, SCD, Vegan

PREP 10 minutes | COOK 5 minutes | TOTAL 15 minutes | SERVES 4-6

I hesitate to call any food my favorite, but I could eat this salad all day, every day. It's dressed with macadamia nut oil and fresh lemon juice, which allows the raw flavors of the other ingredients to shine through. The sautéed and seasoned almonds add just the right amount of additional flavor. This salad is fresh and crunchy and oh so good!

INGREDIENTS

2 teaspoons olive oil

2/3 cup raw slivered almonds

1/4 teaspoon sea salt

1 teaspoon cumin

3 cups chopped kale

3 cups chopped spinach

1 avocado

2 cups broccoli florets

1/4 cup hemp seeds

Macadamia nut oil, about 2 Tablespoons

1 lemon

Sea salt

Black pepper

DIRECTIONS

1. Place the olive oil in a small sauté pan over medium heat.
2. Add the almonds and begin to toast, stirring frequently.
3. Sauté until golden, adding the salt and cumin when almost done.
4. Set the almonds aside.
5. Place the kale and spinach in a salad bowl.
6. Dice the avocado and add it to the bowl.
7. Cut the broccoli florets into small pieces and add them to the bowl.
8. Add the toasted almonds and hemp seeds.
9. Drizzle the macadamia nut oil over the salad.
10. Cut the lemon in half and squeeze the juice from both halves over the salad.
11. Toss salad and season with salt and pepper to taste.

MEDITERRANEAN QUINOA SALAD

Dairy-Free, Gluten-Free, Vegan (Adaptable for Grain-Free, Paleo, SCD)

PREP 10 minutes | COOK 20 minutes | TOTAL 30 minutes | SERVES 4-6

This fresh, light salad was inspired by the popular Mediterranean-Middle Eastern tabouli, which is traditionally prepared using bulgur wheat. In this recipe, the bulgur is replaced by quinoa, creating a gluten-free version. Quinoa is higher in fiber than most grains and one of the few plant foods that contains all nine essential amino acids, making it a complete protein. The fresh tomatoes, cucumber, green onions, parsley and lemon juice add up to the perfect summer dish. Serve it on its own or with grilled chicken, lamb or feta cheese. To adapt for grain-free, paleo and SCD, substitute lightly blanched or sautéed cauliflower rice for quinoa.

INGREDIENTS

2 cups water

1 cup quinoa, rinsed

1 1/2 cups chopped Roma tomatoes

1 cup chopped cucumber

1 cup chopped green onion

1 cup chopped parsley

1/3 cup olive oil

1/3 cup fresh lemon juice

1/2 teaspoon sea salt

1/2 teaspoon black pepper

DIRECTIONS

1. In a small saucepan bring 2 cups of water to a boil.
2. Stir in the quinoa, then turn the heat down to low.
3. Cover and simmer until all the liquid is absorbed, about 15 minutes.
4. Use a fork to fluff and separate the grains.
5. Place the cooked quinoa in a large bowl.
6. Add the tomato, cucumber, green onion and parsley.
7. Add the olive oil, lemon juice, salt and pepper and stir well.
8. Serve warm, room temperature or chilled.

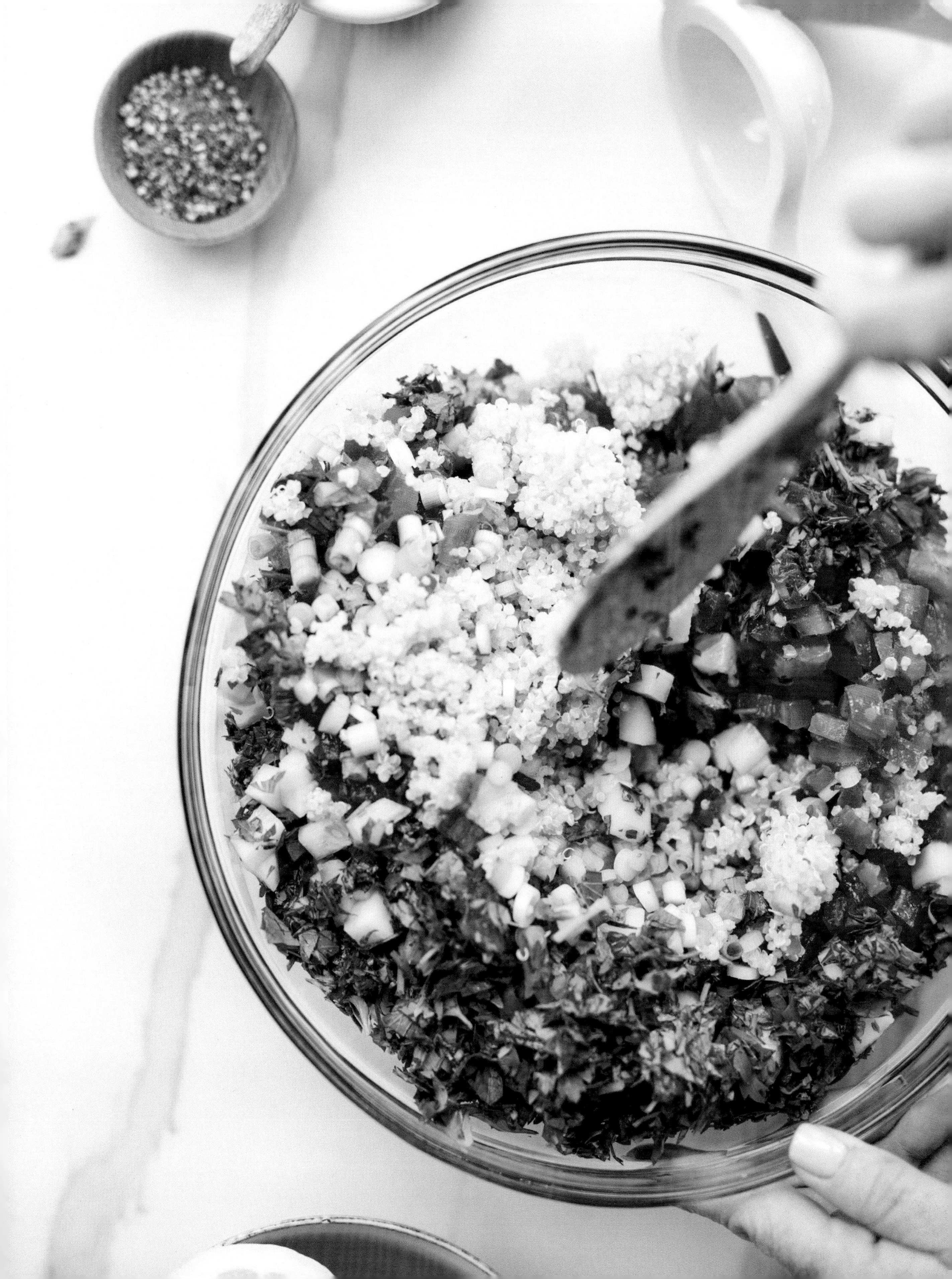

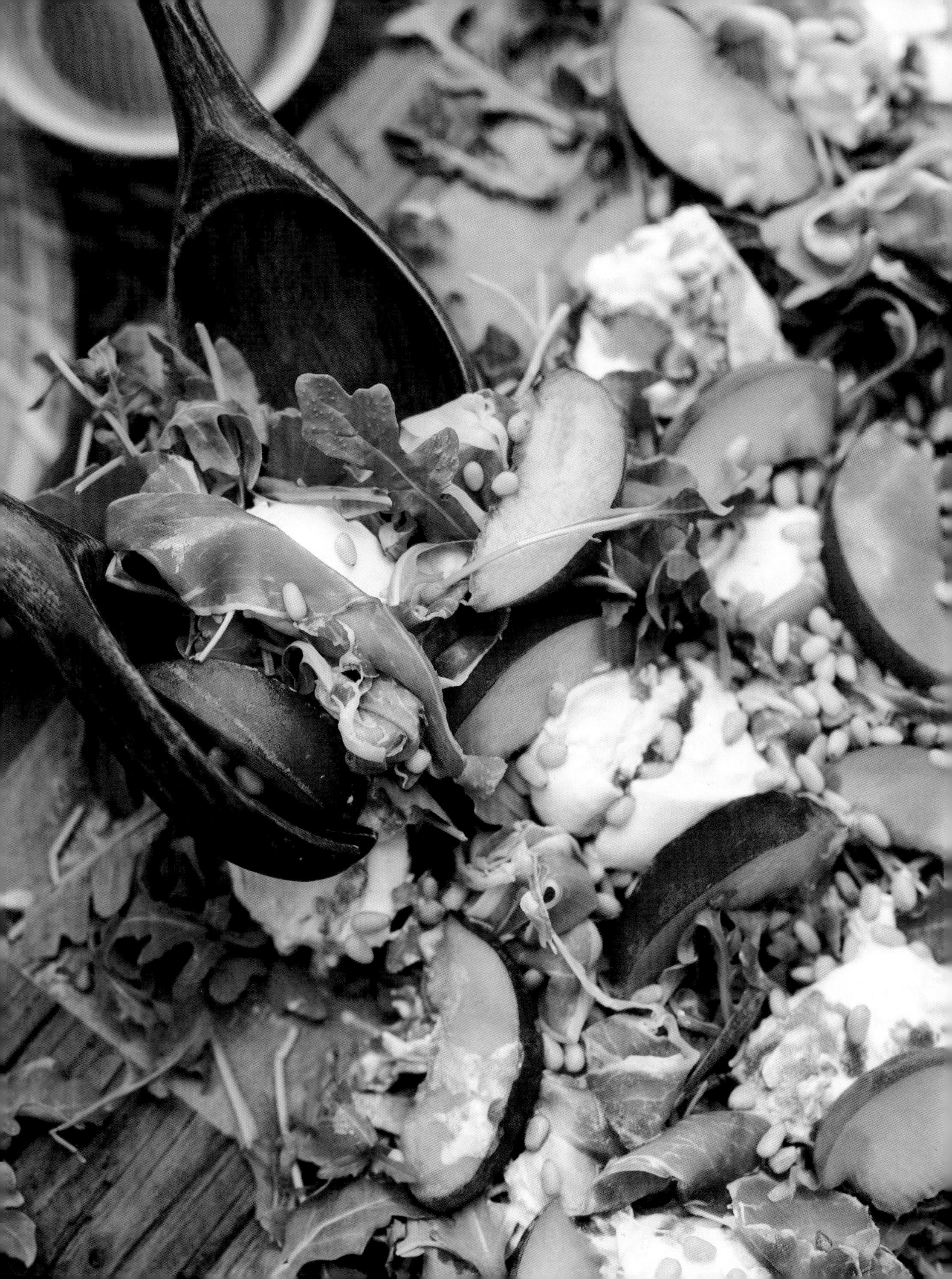

PEACH AND BURRATA SALAD

Gluten-Free, Grain-Free

PREP 10 minutes | COOK 0 minutes | TOTAL 10 minutes | SERVES 4-6

This salad reminds me of Italy because all of the meals I ate there were made with a few simple and fresh ingredients. The dishes didn't need much added to them because of their high-quality components. This salad is easy to assemble and looks beautiful. It's a great one to serve outside with friends and a good bottle of wine.

INGREDIENTS (SALAD)

5 ounces arugula

8 ounces burrata

3 ounces prosciutto

1-2 peaches

1/4 cup pine nuts

INGREDIENTS (DRESSING)

1/4 cup good-quality olive oil

1/8 cup good-quality balsamic vinegar

1 teaspoon Dijon mustard

1/2 teaspoon honey

1/4 teaspoon sea salt

DIRECTIONS

1. Place the arugula on a large board, tray or bowl.
2. Cut the burrata into 8 pieces and place on top of the arugula.
3. Arrange pieces of the prosciutto around the burrata.
4. Slice the peaches and add to the salad.
5. Sprinkle the pine nuts on top.
6. Whisk together the olive oil, balsamic vinegar, Dijon mustard, honey and salt.
7. Drizzle the dressing over the salad and serve.

BLUEBERRY GOAT CHEESE SALAD WITH HONEY WALNUTS

Gluten-Free, Grain-Free

PREP 10 minutes | COOK 6 minutes | TOTAL 16 minutes | SERVES 2-4

I love the combination of flavors and textures in this salad. The soft sweet burst of blueberries with the crunchy walnuts and velvety goat cheese is so satisfying. Adding the freshly toasted walnuts with honey melts the goat cheese and creates a creamy dressing with the olive oil and lemon juice. It is so flavorful you won't even realize you are eating spinach.

INGREDIENTS (SALAD)

6 cups of fresh spinach, chopped

1 pint of fresh blueberries

4 ounces goat cheese, crumbled

INGREDIENTS (DRESSING)

2 Tablespoons olive oil, divided

1 cup walnut halves and pieces

1 Tablespoon honey

1 lemon, juiced

Sea salt to taste

DIRECTIONS

1. Place the chopped spinach in a large salad bowl.
2. Place the blueberries and the goat cheese on top of the spinach.
3. In a large sauté pan over medium-high heat, add 1 Tablespoon olive oil.
4. When the oil is hot, add the walnuts and sauté for 2 minutes, stirring occasionally.
5. Add the honey and sauté and stir the walnuts for an additional 1-2 minutes until the walnuts are golden brown.
6. Pour the warm honey walnuts over the salad and stir quickly to melt the goat cheese.
7. Add 1 Tablespoon of olive oil, juice from 1 lemon and a pinch of sea salt and toss.
8. Adjust salt to taste.

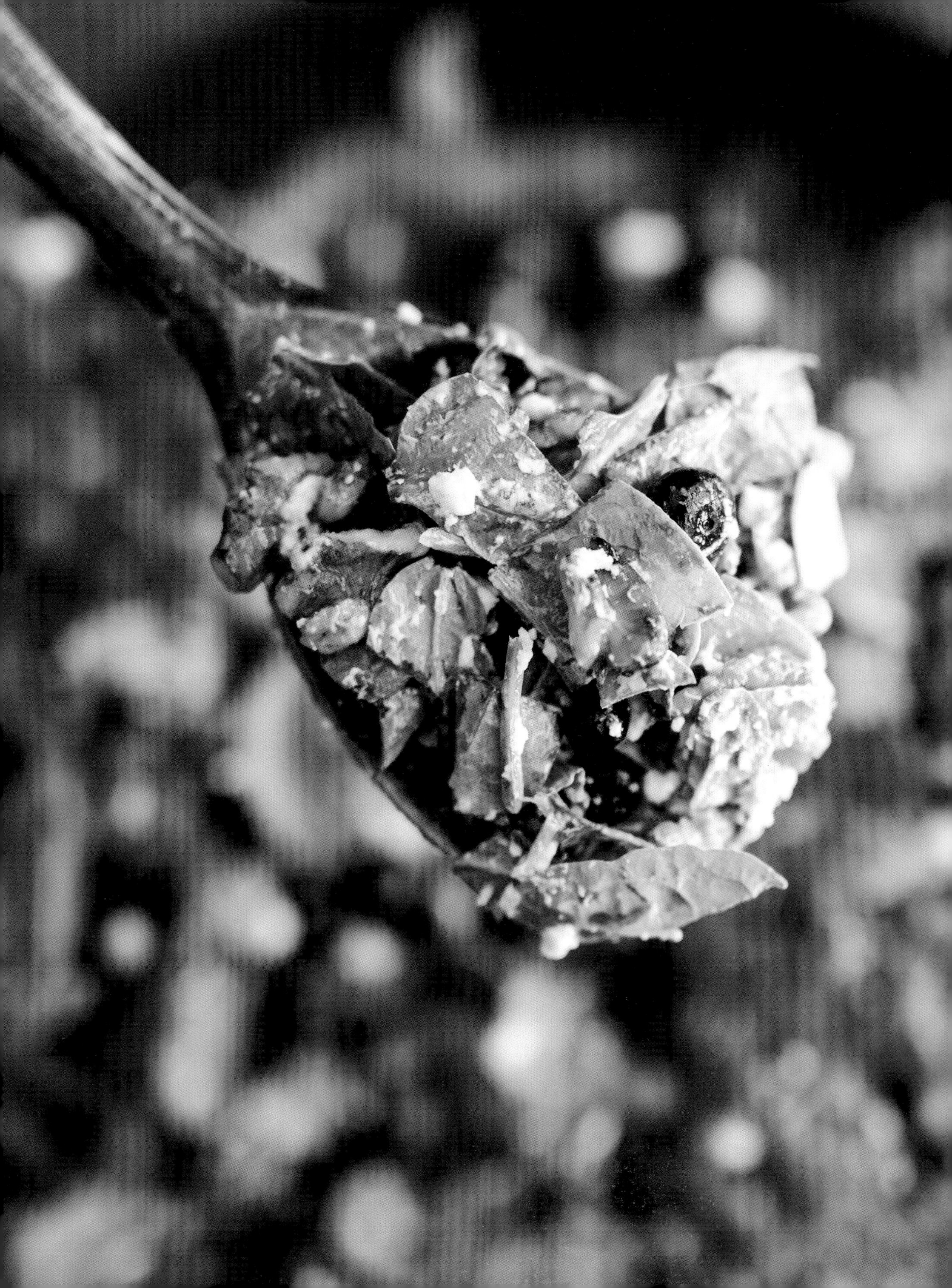

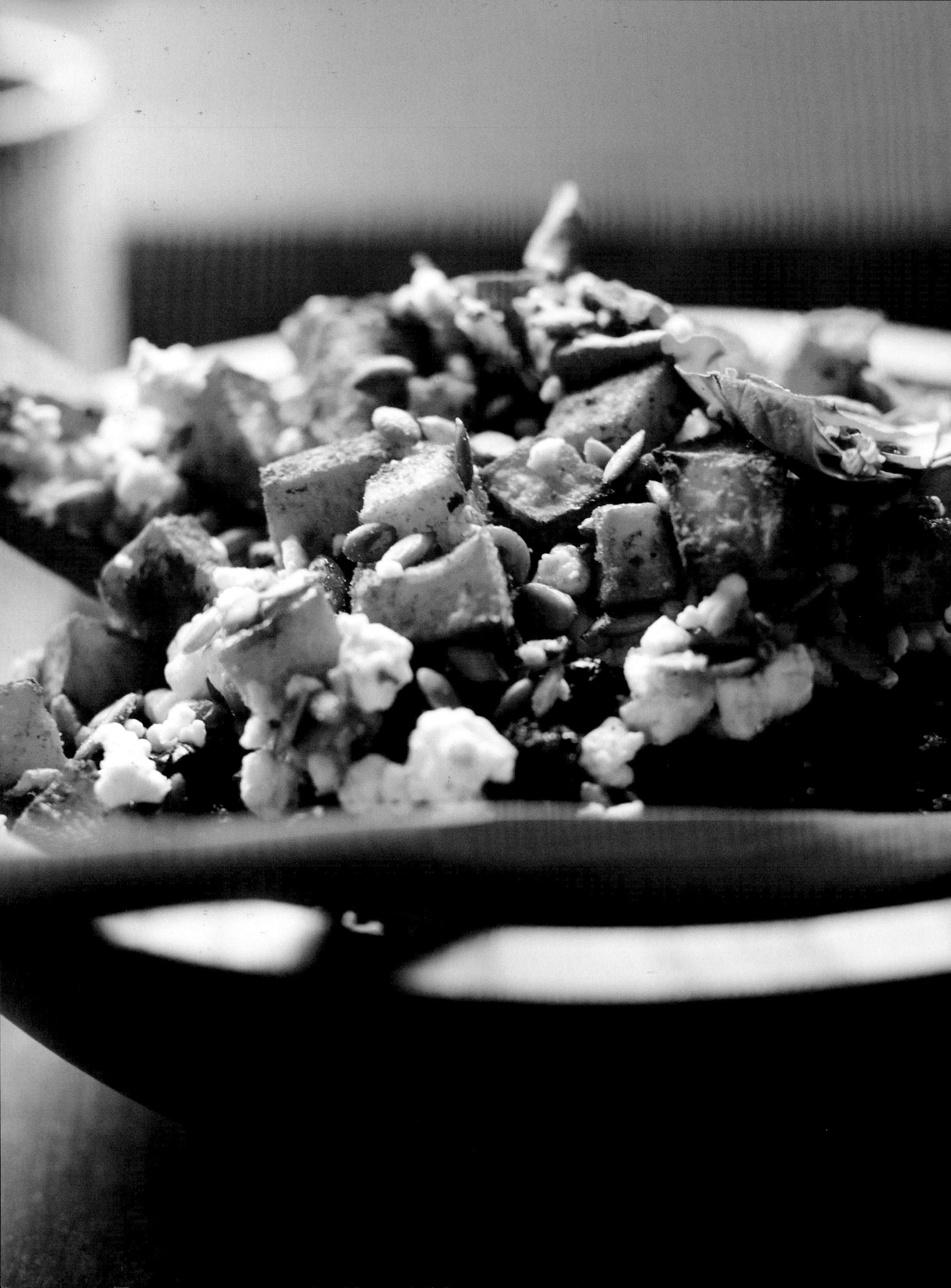

ROASTED PUMPKIN AND QUINOA SALAD

Gluten-Free (Adaptable for Dairy-Free, Vegan)

PREP 40 minutes | COOK 50 minutes | TOTAL 1 hour 30 minutes
SERVES 2 as an entree or 4-6 as a side salad

This roasted pumpkin salad is festive with colorful ingredients that look and taste like fall. The salad is hearty and can be served as an entree or a side dish. To adapt for dairy-free and vegan, omit the goat cheese.

INGREDIENTS (SALAD)

1 small pie or sugar pumpkin

2 Tablespoons olive oil

1 teaspoon sea salt

1 teaspoon paprika

1 teaspoon cumin

1/4 teaspoon cayenne

1/2 cup red quinoa, uncooked

1 cup water

6 cups spinach, chopped

2 ounces crumbled goat cheese

1/2 cup dried cranberries sweetened with apple juice

1/2 cup roasted and salted pepitas

INGREDIENTS (DRESSING)

3 Tablespoons olive oil

1 Tablespoon apple cider vinegar

1 teaspoon pure maple syrup

1 teaspoon Dijon mustard

1/4 teaspoon sea salt

DIRECTIONS

1. Preheat the oven to 400 degrees.
2. Cut the pumpkin in half.
3. Using a large spoon, scrape out the seeds and fibrous strands.
4. Cut the pumpkin into wedges and remove the skin.
5. Cut the wedges into cubes.
6. In a medium bowl, place the pumpkin cubes, olive oil, sea salt, paprika, cumin and cayenne and mix well.
7. Spread the pumpkin on a parchment-lined sheet pan and roast for 40-50 minutes, stirring halfway through.
8. Meanwhile, rinse the quinoa and place in a small saucepan with 1 cup of water.
9. Bring to a boil and then reduce to a simmer and cover.
10. Cook the quinoa until all the water is absorbed, about 10-15 minutes.
11. Fluff with a fork and set aside.
12. Place chopped spinach in a salad bowl.
13. Top spinach with quinoa.
14. Add the roasted pumpkin.
15. Add the goat cheese, cranberries and pepitas.
16. Place ingredients for the dressing in a small jar and shake well.
17. Pour the dressing over the salad and toss well.

BUTTER LEAF SALAD WITH GOAT CHEESE MEDALLIONS

Gluten-Free, Grain-Free

PREP 20 minutes | COOK 20 minutes | TOTAL 40 minutes | SERVES 4

The combination of butter leaf lettuce and warm goat cheese makes for a perfect salad. Slices of goat cheese are coated in egg and an almond flour mixture and lightly fried. The goat cheese medallions are placed on tender lettuce leaves along with toasted walnuts and pomegranate seeds. Serve it with my EFK Shallot Vinaigrette on page 230.

INGREDIENTS

3/4 cup walnut halves and pieces

2 heads butter leaf lettuce

1/2 cup pomegranate seeds

6 ounces goat cheese, chilled

1 egg

1/2 cup almond flour

1/4 teaspoon garlic powder

1/4 teaspoon salt

Olive oil

EFK Shallot Vinaigrette (page 230)

DIRECTIONS

1. Preheat the oven to 350 degrees.
2. Spread the walnuts on a parchment-lined sheet pan.
3. Toast the walnuts in the oven for 8-10 minutes or until browned, shaking halfway through.
4. Set aside to cool.
5. Split the butter leaf lettuce heads in half and arrange on four salad plates.
6. Top the greens with toasted walnuts and pomegranate seeds.
7. Using dental floss, cut the goat cheese into 8 slices.
8. In a small bowl, whisk the egg until blended.
9. In another small bowl, combine the almond flour, garlic powder and salt.
10. Dip a slice of goat cheese in the egg and then toss in the almond flour mixture.
11. Repeat with remaining goat cheese and place the medallions on a small plate or tray.
12. Put the goat cheese medallions in the freezer for 15 minutes.

(Continued)

13. Pour the olive oil into a medium sauté pan until it reaches up about 1/4 inch on the side of the pan.
14. Heat oil over medium heat.
15. Gently fry the medallions until golden brown, flipping once.
16. Place 2 medallions on each salad.
17. Drizzle with EFK Shallot Vinaigrette.
18. Serve while goat cheese is warm.

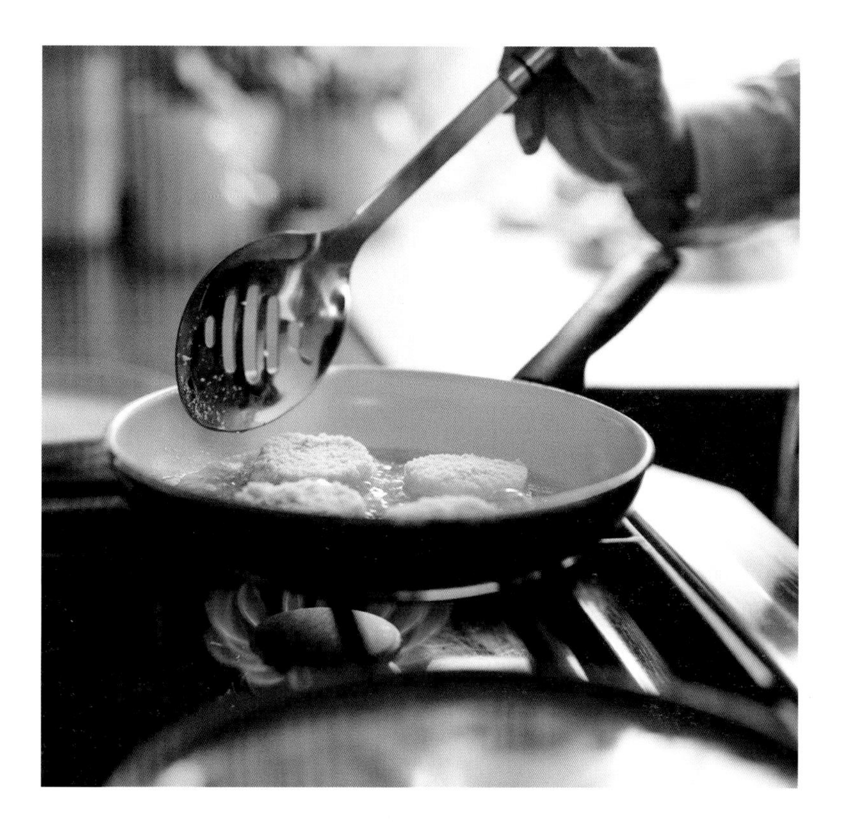

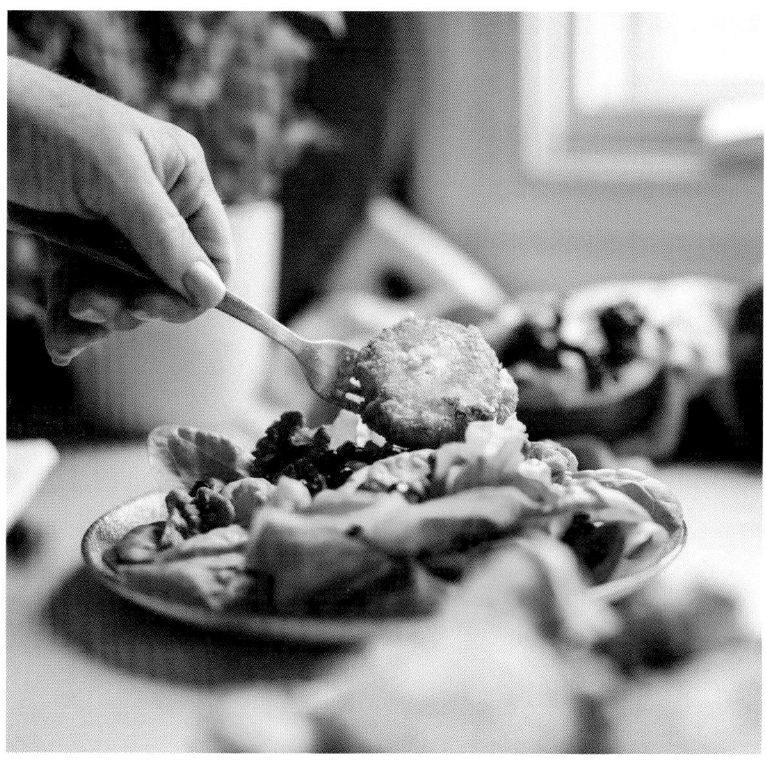

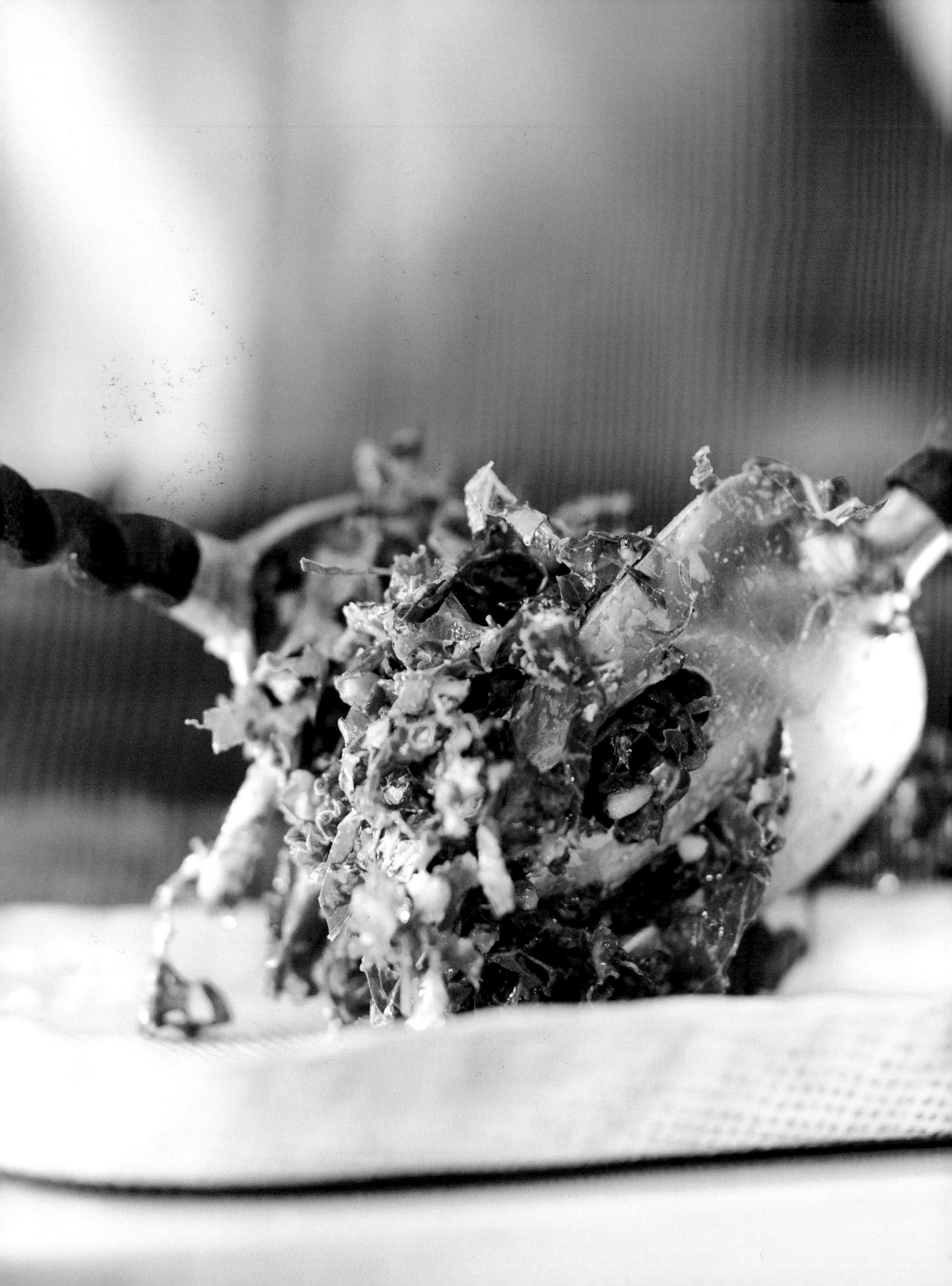

KALE SALAD WITH GARLIC DRESSING

Gluten-Free, Grain-Free, SCD (Adaptable for Dairy-Free, Paleo, Vegan)

PREP 10 minutes | COOK 0 minutes | TOTAL 10 minutes | SERVES 2-4

I'll be honest here: Kale was not one of my favorite vegetables. It is, however, a nutritional powerhouse loaded with vitamins, minerals, essential amino acids and fiber, making it very worthy of consumption. Because of the nutritional benefits, I used to throw kale in my smoothies to ensure I was getting it in my diet. Then I started including kale in my salads, adding more each time. I found that massaging the leaves with a little olive oil makes it more palatable. The taste and texture continued to grow on me and now I love it. To adapt for dairy-free, paleo and vegan, omit the Parmesan cheese.

INGREDIENTS (SALAD)

1 bunch fresh kale

2 teaspoons olive oil

1/3 cup pine nuts, toasted

1/4 cup freshly grated Parmesan cheese

INGREDIENTS (DRESSING)

3 cloves garlic, minced

2 Tablespoons Dijon mustard

Juice from 1 lemon

1/4 teaspoon salt

1/2 cup olive oil

DIRECTIONS

1. Wash kale, remove the center rib and trim off the ends.
2. Chop the kale into thin strips, then chop crosswise into small pieces and place in a salad bowl.
3. Drizzle the kale with 2 teaspoons of olive oil and rub the kale with your hands to massage it, making sure to get all of the pieces for about 2-3 minutes.
4. Place the toasted pine nuts and Parmesan cheese on top of the kale.
5. Place garlic, Dijon mustard, lemon juice and salt in a mini food processor and blend well.
6. With food processor running, slowly add olive oil until combined. It will be thick.
7. Add half of the dressing and toss.
8. Taste the salad and add more dressing if needed.
9. Store leftover dressing in an airtight container in the refrigerator for up to 5 days.

SHAVED BRUSSELS SPROUT SALAD

Gluten-Free, Grain-Free, SCD (Adaptable for Dairy-Free, Paleo, Vegan)

PREP 10 minutes | COOK 0 minutes | TOTAL 10 minutes | SERVES 3-4

This salad was inspired by a dish I had at a restaurant called Biscuit Love in Nashville. While there for breakfast with girlfriends, we decided to order something healthier to balance out the indulgent biscuit dishes we were sampling. It came topped with poached eggs and ended up being as delicious as the restaurant's famous biscuits. When I returned home, I was craving the crunch and lemony flavor of the salad, so I created my own version. I omit the eggs and add avocado, fresh basil, dried blueberries and chopped marcona almonds and toss in a grainy mustard vinaigrette. You can shave the Brussels sprouts yourself in a food processor or buy them shaved and ready to go. To adapt for dairy-free and paleo, omit the Parmesan cheese. To adapt for vegan, omit the Parmesan cheese and substitute pure maple syrup for honey.

INGREDIENTS (SALAD)

10-12 ounces shaved Brussels sprouts

1 cup fresh basil, sliced chiffonade

1/2 cup marcona almonds, roughly chopped

1 avocado, diced

1/3 cup dried blueberries, unsweetened or sweetened with juice if possible

1/3 cup shredded Asiago or Parmesan cheese

INGREDIENTS (DRESSING)

1/4 cup olive oil

1 Tablespoon whole-grain Dijon mustard

1 Tablespoon fresh lemon juice

1/2 teaspoon honey

1/4 teaspoon salt

DIRECTIONS

1. Place the shaved Brussels sprouts in a salad bowl.
2. Add the remaining salad ingredients.
3. In a small bowl, whisk together the olive oil, mustard, lemon juice, honey and salt.
4. Pour the dressing over the salad and toss well.

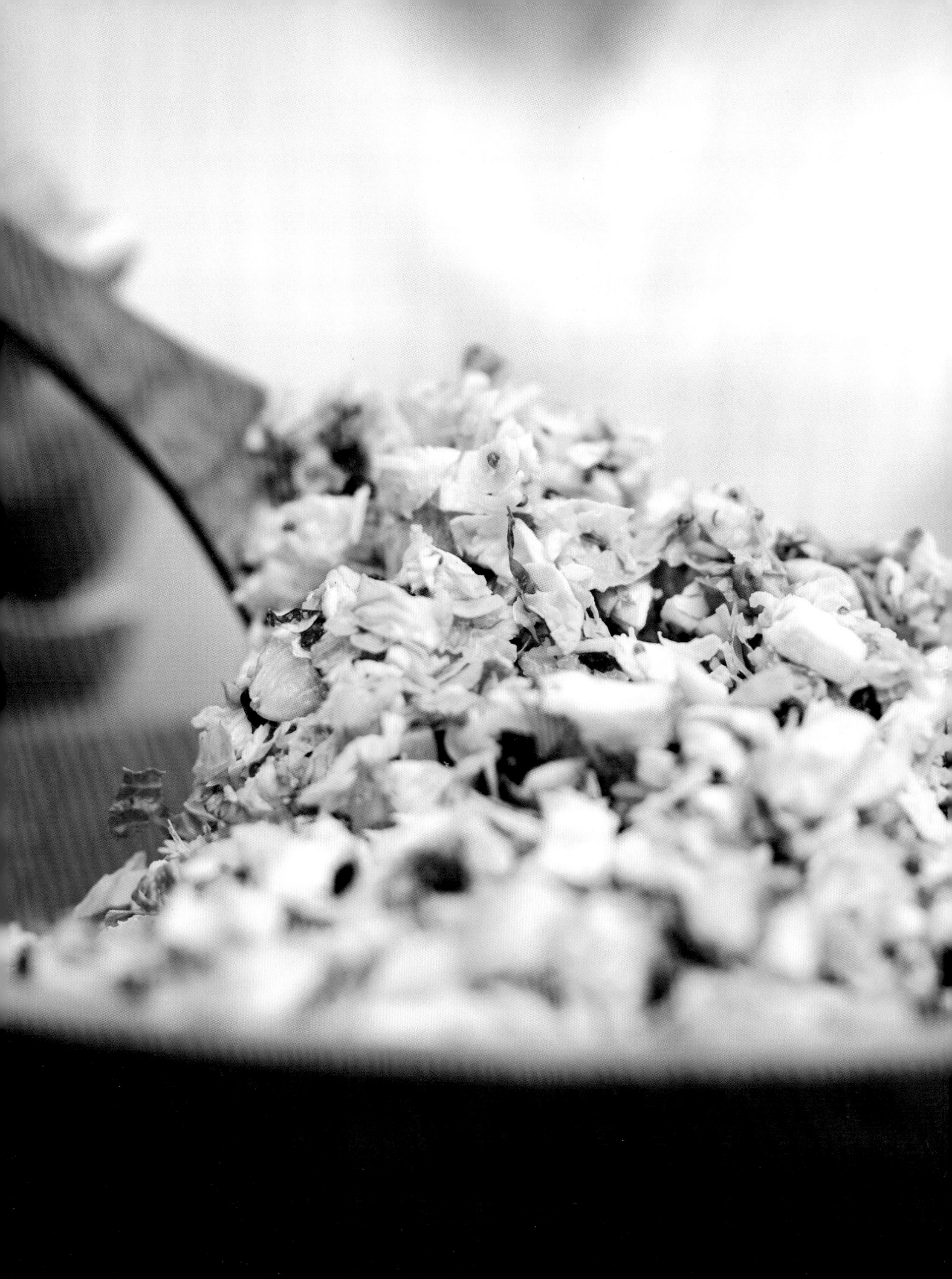

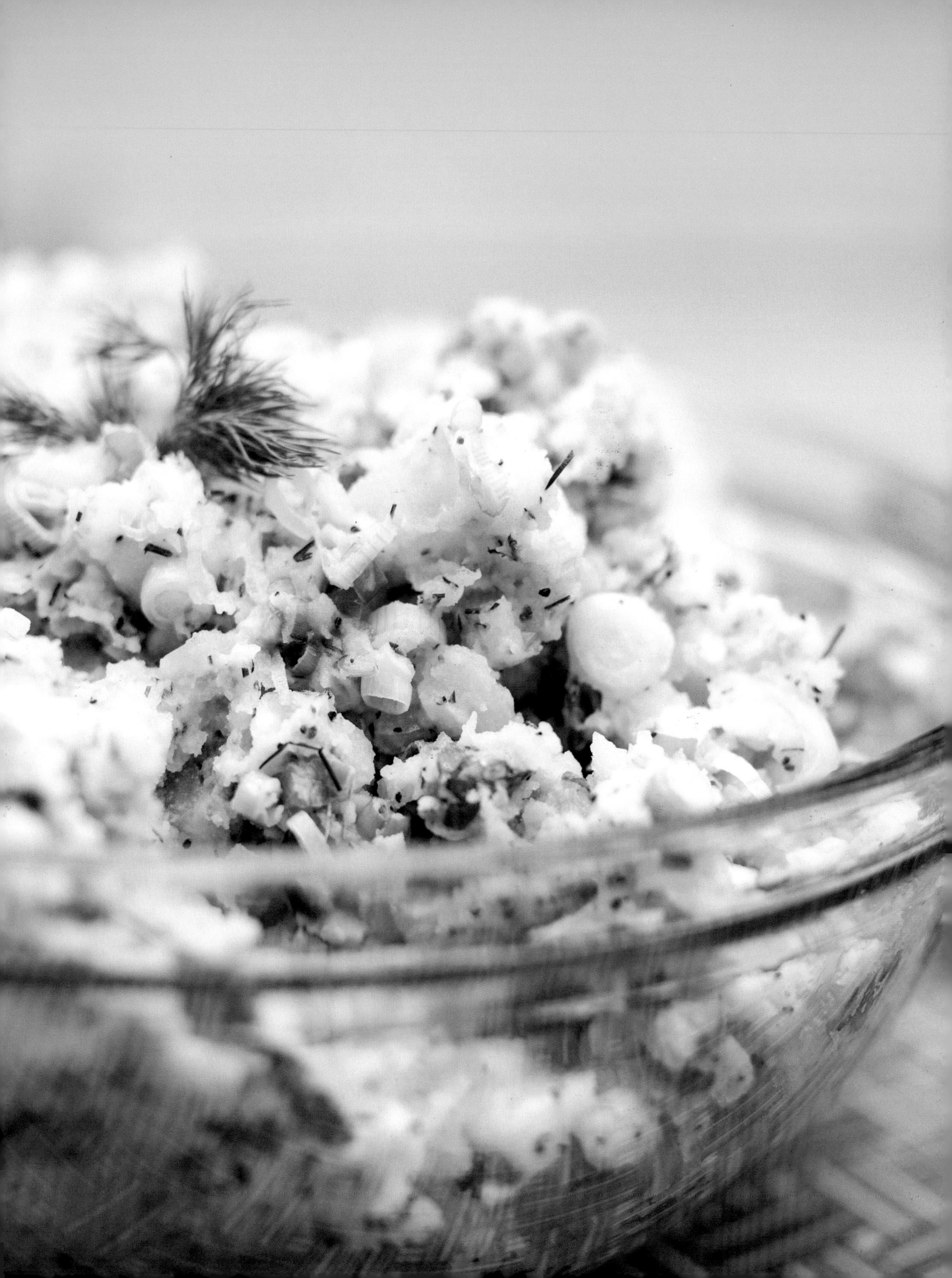

RED POTATO SALAD

Dairy-Free, Gluten-Free, Grain-Free, Paleo (Adaptable for Vegan)

PREP 20 minutes | COOK 30 minutes | TOTAL 50 minutes | SERVES 10-12

Potato salad is an American picnic and potluck staple. It always seems to be the first side dish to disappear at summer gatherings. This recipe is based on the one my mom made when I was growing up. The ingredients are simple but delicious when combined. I recommend using homemade or high-quality mayonnaise—it makes all the difference. My favorite brand is Sir Kensington's made with avocado oil and cage-free eggs. To minimize time chopping, I boil the potatoes whole and break them apart with a potato masher once cooked. I also like how the ingredients meld together when the potatoes are prepared this way. To adapt for vegan, use vegan mayonnaise.

INGREDIENTS

3 pounds red potatoes, scrubbed

1 teaspoon salt

1 1/2 cups chopped celery

3 bunches green onions, chopped

1 cup of homemade or good-quality mayonnaise

2 Tablespoons minced fresh dill

2 teaspoons celery seed

1 1/2 teaspoons salt

1 teaspoon black pepper

DIRECTIONS

1. Place the potatoes in a large pot and cover with water and 1 teaspoon salt.
2. Bring to a boil and cook for 25-30 minutes or until tender.
3. Drain the potatoes and place in a large bowl.
4. Allow the potatoes to cool for 10 minutes.
5. Using a potato masher or a large spoon, break the potatoes into small pieces.
6. Add the remaining ingredients and mix well.
7. Serve warm or chilled.
8. Store leftover salad in an airtight container in the refrigerator for 3-4 days.

MEXICAN STREET CORN SALAD

Gluten-Free

PREP 18 minutes | COOK 12 minutes | TOTAL 30 minutes | SERVES 4-6

I love Mexican street corn and I also love a good green salad. I was craving both one day so I decided to combine the two in one dish. The recipe that resulted has become the most requested menu item in my house this summer. It is simple to make and full of great flavor.

INGREDIENTS (SALAD)

1 large or 2 small heads of romaine, washed and dried

4 cobs of corn

2 teaspoons olive oil

1 cup diced onion

1/2 teaspoon salt

1/8 teaspoon cayenne

4 ounces cotija cheese, crumbled

1 bunch fresh cilantro, chopped

1/3 cup roasted and salted pepitas

1 jalapeño, sliced crosswise

INGREDIENTS (DRESSING)

1/3 cup homemade or good-quality mayonnaise

1/3 cup Mexican crema or sour cream

Juice from 1 lime

1/2 teaspoon salt

1/4 teaspoon cayenne

DIRECTIONS

1. Chop the romaine lettuce and place in a large salad bowl or platter.
2. Cut the corn kernels off of the cob.
3. In a large sauté pan, heat the olive oil.
4. Add the diced onions and corn kernels to the pan and sauté over medium heat, stirring occasionally.
5. Add the salt and cayenne pepper and cook for about 10-12 minutes or until some of the corn and onions are caramelized and golden brown.
6. Meanwhile, whisk together the dressing ingredients and set aside.
7. Place the corn and onion mixture over the romaine lettuce.
8. Sprinkle the cotija cheese and cilantro on top of the corn.
9. Drizzle the dressing over the salad and then top with the pepitas and sliced jalapeños.

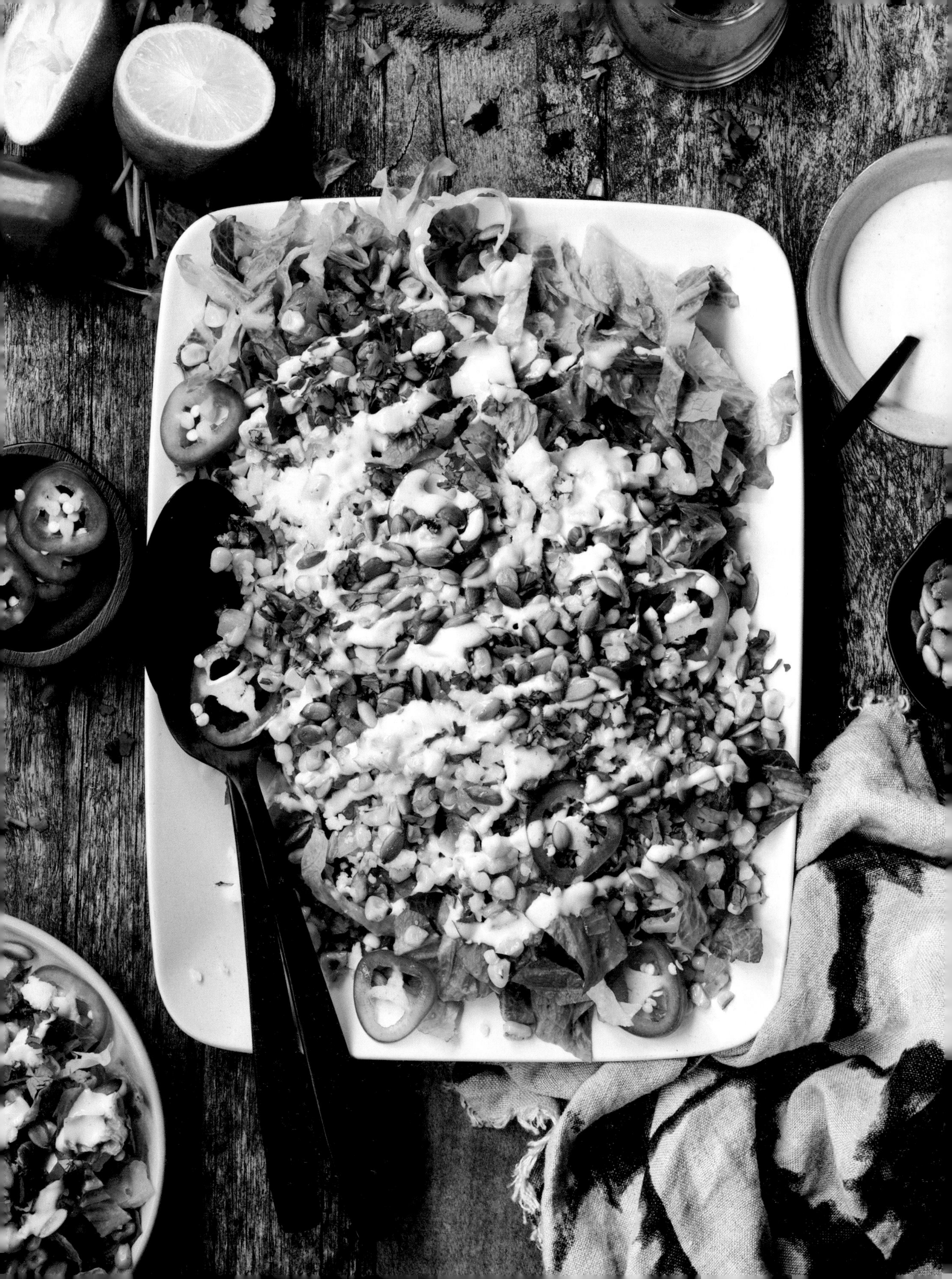

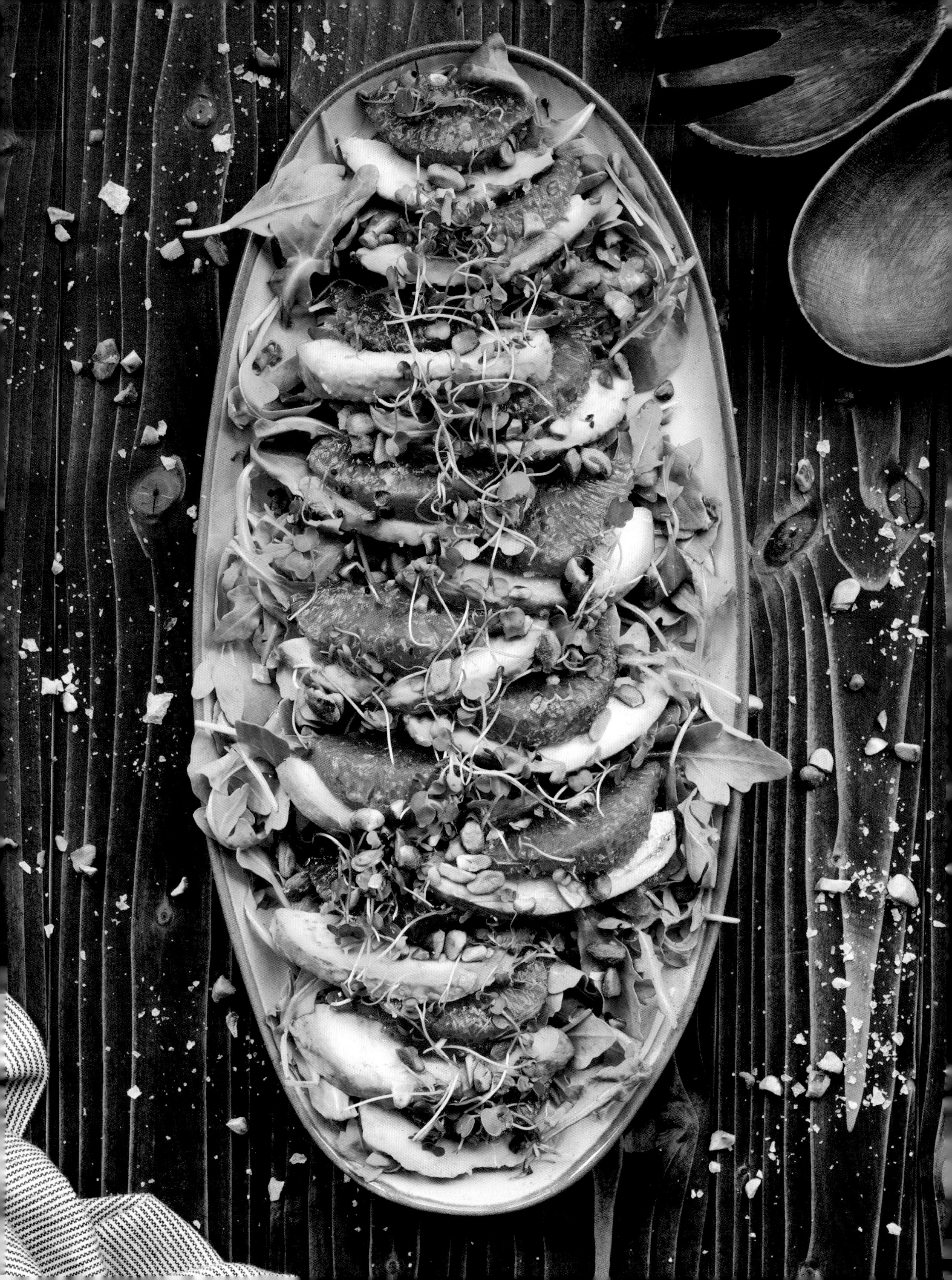

GRAPEFRUIT AND AVOCADO SALAD

Dairy-Free, Gluten-Free, Grain-Free, Paleo, SCD, Vegan

PREP 10 minutes | COOK 0 minutes | TOTAL 10 minutes | SERVES 4

This simple salad is as delicious as it is gorgeous. The bright grapefruit and creamy avocado complement each other impeccably well. To preserve the individual flavors of each fruit, I keep the dressing simple using only olive oil and Maldon sea salt. The microgreens add an additional boost of nutrients, and the pistachios give it a delightful crunch. This salad is a beautiful accompaniment to any brunch, lunch or dinner table.

INGREDIENTS

2 ruby red grapefruits

2 ripe but firm avocados

3 cups arugula

Olive oil for drizzling

Maldon sea salt or other coarse sea salt flakes

1/2 cup of microgreens

1/3 cup pistachios, roughly chopped

DIRECTIONS

1. Using a sharp knife, trim off the ends of a grapefruit and place it with the cut side up.
2. Cut off the rind and pith following the shape of the fruit, taking care not to remove too much of the flesh.
3. Slice lengthwise between a section of the grapefruit and the membrane. Repeat on the other side of the segment.
4. Repeat until all of the grapefruit segments are cut and removed.
5. Repeat with the second grapefruit.
6. Cut an avocado in half lengthwise and remove the pit.
7. Using a large spoon, scoop out the flesh of the avocado in one piece.
8. Place the avocado with the cut side down on a cutting board and slice lengthwise.
9. Repeat with the second avocado.
10. Place the arugula on a medium platter or in a shallow bowl.
11. Arrange the grapefruit sections and avocado over the arugula, alternating between fruits.
12. Drizzle olive oil over the salad.
13. Sprinkle sea salt flakes over the salad.
14. Top with the microgreens.
15. Sprinkle the pistachio nuts on top of the salad.

BIRCH'S SALAD

Gluten-Free

PREP 10 minutes | COOK 20 minutes | TOTAL 30 minutes | SERVES 2-4

We have a wonderful restaurant close to our home called Birch's on the Lake. It is one of those places that has a neighborhood feel and everything on the menu is great. There is one salad it serves that I particularly love made with crisp lettuce, quinoa, chèvre, avocado, red onion, pistachios and a lovely green goddess dressing. I find myself craving it at times. When the pandemic hit and restaurants temporarily closed, I recreated the salad at home using my EFK Avocado Herb Dressing on page 225.

INGREDIENTS

6 cups butter lettuce pieces

1 1/2 cups tricolor quinoa, cooked

1/2 cup sliced red onion

1 avocado, sliced

1/2 cup pistachios

4 ounces chèvre

EFK Avocado Herb Dressing (page 225)

DIRECTIONS

1. In a large salad bowl, layer the butter lettuce, quinoa, red onion, avocado and pistachios.
2. Break the soft chèvre into small pieces and place on top of the salad.
3. Serve with EFK Avocado Herb Dressing.

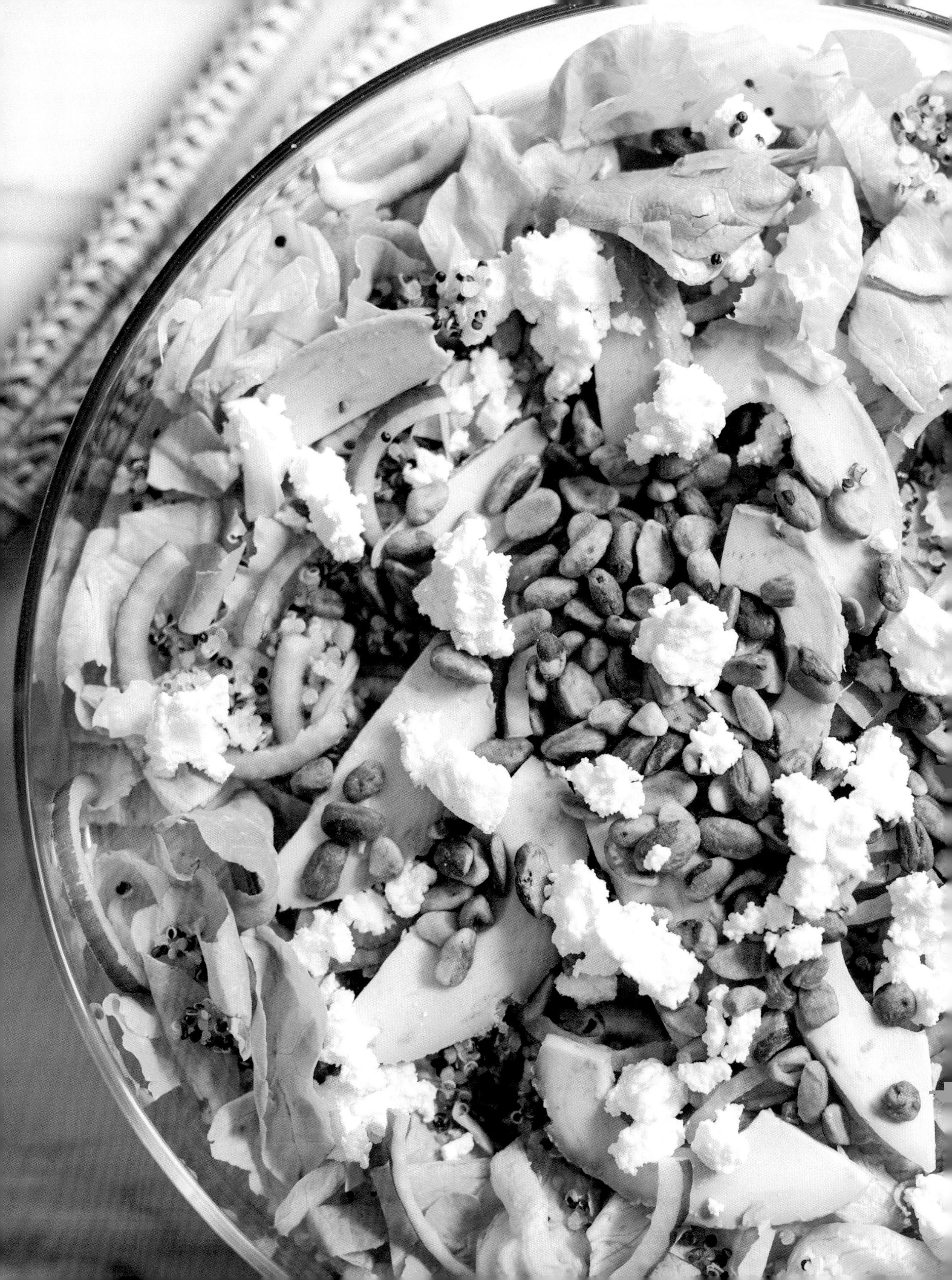

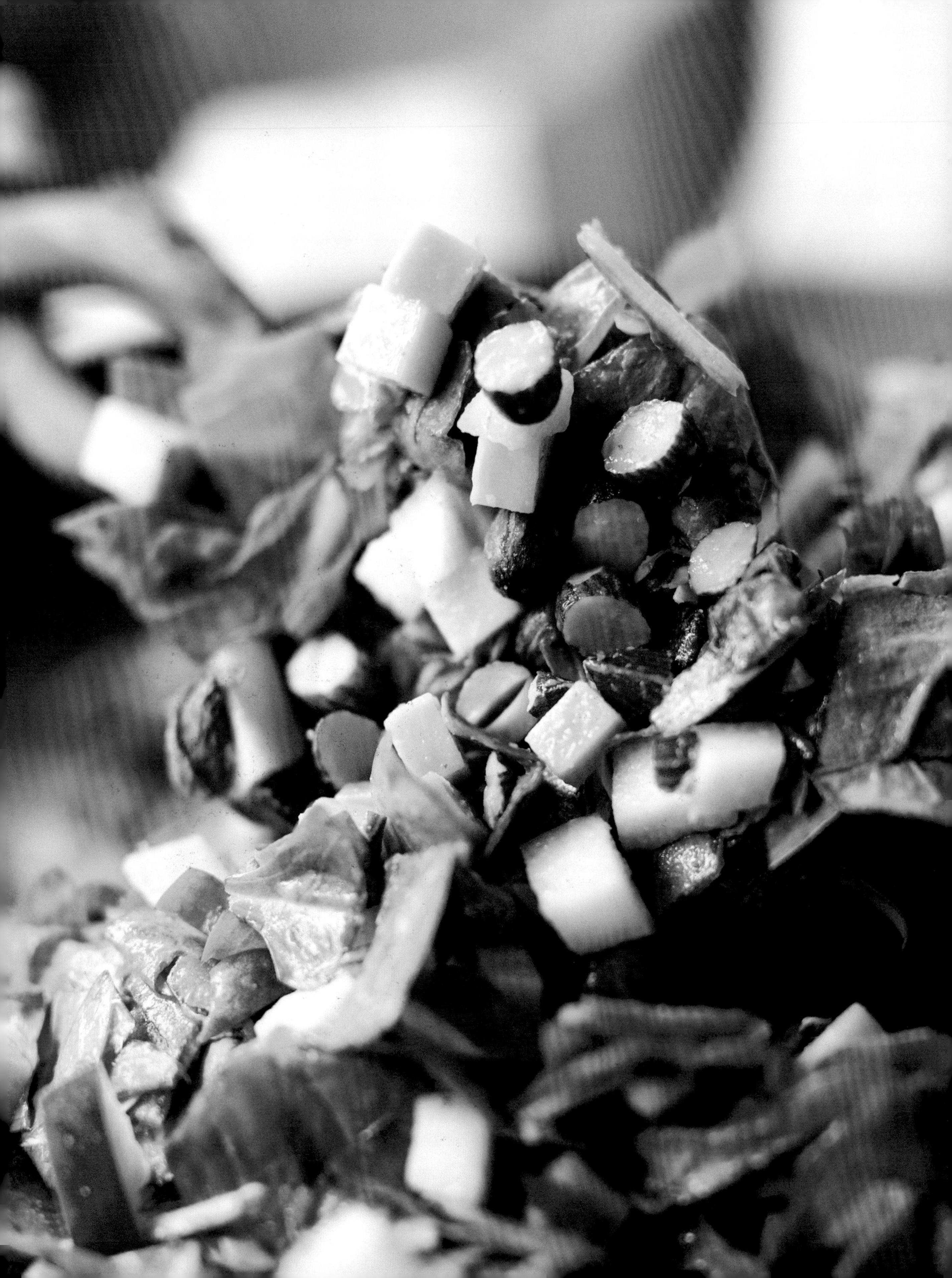

APPLE, CHEDDAR AND SMOKED ALMOND SALAD

Gluten-Free, Grain-Free (Adaptable for SCD)

PREP 15 minutes | COOK 0 minutes | TOTAL 15 minutes | SERVES 4

I love the combination of apples, cheddar cheese and smoked almonds. Adding these ingredients to fresh spinach and topping it with a simple honey Dijon mustard dressing makes a delicious salad. This recipe couldn't be easier to prepare and it is always a crowd pleaser. To adapt for SCD, use SCD-approved almonds.

DIRECTIONS

1. Chop the fresh spinach and place in a large salad bowl.
2. Cut the cheddar cheese into small cubes and place on top of the spinach.
3. Core and dice the apple and add to the salad.
4. Add the smoked almonds.
5. In a small jar, add the olive oil, vinegar or lemon juice, Dijon mustard, honey and sea salt.
6. Place a lid on the jar and shake until combined.
7. Pour over the salad and toss well.

INGREDIENTS (SALAD)

4 cups of fresh spinach

4 ounces sharp cheddar cheese

1 apple (I like Honeycrisp, but any variety will do)

1/2 cup chopped smoked almonds

INGREDIENTS (DRESSING)

3 Tablespoons olive oil

1 Tablespoon white balsamic vinegar or fresh lemon juice

1 Tablespoon Dijon mustard

1 teaspoon honey

1/4 teaspoon sea salt

WILD RICE SALAD WITH CHICKEN

Dairy-Free, Gluten-Free (Adaptable for Vegan)

PREP 10 minutes | COOK 55 minutes | TOTAL 1 hour 5 minutes | SERVES 6

This is a wonderful recipe that my mother has made for years. It's great to serve for lunch when entertaining family or friends. I love the nuttiness of the wild rice, the creaminess of the avocado and the crunch of the pecans. This salad is great without the chicken too. To adapt for vegan, omit the chicken, substitute pure maple syrup for honey and add extra red peppers and snow peas.

INGREDIENTS (SALAD)

2 cups wild rice

6 cups water

1 teaspoon sea salt

1/2 lemon, juiced

2 cooked chicken breasts, cubed

1 red pepper, diced

4 green onions, chopped

3 ounces snow peas, cut in 1-inch pieces

1-2 avocados, diced

1 cup of toasted pecan halves

INGREDIENTS (DRESSING)

2 cloves garlic, minced

1 Tablespoon Dijon mustard

1/2 teaspoon sea salt

1/2 teaspoon honey

1/4 teaspoon black pepper

1/4 cup rice vinegar

1/3 cup olive oil

DIRECTIONS

1. Place wild rice, 6 cups of water and sea salt in a saucepan and place over high heat.
2. Bring to a boil and stir.
3. Turn the heat down to low and cover.
4. Simmer for 40-45 minutes or until tender.
5. Drain the excess liquid and cool.
6. In a large bowl, toss the wild rice with the lemon juice.
7. Add the chicken, red pepper, green onions and snow peas.
8. In a small food processor, combine the garlic, Dijon mustard, sea salt, honey, black pepper and rice vinegar and blend well.
9. With the food processor running, slowly add the olive oil to make the dressing.
10. Add the dressing to the salad and toss well.
11. Right before serving, add the avocados and toasted pecan halves and lightly toss.

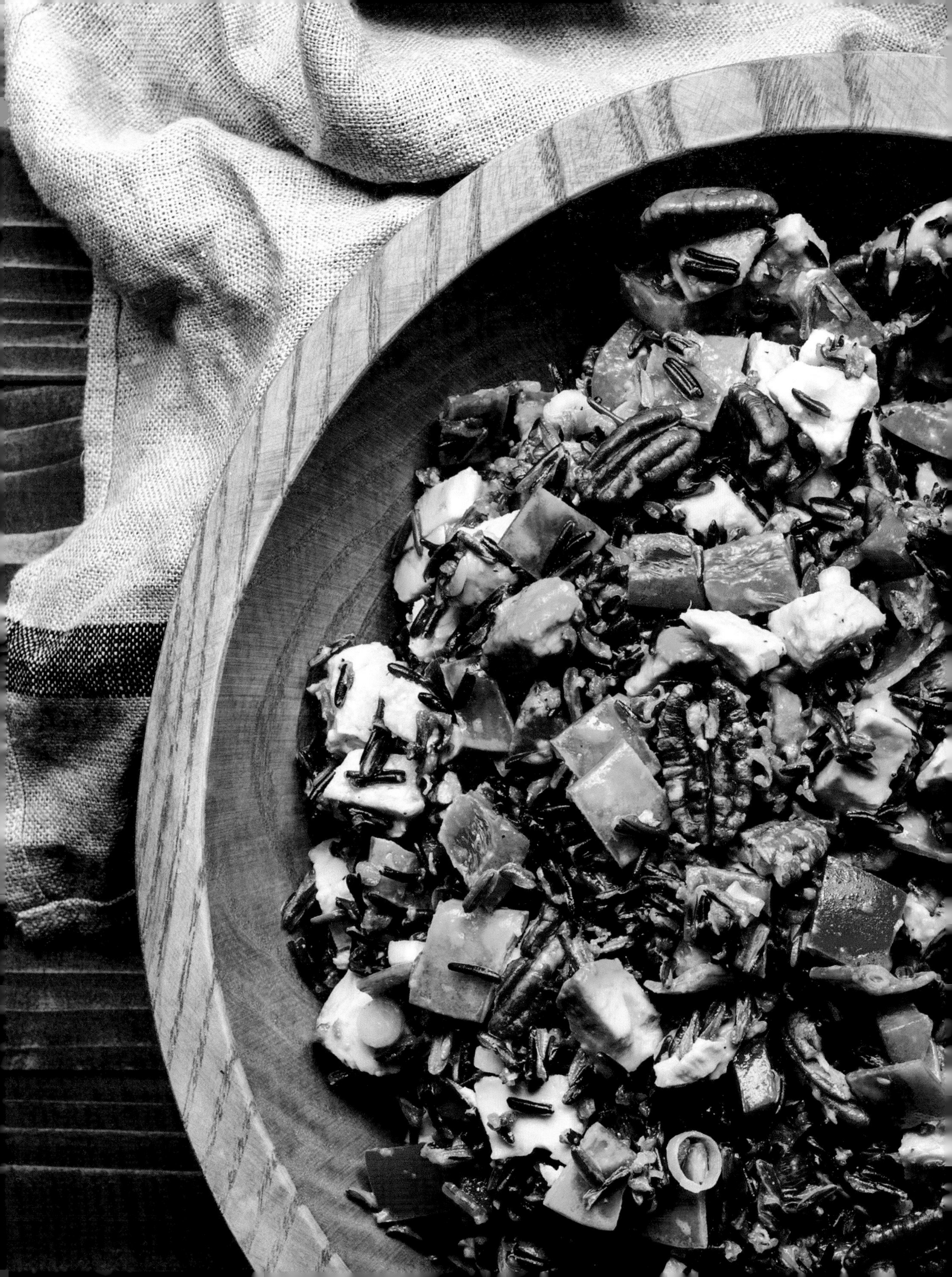

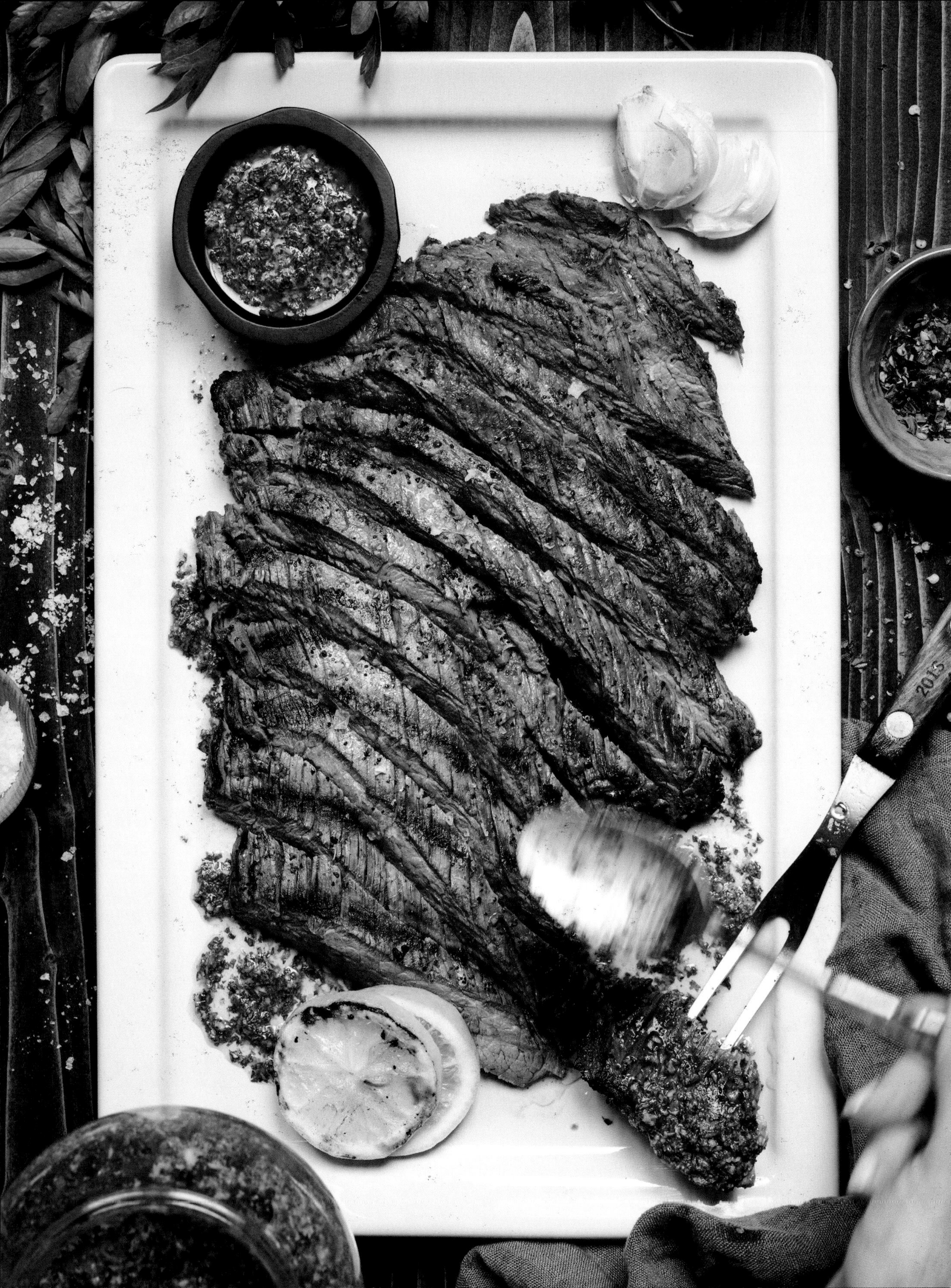

MAIN DISHES

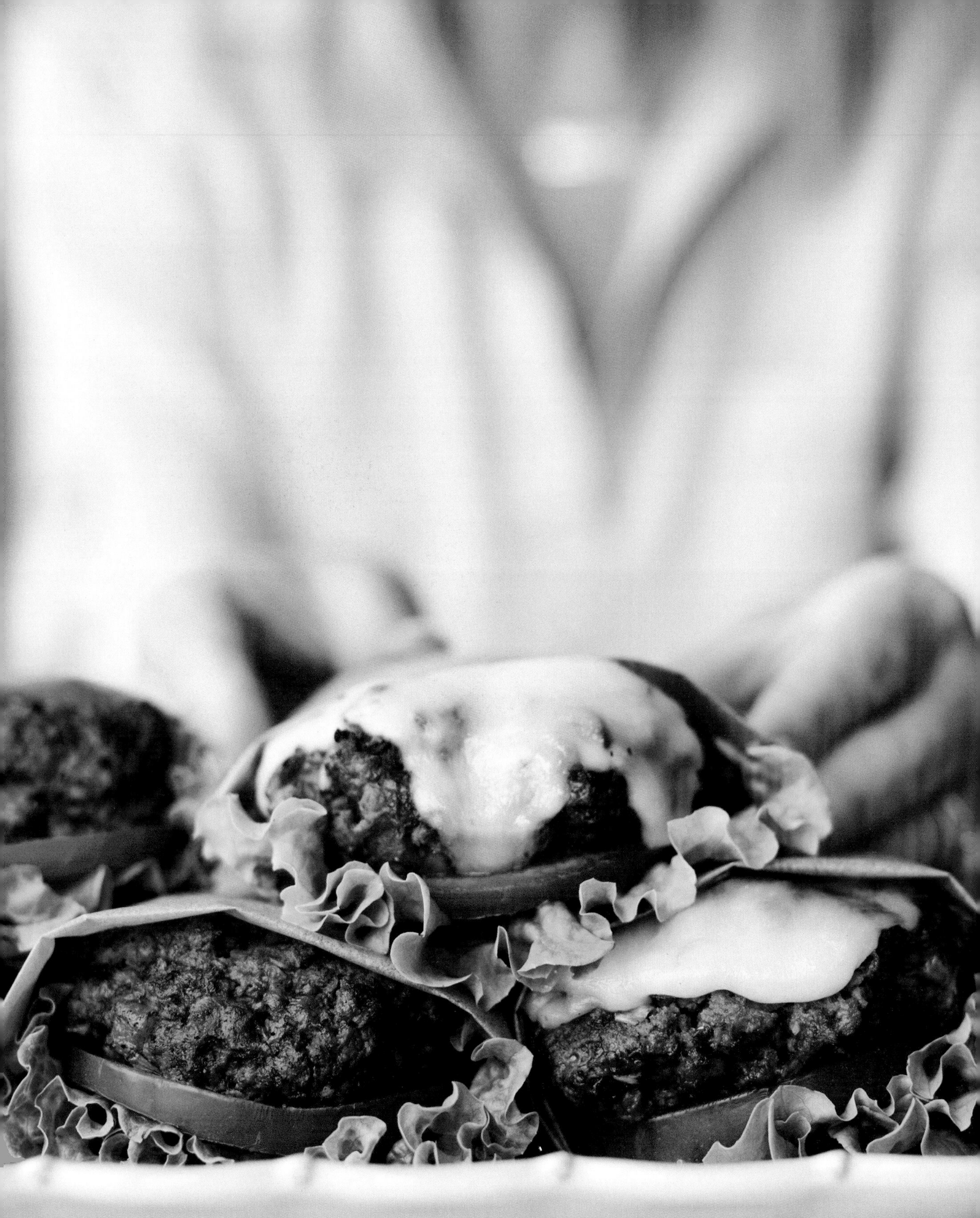

AVOCADO BURGERS

Dairy-Free, Gluten-Free, Grain-Free, Paleo, SCD

PREP 15 minutes | COOK 15 minutes | TOTAL 30 minutes | SERVES 8

These are honestly the best burgers. I have yet to meet someone who has not loved them. My mother made these often when we were growing up, and they are still a favorite for everyone in my family. Be sure to use 90 percent lean ground beef. A higher fat content than that will cause the burgers to fall apart on the grill. If you like more fat in your ground beef, don't worry. The avocado adds enough fat to keep them tender and juicy. At my house, we like to eat these wrapped in lettuce with tomato. If you eat bread, they are also incredible on a toasted, buttered bun.

INGREDIENTS

2 pounds grass-fed ground beef, 90% lean

1 avocado, mashed

1 4-ounce can diced green chiles

1/4 cup chopped green onions

2 cloves garlic, minced

1 Tablespoon lemon pepper

1 teaspoon salt

Large lettuce leaves or buttered and toasted hamburger buns, Monterey Jack cheese and sliced tomatoes, for serving

DIRECTIONS

1. In a large bowl, combine the burger ingredients and mix well.
2. Form the mixture into 8 patties and grill over medium heat for 5-7 minutes on each side or until desired doneness.
3. If using cheese, top burgers for last minute of cooking.
4. Wrap the burgers in a lettuce leaf with tomato if not using buns.
5. If you are serving on a bun, place hamburger buns open facedown on the grill for 1-2 minutes to toast.
6. Butter and top the buns with burger, lettuce and tomato.

GRILLED ASIAN CHICKEN THIGHS

Dairy-Free, Gluten-Free, Grain-Free (Adaptable for Paleo)

PREP 8 minutes | COOK 12 minutes | TOTAL 20 minutes* | SERVES 4-6

These chicken thighs are on the dinner rotation at my house year-round and are a guaranteed hit. I always make extra to add to salads or wraps for my family's lunches the next day. This is a great recipe to multiply and grill for a crowd. It is simple, delicious, and a change of pace from the usual burgers and brats served at large gatherings. To adapt for paleo, substitute coconut aminos for tamari.

**Does not include marinating or resting times, which are noted in the directions.*

INGREDIENTS

4 green onions

1/3 cup olive oil

1/3 cup tamari

3 Tablespoons Dijon mustard

2 teaspoons fresh garlic, minced

1 1/2 teaspoons fresh ginger, grated

1 1/2 teaspoons fresh lime juice

2 pounds boneless, skinless chicken thighs

DIRECTIONS

1. Chop the green onions, using the white and light green parts for the marinade and reserving the dark green part for garnish.
2. Whisk together the olive oil, tamari, Dijon mustard, white and light green parts of chopped onion, garlic, ginger and lime juice.
3. Add the chicken thighs to the marinade and refrigerate for 4-24 hours.
4. Remove the chicken from the refrigerator and let it sit at room temperature 30 minutes before grilling.
5. Grill the chicken over medium-high heat for 5-6 minutes per side or until cooked through.
6. Sprinkle with the reserved green onion.

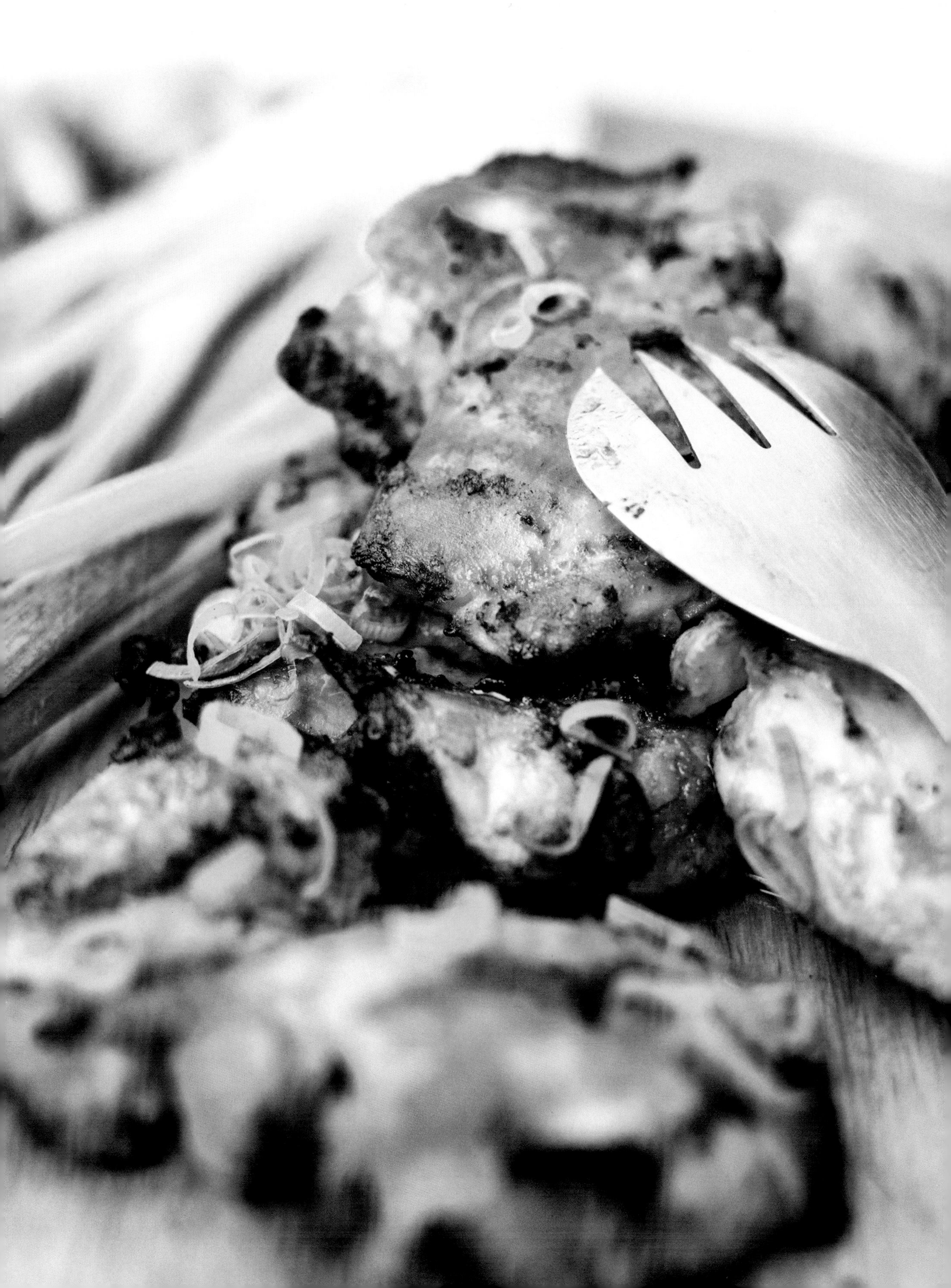

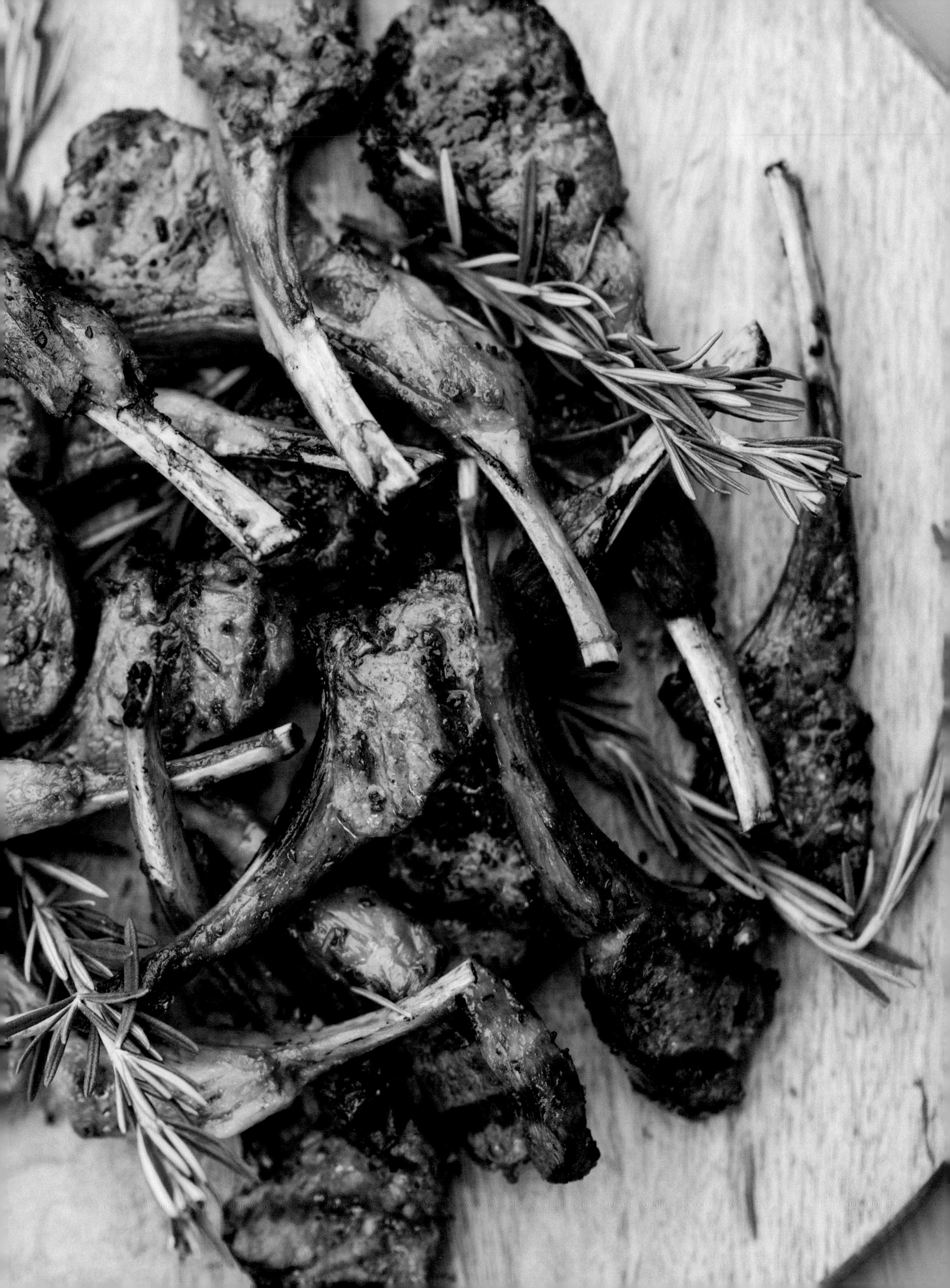

GRILLED LAMB LOLLIPOPS

Dairy-Free, Gluten-Free, Grain-Free, Paleo, SCD

PREP 20 minutes | COOK 6 minutes | TOTAL 26 minutes* | SERVES 4

This recipe is on repeat at our house in the summer. I fire up the grill as often as I can after our long Minnesota winters. These little lamb lollipops cook up quickly and are always a crowd pleaser. I wrap the bones in foil before grilling to prevent them from burning. Once they are ready, I remove the foil before arranging them on a platter with sprigs of rosemary for serving.

**Does not include marinating or resting times, which are noted in the directions.*

INGREDIENTS

3/4 cup olive oil

2 lemons, juiced

1/4 cup chopped fresh rosemary

4 cloves garlic, minced

2 teaspoons salt

2 teaspoons black pepper

2 Frenched lamb racks, about 3 pounds or 16 chops total

Sprigs of rosemary, for serving

DIRECTIONS

1. In a small bowl, combine the olive oil, lemon juice, rosemary, garlic, salt and pepper. Set aside.
2. Trim the silver skin off the underside of the lamb racks. This is the thin, white or silvery connective tissue attached to the meat.
3. Cut the racks into individual chops.
4. Wrap the bone end of the chop with a small piece of foil.
5. Dip the meat side of the chop in the marinade, making sure to get the pieces of garlic and rosemary on each chop.
6. Set in a dish to marinate.
7. Refrigerate the lamb chops for 3-24 hours.
8. Remove from the refrigerator and let sit at room temperature for 30 minutes before grilling.
9. Preheat grill to medium-high heat.
10. Grill the lamb for 2-3 minutes on each side.
11. Remove foil wraps and place on a serving tray with sprigs of rosemary.

BARBECUE BACON-WRAPPED SHRIMP

Dairy-Free, Gluten-Free, Grain-Free, Paleo, SCD

PREP 20 minutes | COOK 20 minutes | TOTAL 40 minutes | SERVES 6

When I was growing up, my family took a few vacations to the Gulf Coast of Florida. Many of the restaurants we went to offered barbecue bacon-wrapped shrimp on their menus. It became a popular entree for members of my family to order. When we returned to Minnesota, my mom would duplicate it at home for us. After I grew up, I started making it for my own family and it became a favorite for them as well.

When I was following the Specific Carbohydrate Diet, I couldn't use bottled condiments and sauces because of the added sugars and other additives. It motivated me to create a barbecue sauce I could use to make these delicious shrimp while adhering to my dietary restrictions. The recipe is on page 218. I still prefer my EFK Barbecue Sauce over bottled sauce, but you can use any barbecue sauce you like with this recipe.

INGREDIENTS

16 strips of bacon

2 pounds 21/25 count raw peeled and deveined shrimp

EFK Barbecue Sauce (page 218)

DIRECTIONS

1. Preheat oven to 350 degrees.
2. Cut strips of bacon into 3 pieces each.
3. Place the bacon pieces on a baking sheet lined with parchment paper.
4. Bake the bacon for 8 minutes.
5. If using bamboo skewers, soak in warm water for 20-30 minutes before using.
6. Wrap a piece of bacon around a shrimp and slide onto a skewer.
7. Repeat with remaining shrimp and bacon to make 6 skewers.
8. Brush each skewer of shrimp with my EFK Barbecue Sauce on both sides.
9. Grill skewers over medium-high heat for 5-6 minutes on each side or until bacon is crisp.

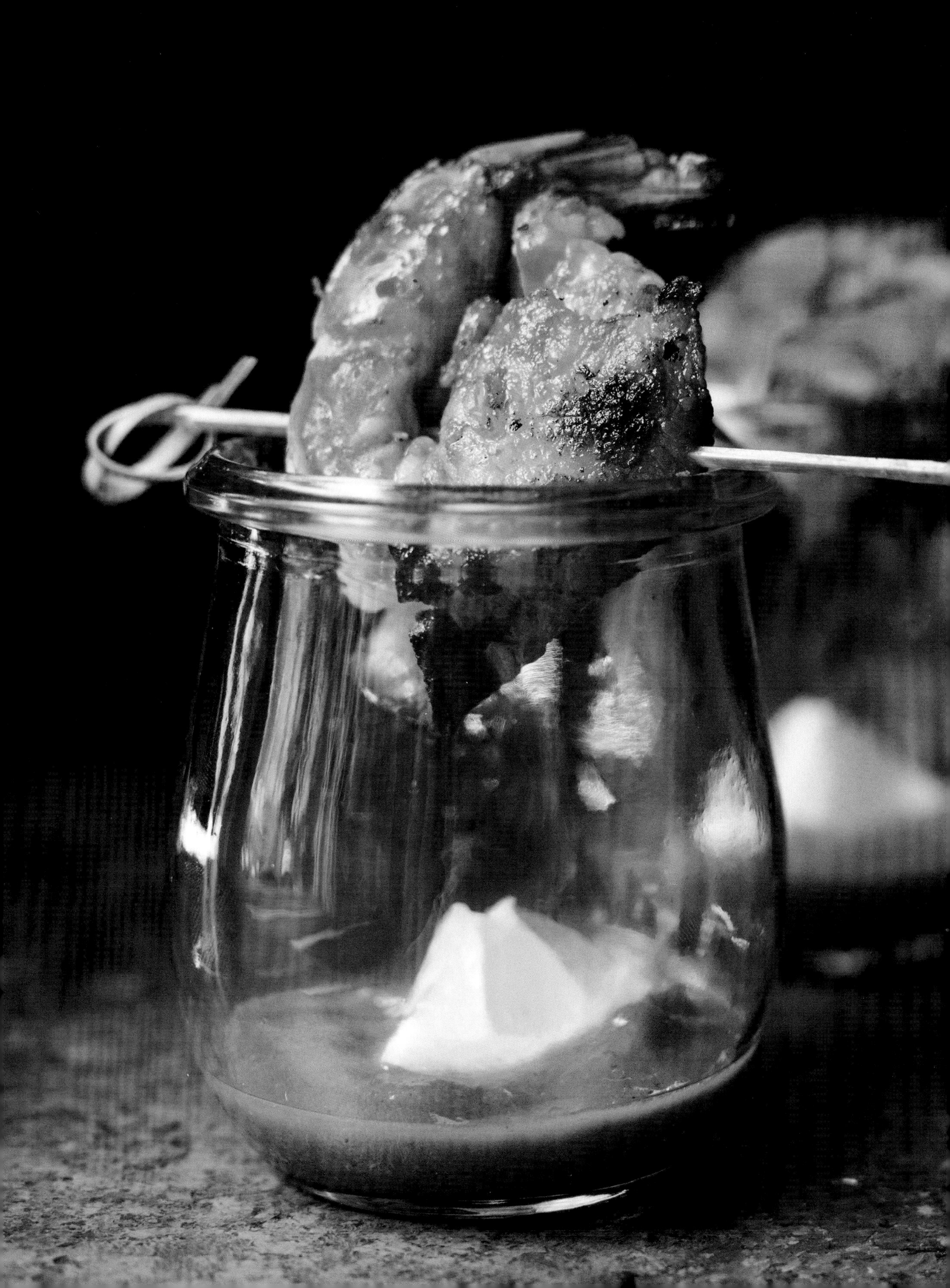

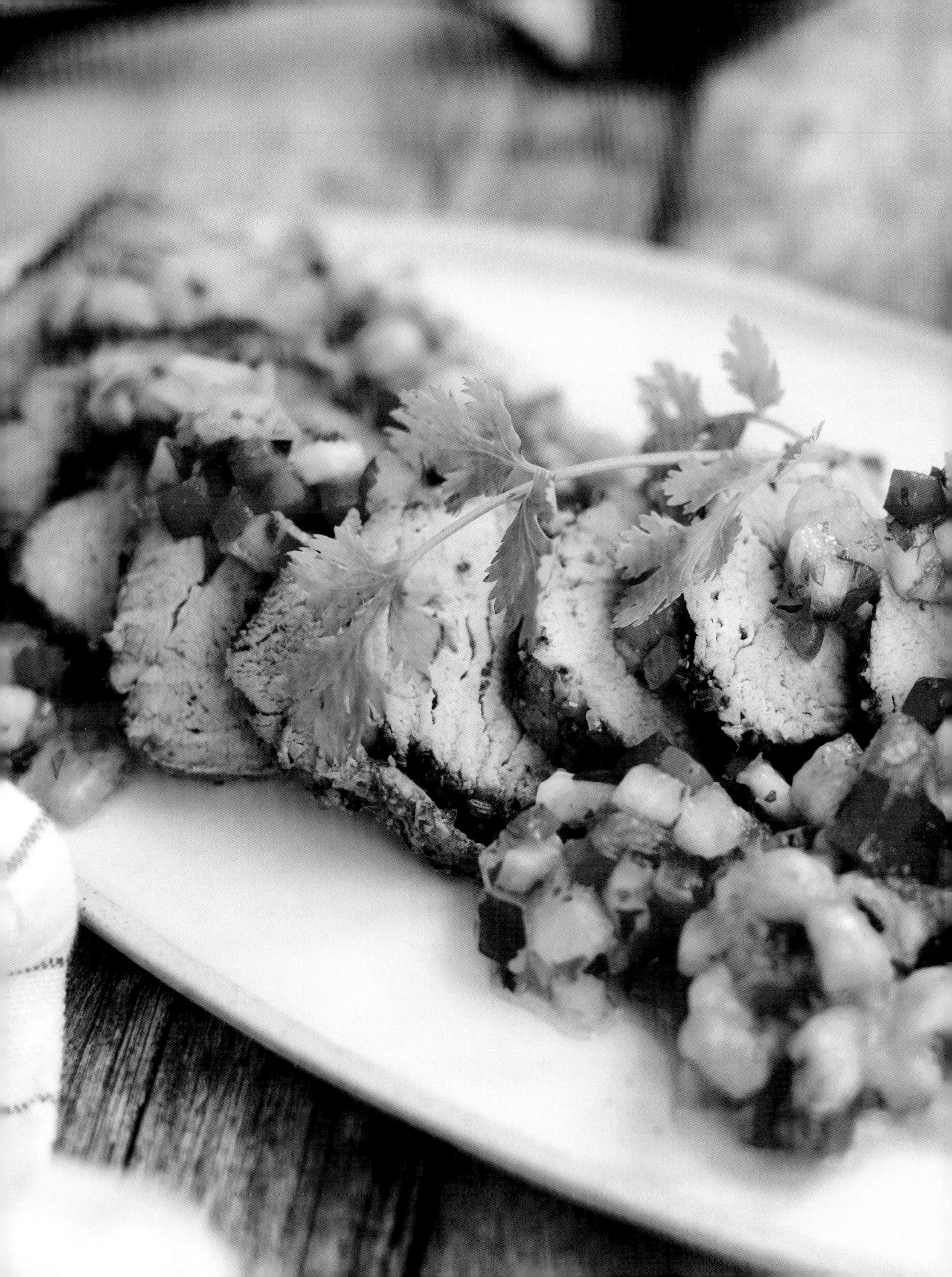

GRILLED PORK TENDERLOIN WITH PEACH SALSA

Dairy-Free, Gluten-Free, Grain-Free, Paleo, SCD

PREP 15 minutes | COOK 25 minutes | TOTAL 40 minutes | SERVES 6

Grilled pork tenderloin with fresh peach salsa is easy to make and full of flavor. Mixing spices to create a dry rub is a great way to add a lot of flavor to grilled or roasted meats without taking the time necessary for a marinade. This combination of seasonings on the pork pairs well with my light and fruity EFK Peach Salsa on page 171. It is a perfect summer dish.

INGREDIENTS

2 pork tenderloins

2 teaspoons black peppercorns

2 teaspoons fennel seeds

2 Tablespoons dried oregano

1 Tablespoon dried minced onion

2 teaspoons granulated garlic

1 teaspoon crushed red pepper flakes

1 Tablespoon sea salt

EFK Peach Salsa (page 171)

DIRECTIONS

1. Remove the silver skin from the pork tenderloins by slipping a boning knife between the silver skin and the meat, using one hand to hold the skin while cutting.
2. Pat the tenderloins dry with a paper towel.
3. Using a mortar and pestle, crush the peppercorns and fennel seeds.
4. Add the oregano, onion, garlic, red pepper and sea salt. Combine well.
5. Rub the seasoning mix generously on the tenderloins, completely coating the meat.
6. Preheat the grill to medium-high.
7. Grill the pork for 20-25 minutes or until done, flipping halfway through.
8. Remove the pork from the grill and let rest for 10 minutes.
9. Slice the pork and place on a platter with my EFK Peach Salsa.

GRILLED CHICKEN BRUSCHETTA

Dairy-Free, Gluten-Free, Grain-Free, Paleo, SCD

PREP 14 minutes | COOK 6 minutes | TOTAL 20 minutes | SERVES 4-6

Nothing says summer like fresh tomatoes, especially if they come from your garden or the local farmers market. One of my favorite ways to eat tomatoes is with fresh basil and garlic. This grilled chicken bruschetta recipe is similar to traditional bruschetta except I skip the toasted bread and use grilled chicken breasts in its place. This dish is a great one to have on repeat during the warm summer months. It is light and packed with flavor. To chiffonade the basil, remove the stems and stack the leaves on top of each other. Roll the basil lengthwise like a cigar. Then slice the roll crosswise into thin strips.

INGREDIENTS

1 pint cherry tomatoes

6 garlic cloves, minced

1 cup basil, cut chiffonade

1/4 cup olive oil

1 teaspoon sea salt

3-4 boneless, skinless chicken breast halves

Additional olive oil and salt for chicken

Balsamic vinegar

DIRECTIONS

1. Slice the cherry tomatoes and place in a mesh strainer to drain excess juice.
2. In a small bowl combine tomatoes, garlic, basil, 1/4 cup olive oil and 1 teaspoon sea salt and set aside.
3. Place one chicken breast half on a cutting board, flat side down.
4. Place the palm of your hand on top of the breast to secure.
5. Using a very sharp knife, slowly cut through the breast horizontally starting with the thicker side.
6. Repeat with the remaining breast halves.
7. Drizzle the chicken with a little olive oil and season with sea salt.
8. Preheat the grill to medium-high.
9. Grill the chicken for 2-3 minutes per side or until cooked through.
10. Place the chicken breasts on a platter and top with the bruschetta mixture.
11. Drizzle with balsamic vinegar.

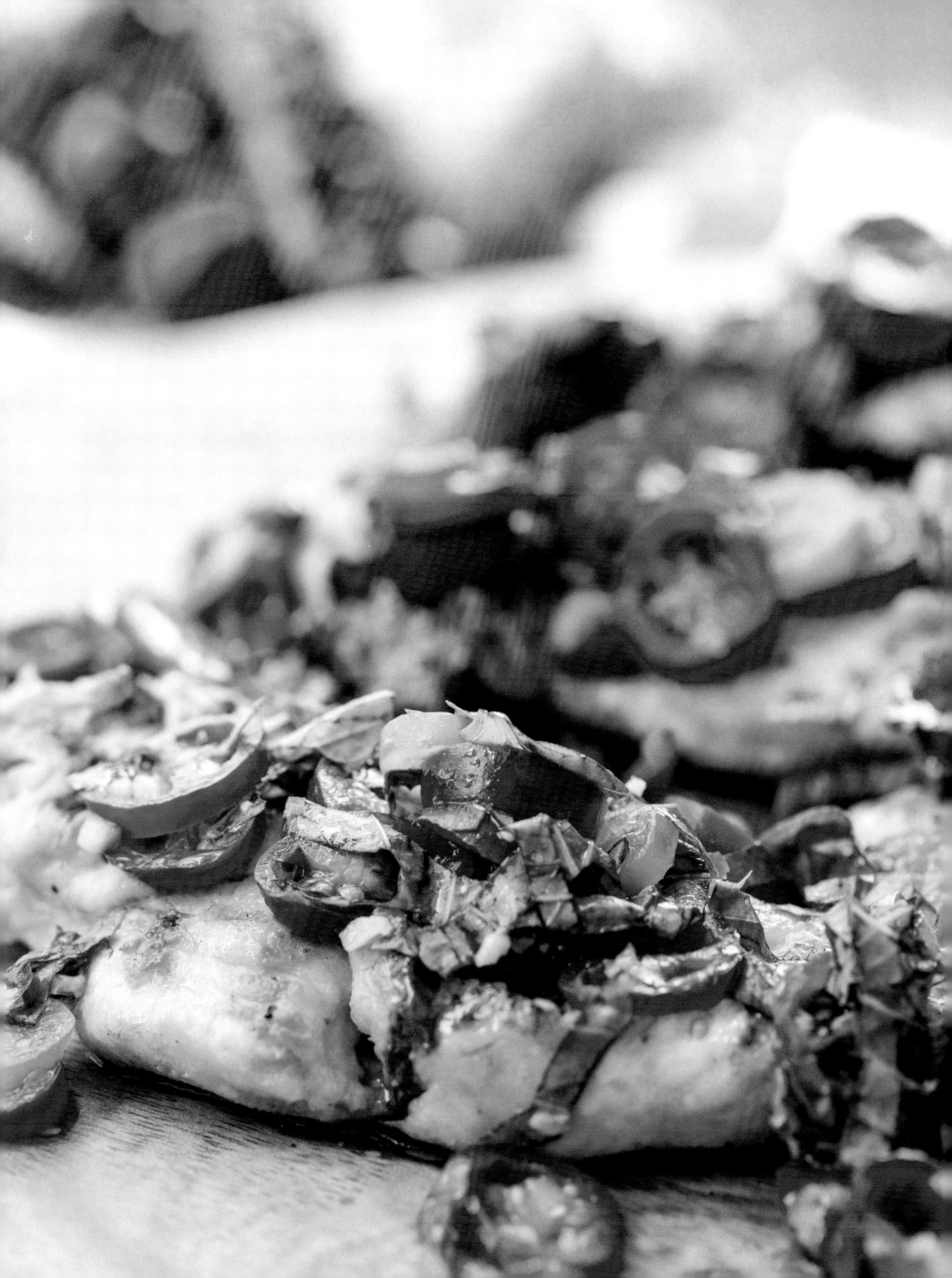

SEARED TUNA BOWLS

Dairy-Free, Gluten-Free (Adaptable for Grain-Free, Paleo)

PREP 40 minutes | COOK 4 minutes | TOTAL 44 minutes* | SERVES 4

When my daughters visit from college, I ask them what meals they want me to prepare while they are home. Their first request is always seared tuna bowls. This dish is light and fresh with a delicious combination of flavors. It is one of those satisfying meals that leaves you feeling full but not stuffed. I usually make the bowls with sushi rice. I use tamari in this recipe, which is a gluten-free soy sauce. You can substitute traditional soy sauce if you prefer. You can also use coconut aminos with a dash of salt if you would like a soy-free version. To adapt for grain-free, substitute lightly blanched or sautéed cauliflower rice for sushi rice. To adapt for paleo, substitute cauliflower rice for sushi rice and coconut aminos for tamari.

**Does not include marinating or resting times, which are noted in the directions.*

INGREDIENTS (MAIN DISH)

1/3 cup toasted sesame oil

1/3 cup tamari

4 teaspoons minced garlic

2 Tablespoons grated ginger

4 teaspoons lime juice

4 ahi or yellowtail tuna steaks, about 2 pounds

2 Tablespoons olive or avocado oil

1 batch of Asian slaw (page 63)

3 cups cooked sushi rice, warm

1 avocado, peeled and diced

1 mango, peeled and diced

1/2 cup chopped green onions

2 Tablespoons sesame seeds, toasted

DIRECTIONS

1. Whisk together the toasted sesame oil, tamari, garlic, ginger and lime juice.
2. Place the tuna steaks in the marinade and turn to coat.
3. Cover and refrigerate for at least 30 minutes and up to 2 hours.
4. Remove the tuna from the fridge and let it sit at room temperature for 20-30 minutes.
5. Place a large sauté pan or skillet over medium-high heat and coat with olive or avocado oil.
6. Cook the tuna steaks for 1-2 minutes per side.
7. Remove from heat and allow to rest.
8. Divide the Asian slaw and cooked sushi rice between 4 bowls.
9. Slice the seared tuna against the grain and add to the bowls.
10. Top with avocado, mango, green onions and sesame seeds.
11. Serve with tamari or soy sauce and mayonnaise (I like Primal Kitchen Chipotle Lime Mayo).

INGREDIENTS (SLAW)

1/2 cup homemade or good-quality mayonnaise

2 Tablespoons toasted sesame oil

2 Tablespoons tamari

2 Tablespoons honey

1 Tablespoon rice vinegar or lime juice

2 teaspoons grated ginger

6 cups shredded cabbage

DIRECTIONS

1. In a medium bowl combine all the ingredients except the shredded cabbage and whisk until smooth.
2. Add the shredded cabbage and stir well.
3. Store in an airtight container in the refrigerator until ready to serve.

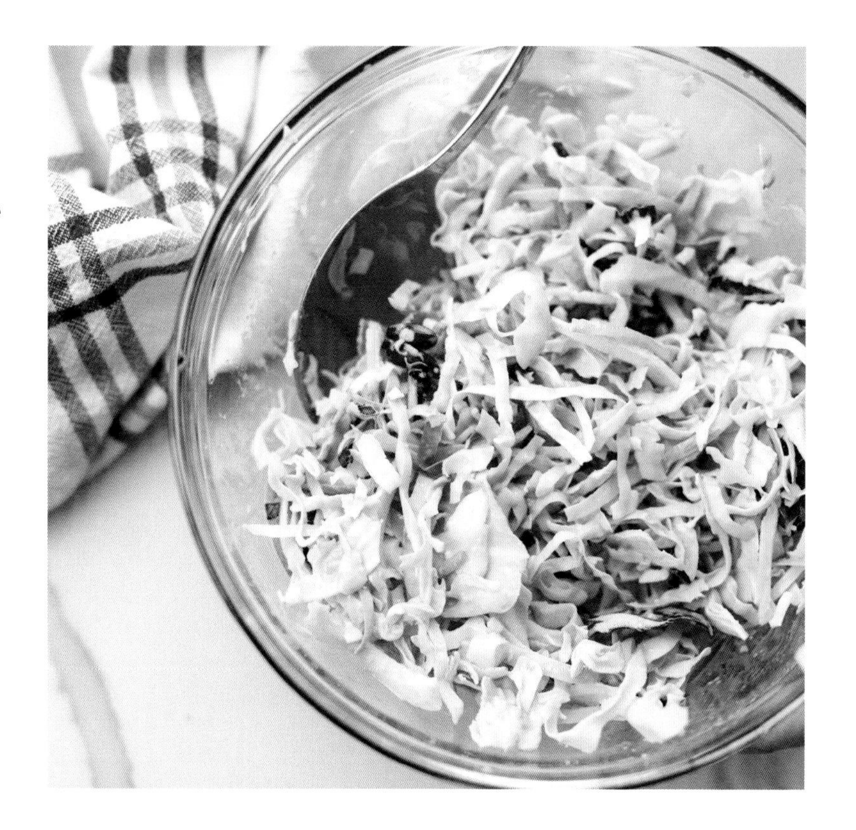

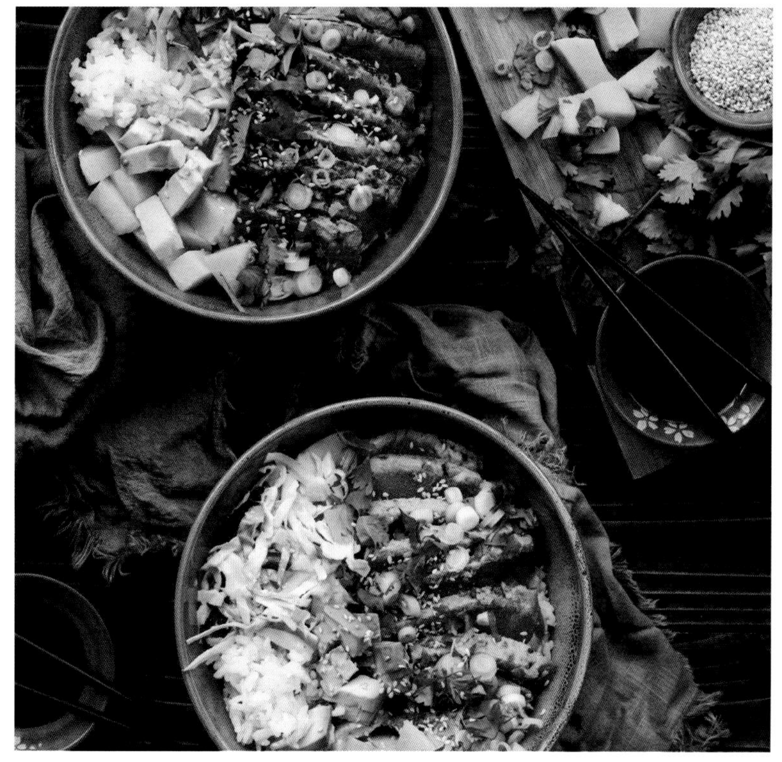

PARMESAN CHICKEN STRIPS

Gluten-Free, Grain-Free, SCD

PREP 12 minutes | COOK 8 minutes | TOTAL 20 minutes | SERVES 4

There are many people today who cannot tolerate gluten or certain grains. It can be difficult to find substitutes for favorite foods, especially for children. Having worked in school food service and having two children of my own, I know how popular chicken strips are with kids. When I was on the Specific Carbohydrate Diet and couldn't have grains of any kind, I was craving something breaded so I came up with this recipe. I can now tolerate grains again, but I still make these chicken strips for my family. My daughters are adults now, but they still love chicken strips. They say they would rather eat these than the ones they can get at a restaurant. The coating is made with almond flour and Parmesan cheese. Whether or not you have a gluten or grain sensitivity, these homemade chicken strips are still a healthier choice.

INGREDIENTS

1 egg

1 Tablespoon water

1 1/2 cups almond flour

1/2 cup Parmesan cheese, grated or shredded

1 1/2 teaspoons salt

1 teaspoon garlic powder

1 1/2 pounds chicken tenders or chicken breasts cut into strips

Avocado, olive or coconut oil

Favorite dipping sauce, for serving

DIRECTIONS

1. In a small bowl whisk together the egg and the water. Set aside.
2. Place the almond flour on a dinner plate or tray.
3. Add the Parmesan cheese, salt and garlic powder and whisk with a fork to combine.
4. Dredge a chicken strip through the egg mixture and then coat it with the almond flour breading.
5. Repeat until all the chicken has been coated.
6. Place oil in a large sauté pan, filling to 1/8 to 1/4 inch high.
7. Place the pan over medium-high heat and add the chicken strips when the oil is hot.
8. Cook the chicken strips for 3-4 minutes on each side.
9. Place the chicken strips on a paper towel-lined plate to absorb any excess oil.
10. Serve with your favorite dipping sauce.

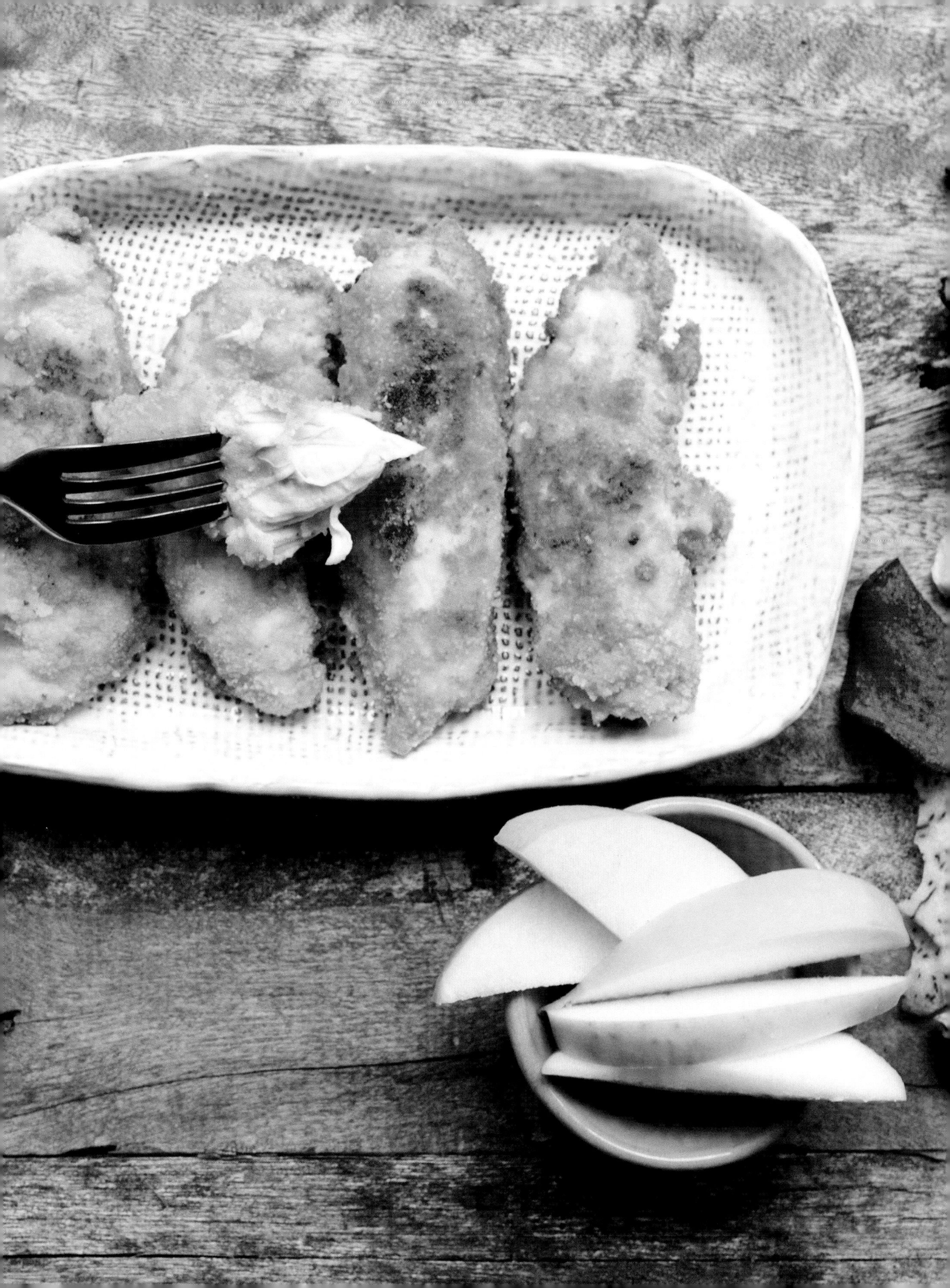

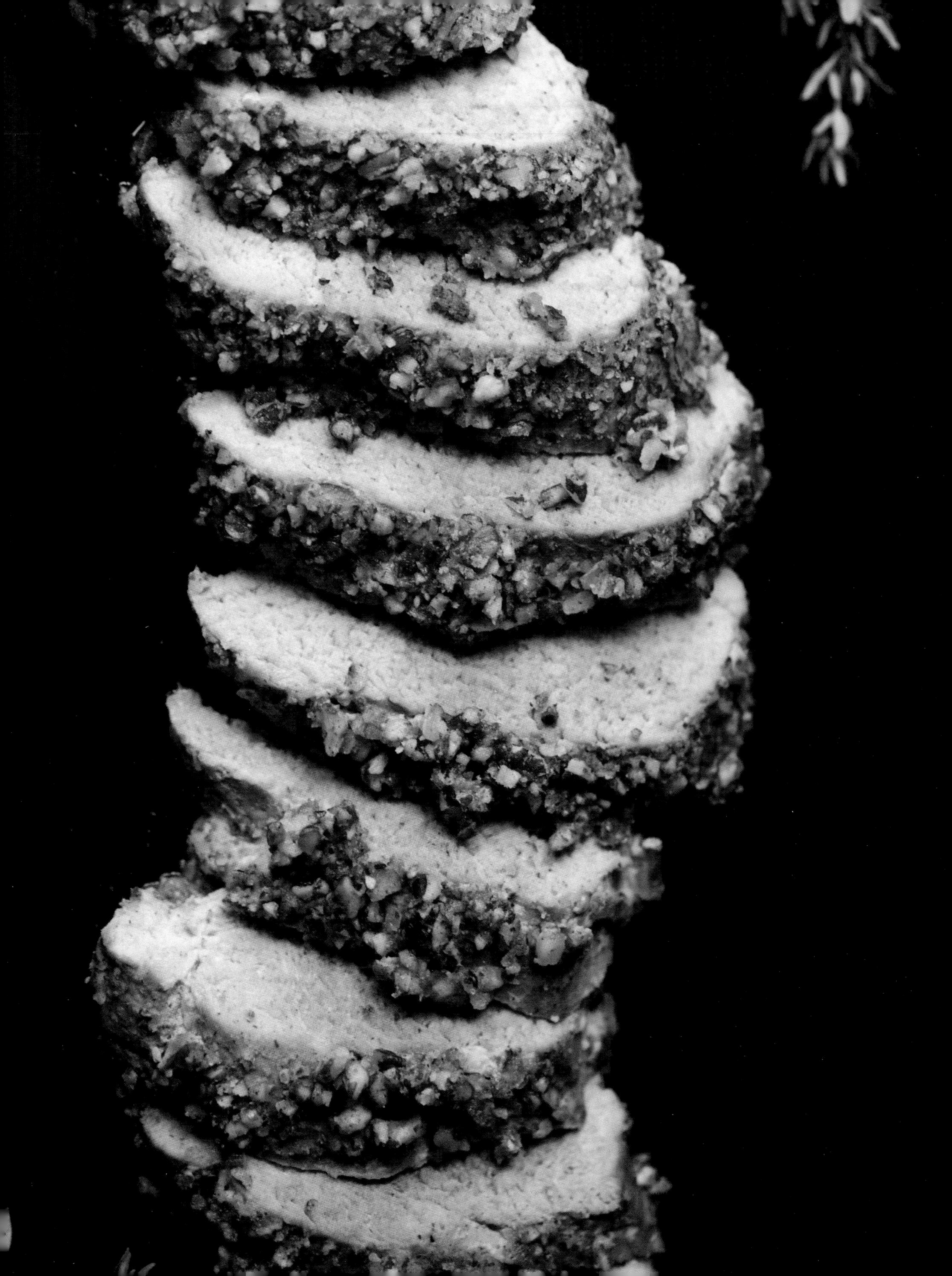

PECAN-CRUSTED PORK TENDERLOIN

Dairy-Free, Gluten-Free, Grain-Free, Paleo, SCD

PREP 15 minutes | COOK 25 minutes | TOTAL 40 minutes* | SERVES 6

I love the combination of flavors in this dish. The Dijon mustard, maple syrup, pecans and cayenne pepper together complement the pork really well. This recipe is quick and easy to make and will bring rave reviews at the dinner table.

**Does not include resting time, which is noted in the directions.*

INGREDIENTS

2 pork tenderloins

1 1/2 cups pecan halves and pieces

1 1/2 teaspoons sea salt

1 teaspoon black pepper

1/4 teaspoon cayenne pepper

1/2 cup Dijon mustard

2 Tablespoons pure maple syrup

DIRECTIONS

1. Preheat the oven to 425 degrees.
2. Remove the silver skin from the pork tenderloins by slipping a boning knife between the silver skin and the meat, using one hand to hold the skin while cutting.
3. Pat the tenderloins dry with a paper towel.
4. Place the pecans in a small food processor and blend until they become a coarse meal.
5. Place the pecan meal in a bowl and stir in the sea salt, black pepper and cayenne pepper.
6. Spread the pecan mixture out onto a sheet pan lined with parchment paper.
7. In a small bowl combine the Dijon mustard and maple syrup.
8. Using a spatula, coat the tenderloins with the mustard mixture.
9. Roll the tenderloins in the pecan mixture until evenly coated.
10. Pat on any extra pecan meal.
11. Place the coated tenderloins on a baking sheet lined with parchment paper.
12. Bake for 25 minutes or until pork reaches an internal temperature of 145 degrees.
13. Remove from the oven and let rest for 10 minutes.
14. Slice the pork and place on a platter for serving.

SALMON KEBABS

Dairy-Free, Gluten-Free, Grain-Free, Paleo, SCD

PREP 10 minutes | COOK 14 minutes | TOTAL 24 minutes* | SERVES 4-6

These healthy salmon kebabs are easy to make and loaded with flavor. I love the peppery punch from the horseradish and the brightness of the lemon and chives in the marinade. The combination is delicious. I suggest using two skewers per kebab because it makes the delicate fish easier to flip on the grill. I like to serve these with my EFK Chopped Green Salad on page 21 for the perfect summer meal.

**Does not include marinating time, which is noted in the directions.*

INGREDIENTS

2 Tablespoons olive oil

1 Tablespoon fresh lemon juice

2 teaspoons minced garlic

1 teaspoon salt

2 teaspoons horseradish

2 teaspoons Dijon mustard

2 Tablespoons chopped fresh chives

1 1/2 pounds wild salmon, skin removed and cut into 1-inch cubes

2 lemons, sliced

DIRECTIONS

1. If using wooden skewers, soak 12 of them in water for 30 minutes or longer.
2. In a medium bowl, combine the olive oil, lemon juice, garlic, salt, horseradish, Dijon mustard and chives and mix well.
3. Add the salmon cubes and stir until well coated.
4. Cover and refrigerate for 15-20 minutes.
5. Thread the salmon cubes on pairs of wooden skewers, alternating with folded lemon slices.
6. Continue until all the salmon has been skewered.
7. Lightly oil a hot grill by putting olive oil on a bunched-up paper towel and using tongs to wipe the grill grate.
8. Grill the salmon over medium-high heat for 5-7 minutes per side or until done.

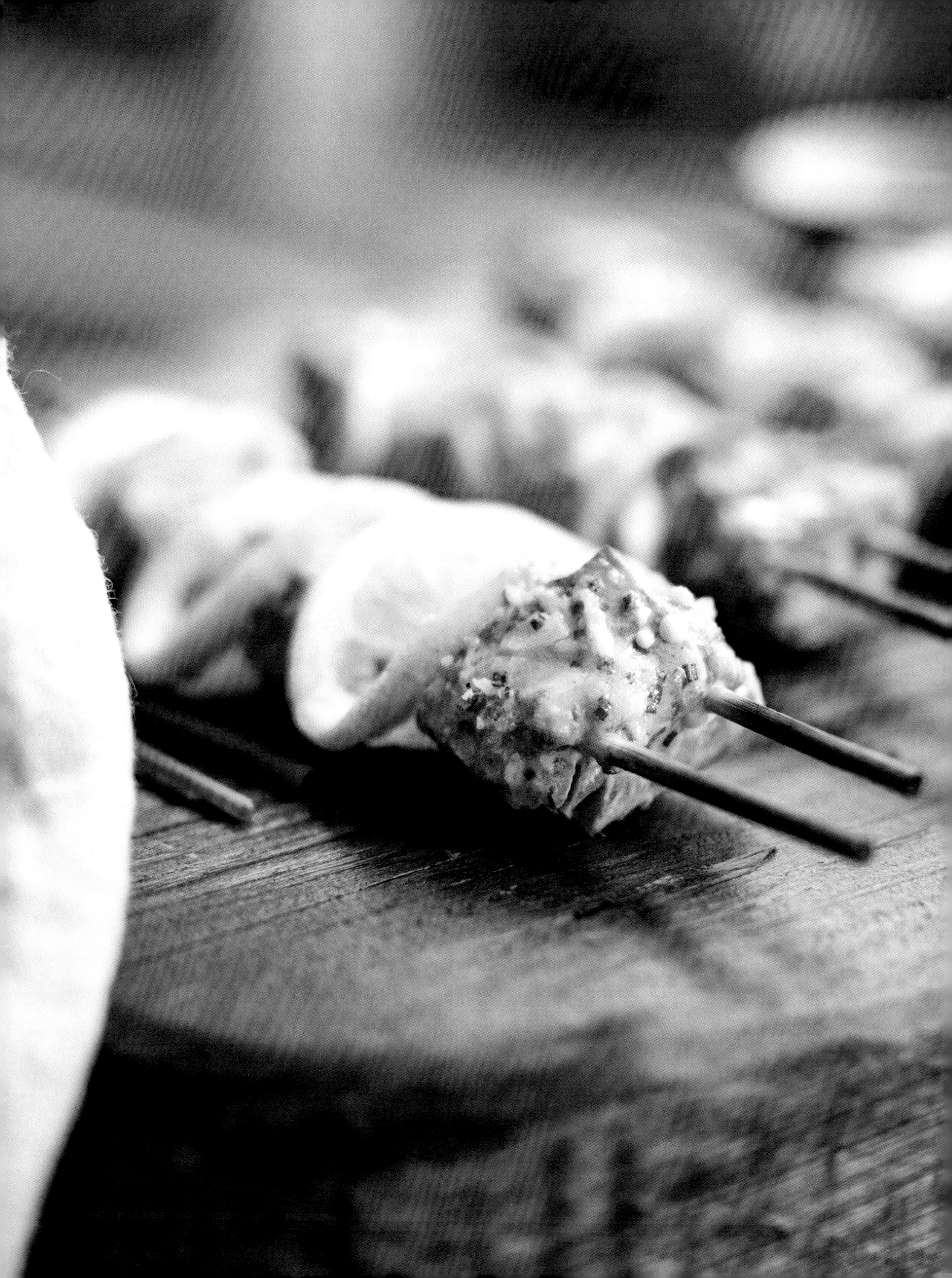

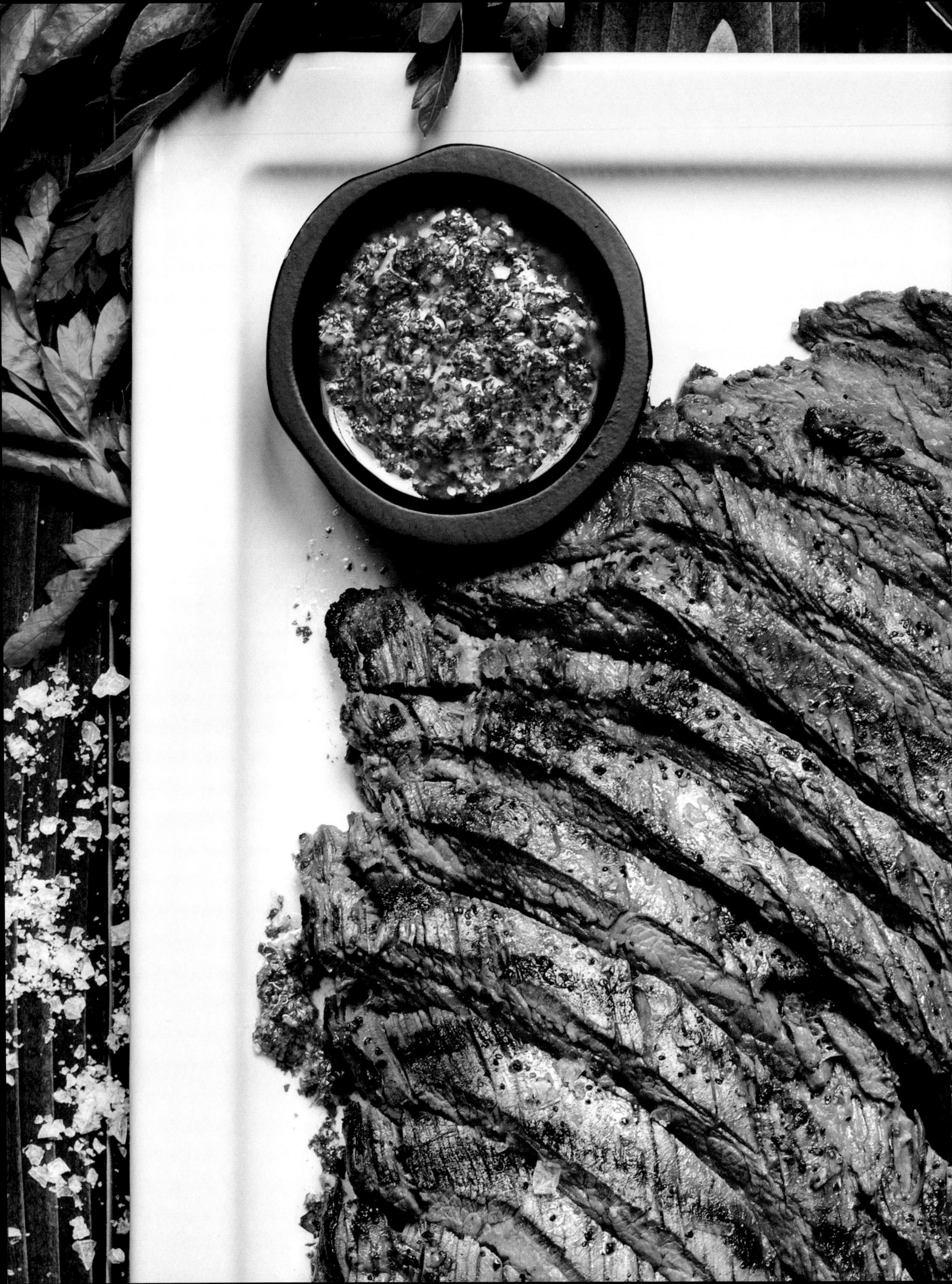

GRILLED FLANK STEAK WITH CHIMICHURRI

Dairy-Free, Gluten-Free, Grain-Free, Paleo, SCD

PREP 5 minutes | COOK 10 minutes | TOTAL 15 minutes* | SERVES 6

Marinating and then searing on a hot grill is a simple way to prepare flank steak. The marinade is easy to make, tenderizes the beef and adds a great boost of flavor. Once grilled, it is important to slice the meat against the grain to avoid a chewy texture. When cut properly, the steak is just as tender as more expensive cuts of beef. Marinated grilled flank steak is great on its own or used as fajita or taco meat. My favorite way to serve it is with chimichurri, a flavorful herb and garlic sauce. It is simple to make and complements the steak very well. Use my EFK Chimichurri recipe on page 214.

**Does not include marinating or resting times, which are noted in the directions.*

INGREDIENTS

1/3 cup olive oil

4 cloves garlic, minced

1 teaspoon salt

1 teaspoon black pepper

2 lemons, juiced

1 flank steak, about 1 1/2-2 pounds

EFK Chimichurri (page 214), for serving

DIRECTIONS

1. Whisk together the olive oil, garlic, salt, pepper and lemon juice in a small bowl.
2. Place the flank steak in a large baking dish.
3. Pour the marinade over the steak and flip to coat both sides.
4. Cover and refrigerate for 2 hours or overnight.
5. Let the steak sit at room temperature for 30 minutes before cooking.
6. Turn the grill on and bring up to medium-high heat.
7. Wipe off excess marinade with a paper towel and place the steak on the hot grill.
8. Grill the steak for 4-5 minutes and then flip.
9. Grill for another 4-5 minutes or until medium-rare.
10. Remove the steak from the grill and allow to rest for 5 minutes.
11. Slice the steak across the grain into thin strips.
12. Serve with my EFK Chimichurri.

MACADAMIA NUT-CRUSTED WALLEYE

Dairy-Free, Gluten-Free, Grain-Free, Paleo, SCD

PREP 15 minutes | COOK 15 minutes | TOTAL 30 minutes | SERVES 4

Walleye is a popular fish in the Great Lakes region of North America. So much so that Minnesota designated walleye as the official state fish. Not only is it a fun fish to catch, it is delicious to eat. My family is fortunate to have good friends who are avid fishermen, so we have been treated to walleye fresh from the lake. It can also be found in the freezer section of most grocery stores throughout the Midwest and in the fresh seafood section on occasion. If you do not have access to walleye, you can substitute another whitefish for this recipe.

As an alternative to traditional walleye batter or breading, I use a blend of macadamia nuts and almond flour to coat the fish, which makes it grain-free and suitable for paleo and keto diets. This mixture complements the sweet mild flavor of walleye very well. It is pan-fried and then finished in the oven to keep it a little lighter. Serve with fresh dill and lemon wedges and my homemade EFK Tartar Sauce on page 222.

INGREDIENTS

1 1/4 cups macadamia nuts

1 1/4 cups almond flour

1 teaspoon sea salt

1/2 teaspoon black pepper

2 eggs

1 1/2 pounds walleye, about 4-6 fillets

Olive oil, coconut oil or ghee

Fresh dill, lemon wedges and EFK Tartar Sauce (page 222), for serving

DIRECTIONS

1. Preheat the oven to 400 degrees.
2. Place the macadamia nuts in a mini food processor and blend until they become a coarse meal.
3. Add the almond flour, salt and pepper to the macadamia nuts and pulse until well blended.
4. Spread the macadamia nut mixture on a dinner plate or tray.
5. In a medium bowl whisk the eggs until well blended.
6. Pat the walleye fillets dry with a paper towel and season with salt.
7. Dredge a fillet through the egg and then coat it with the nut mixture.
8. Place the fillet on a clean dinner plate or tray and repeat with remaining fillets.

(Continued)

9. Heat 1/4 inch of oil or ghee in a cast iron pan or large skillet over medium-high heat until hot.
10. Place 2 fillets in the pan and fry until the underside is golden, about 3-4 minutes.
11. Gently flip the fillets and repeat on the other side.
12. Place the browned fillets on a sheet pan lined with parchment paper and repeat with the remaining fillets.
13. Bake for 10-12 minutes or until cooked through.
14. Garnish with fresh dill and serve with lemon wedges and EFK Tartar Sauce.

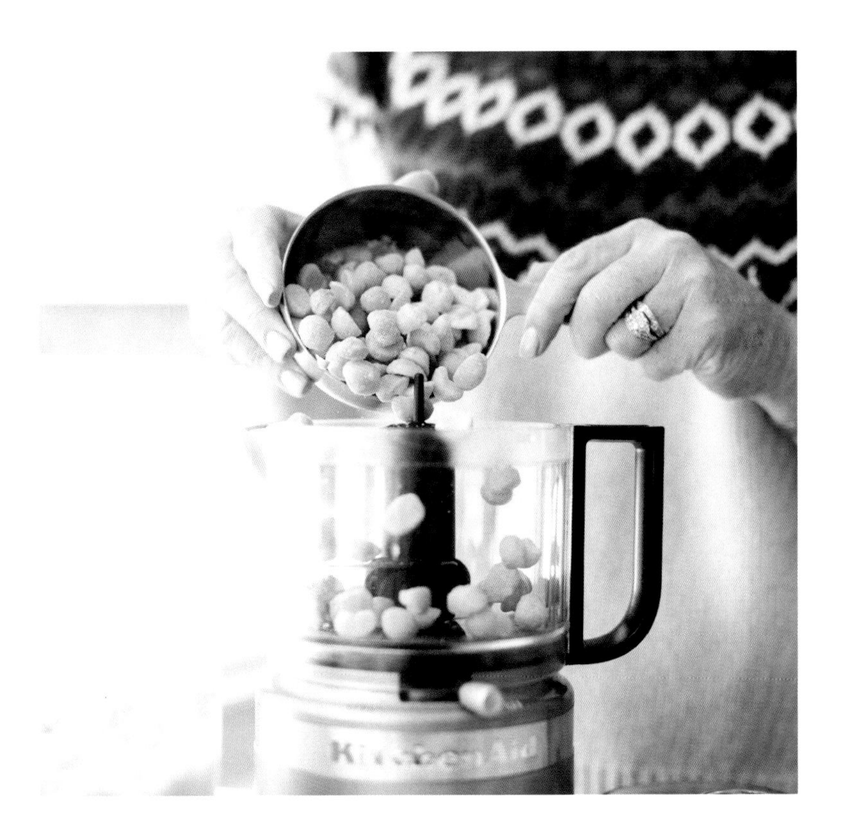

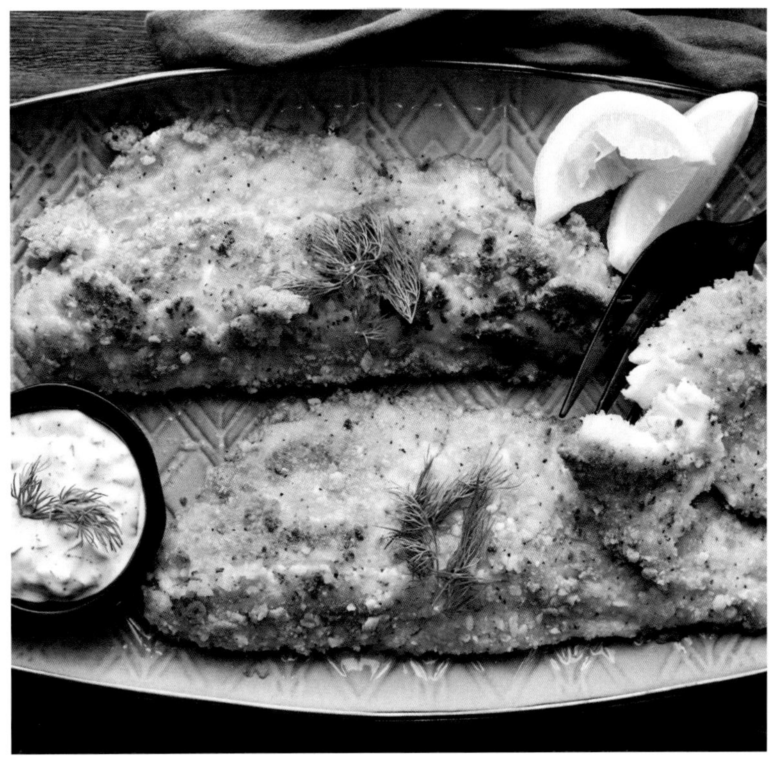

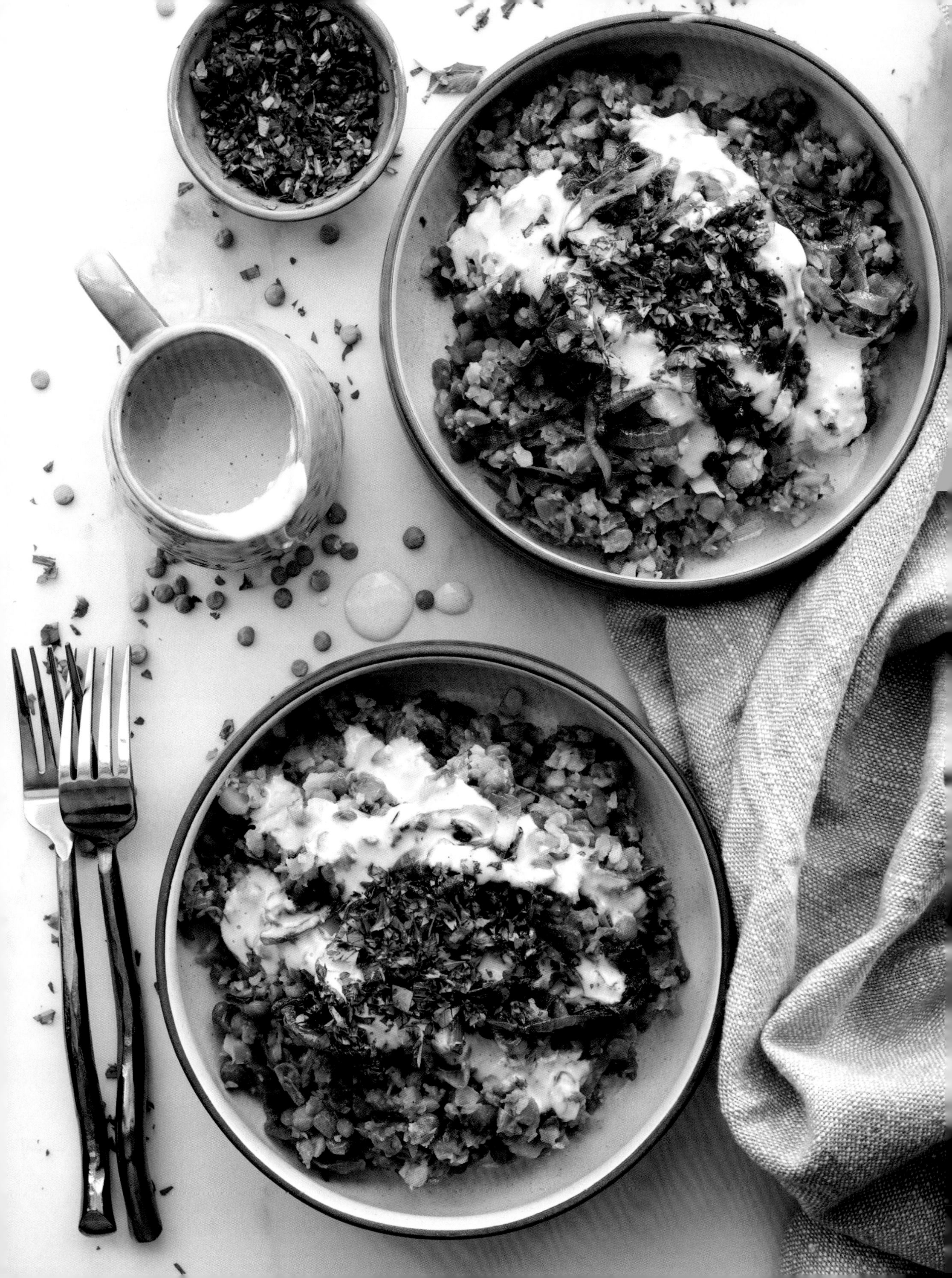

LENTIL AND CAULIFLOWER RICE BOWLS

Dairy-Free, Gluten-Free, Grain-Free, SCD, Vegan

PREP 10 minutes | COOK 30 minutes | TOTAL 40 minutes | SERVES 2-4

This is one of my all-time favorite meatless dishes. It is inspired by Mujadara, which is a Lebanese dish made of lentils, rice and caramelized onions. In this recipe, I substitute cauliflower rice for regular rice and top the mixture with my EFK Lemon Garlic Tahini on page 221. It is the ultimate comfort food and perfect for enjoying on a cold winter day.

INGREDIENTS

2 large onions

4 Tablespoons olive oil, divided

1 1/2 cups green or brown lentils

3 cups of water or broth

4 cups of riced cauliflower

1 teaspoon sea salt

1 Tablespoon cumin

EFK Lemon Garlic Tahini (page 221) and fresh chopped parsley, for serving

DIRECTIONS

1. Cut the onions in half and thinly slice them.
2. In a large sauté pan heat 2 Tablespoons olive oil.
3. Add the onions and cook over medium-high heat, stirring occasionally.
4. Rinse the lentils.
5. In a medium saucepan, combine the lentils and water or broth and bring to a boil.
6. Reduce the heat and simmer for 20-25 minutes or until tender.
7. Drain any excess liquid and return to the pan.
8. When the onions are a deep brown, remove half of them from the pan and set aside.
9. Add 1-2 Tablespoons of olive oil to the pan with the remaining onions.
10. Add the cauliflower rice to the olive oil and onions and sauté for 3-5 minutes.
11. Add the lentils, sea salt and cumin to the mixture and combine well.
12. Divide the lentil mixture between 2-4 bowls.
13. Top each bowl with the extra caramelized onions.
14. Drizzle with my EFK Lemon Garlic Tahini.
15. Top with chopped parsley.

SPICY BAKED YUCATAN SHRIMP

Gluten-Free, Grain-Free, Paleo, SCD

PREP 7 minutes | COOK 15 minutes | TOTAL 22 minutes | SERVES 6-8

My family vacationed at the Gulf Coast of Florida when I was growing up. At restaurants there, we often ordered shrimp because it was so fresh. One of our favorite shrimp dishes was a spicy Yucatan peel-and-eat version. In this recipe, I recreate the flavors of that dish, but I bake already-peeled shrimp to eliminate the mess when eating. The restaurant serves it with crusty bread to soak up the wonderful spicy sauce. I like to serve mine with cauliflower rice, which also absorbs all the great flavor.

INGREDIENTS

2 pounds 21/25 count raw peeled and deveined shrimp

1/2 cup ghee

2 Tablespoons garlic, minced

3-4 teaspoons chili garlic sauce (I like Yai's Thai brand because it doesn't have any added sugar)

2 teaspoons salt

1 teaspoon black pepper

4 large limes, juiced, and fresh chopped cilantro, for serving

DIRECTIONS

1. Preheat the oven to 400 degrees.
2. Arrange the shrimp in one layer in an oven-proof baking dish, with only the tails overlapping.
3. In a medium saucepan melt the ghee.
4. Add the garlic, chili garlic sauce, salt and pepper and simmer for one minute.
5. Pour the seasoned ghee over the shrimp.
6. Bake for 12-15 minutes or until pink.
7. Top with the fresh lime juice and cilantro.

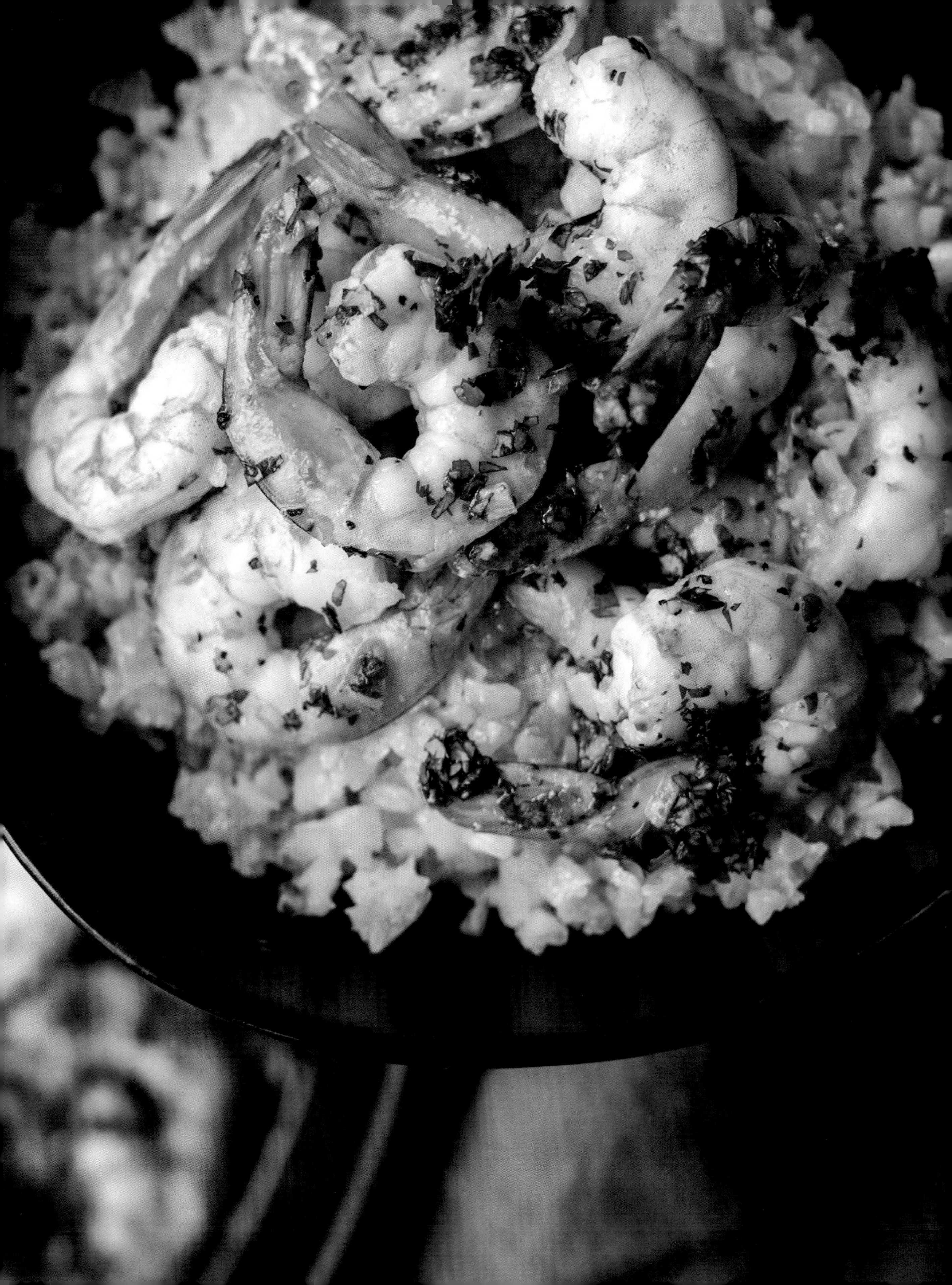

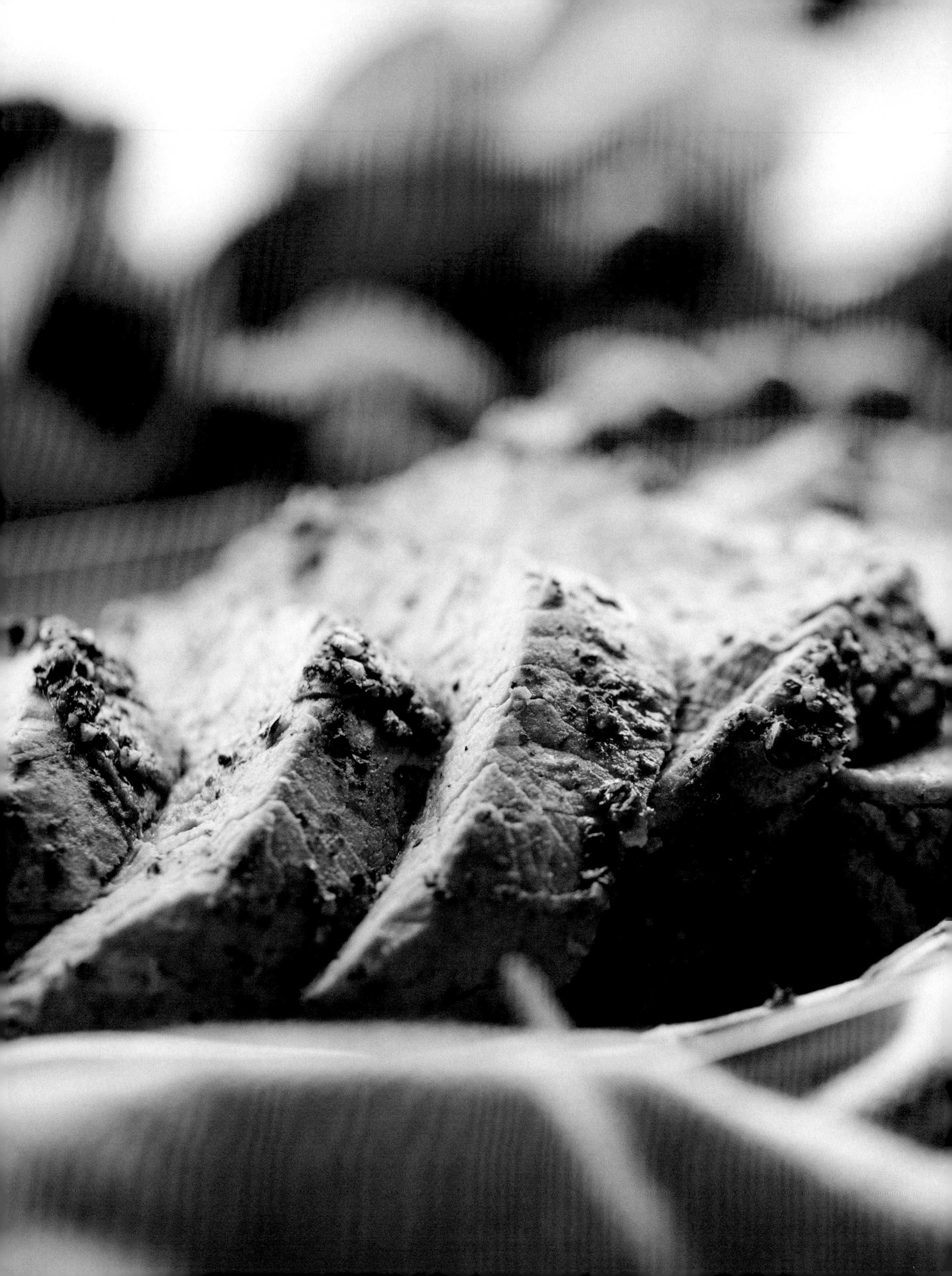

MAKE-AHEAD BEEF TENDERLOIN

Gluten-Free, Grain-Free, Paleo, SCD

PREP 5 minutes | COOK 35 minutes | TOTAL 40 minutes | SERVES 8-10

Roast beef tenderloin is a special occasion dish that's perfect to serve during the holidays. It is the most tender cut of beef and always a crowd pleaser. With this recipe you can roast the meat a few hours ahead of time and store it in a cooler until you are ready to serve it. It will hold its temperature. This works great if you are entertaining and plan to serve dinner immediately following a church service or program. It also works well if you are bringing a dish to a friend or family member's house. Tenderloin works well as an entree, but it can also be served as a heavy appetizer with soft rolls. Horseradish sauce or grainy mustard make great condiments.

INGREDIENTS

1 whole beef tenderloin trimmed, 4-5 pounds

4 Tablespoons ghee

1 Tablespoon salt

2 teaspoons freshly cracked black pepper

DIRECTIONS

1. Preheat oven to 475 degrees.
2. Place the tenderloin on a parchment-lined baking sheet.
3. Spread ghee all over the tenderloin.
4. Sprinkle generously with salt and pepper.
5. Roast the beef for 30-40 minutes or until thermometer reads 135 for medium-rare.
6. Remove from the oven and wrap tightly in aluminum foil.
7. Place the wrapped tenderloin in a cooler.
8. The tenderloin will hold for up to 2 hours in the cooler.
9. When you are ready to serve, unwrap the tenderloin and slice.
10. If serving right away, allow the meat to rest for 10 minutes before slicing.

GRILLED CHICKEN TACOS WITH GUACAMOLE

Dairy-Free, Gluten-Free, Grain-Free, Paleo, SCD

PREP 5 minutes | COOK 14 minutes | TOTAL 19 minutes* | SERVES 4-8

We eat a lot of tacos at our house. All varieties—shrimp, carnitas, fish, veggie. They are all delicious and everyone loves them. These grilled chicken tacos with guacamole are one of our favorites. The marinade for the chicken has all the traditional flavors, including lime, cilantro, garlic and cumin. Plus, nothing beats freshly made guacamole—taco or no taco. Guacamole is everything! My EFK Guacamole recipe is on page 168.

**Does not include marinating or resting times, which are noted in the directions.*

INGREDIENTS

1 cup fresh cilantro

2 garlic cloves, minced

3 limes, juiced

1 teaspoon cumin

1 teaspoon sea salt

1 cup olive oil

4-8 boneless, skinless chicken breasts

Large lettuce leaves or tortillas and EFK Guacamole (page 168), for serving

DIRECTIONS

1. Place the cilantro, garlic, lime juice, cumin and sea salt in a food processor.
2. Blend on high until well combined.
3. Slowly add the olive oil through the top opening of the food processor while it is running until well combined.
4. Pour the marinade over the chicken breasts in a large bowl.
5. Cover the bowl and refrigerate for 4-24 hours.
6. When you are ready to grill, take the chicken out of the refrigerator and let it sit for 30 minutes at room temperature.
7. Preheat the grill to medium-high.
8. Grill the chicken for 6-7 minutes per side or until done.
9. Let the chicken rest for 5-10 minutes and then slice.
10. Serve with lettuce leaves or tortillas of choice and my EFK Guacamole.

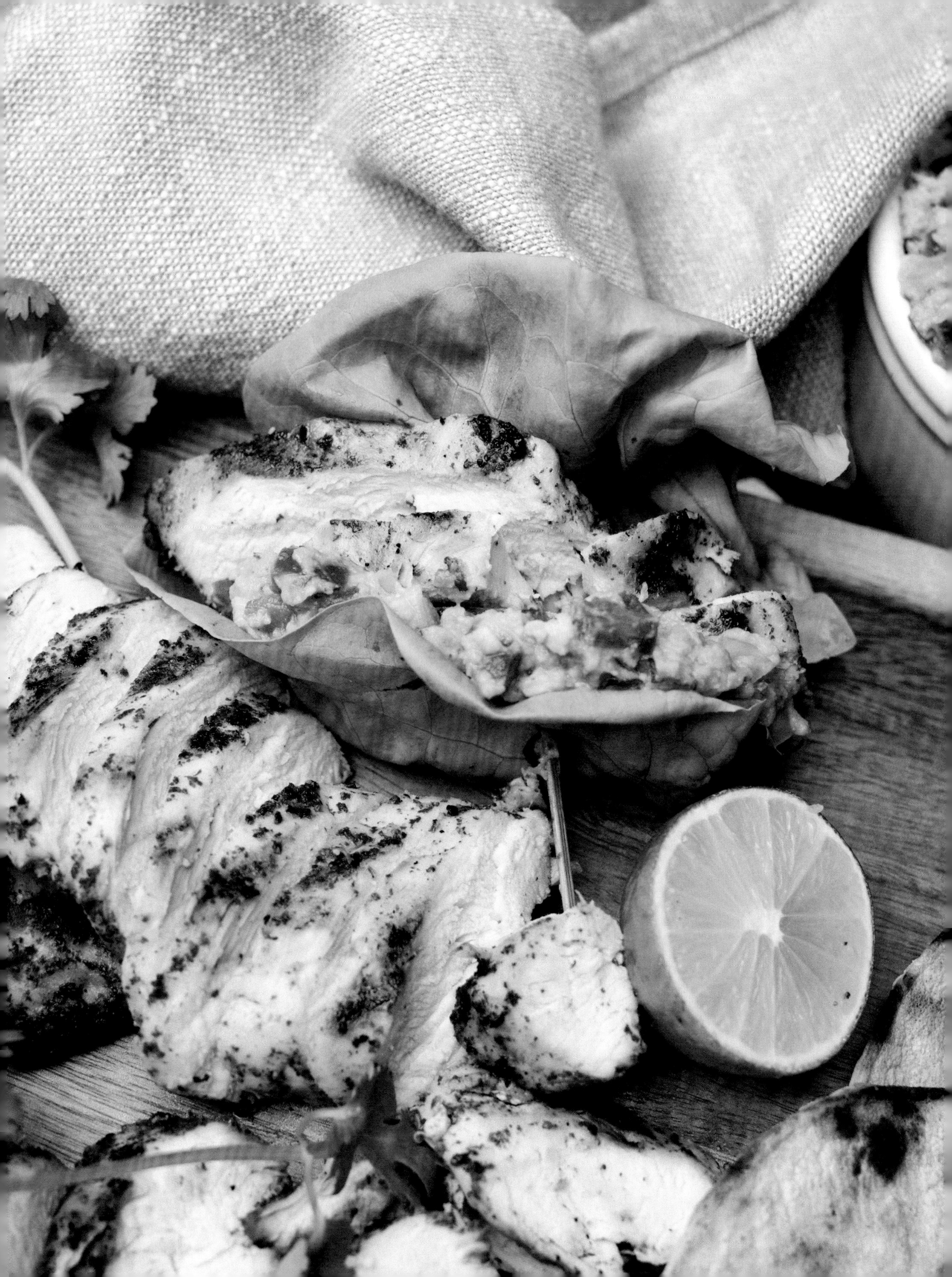

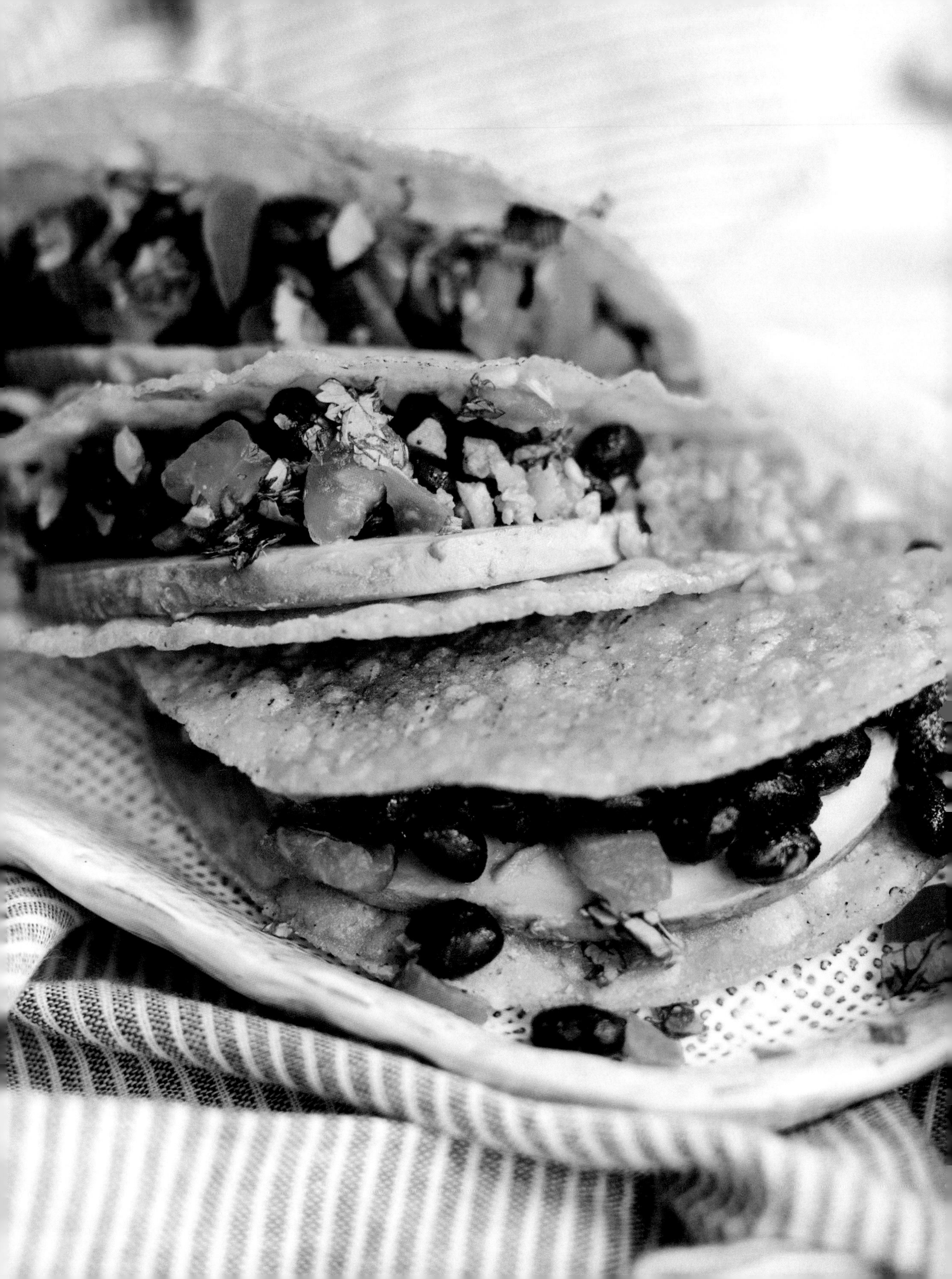

BLACK BEAN AND CAULIFLOWER TACOS

Dairy-Free, Gluten-Free, Grain-Free, Vegan

PREP 7 minutes | COOK 8 minutes | TOTAL 15 minutes | SERVES 4

Cauliflower has to be the most versatile vegetable. It is used as a replacement for rice, mashed potatoes, pasta, meat—and even pizza crust. In addition to being so adaptable, cauliflower has many nutritional and health benefits. It's packed with vitamin C, fiber and disease-fighting antioxidants. Its mild flavor makes it a blank canvas in the kitchen.

In this recipe, I use cauliflower as a substitute for taco meat. When lightly sautéed and seasoned with the right spices, the taste and texture is similar to the traditional version made with beef. I like to serve these tacos with black beans, avocado, pico de gallo and fresh cilantro in a crunchy taco shell. This recipe is a great way to mix up your Taco Tuesday and add more vegetables to your diet.

DIRECTIONS

1. Heat 1 Tablespoon olive oil in a medium saucepan.
2. Add the minced garlic and jalapeño and cook for 2 minutes.
3. Add the black beans, 1 Tablespoon EFK Taco Seasoning and juice from half of the lime and mix well.
4. Let the beans simmer on low heat while you prepare the cauliflower.
5. In a large sauté pan, heat 3 Tablespoons olive oil.
6. Add onions and sauté until translucent.
7. Add the cauliflower rice and 2 Tablespoons EFK Taco Seasoning and mix well.
8. Add juice from the other half of the lime and sauté for 3-4 minutes or until the cauliflower is cooked but still firm.
9. Spoon the cauliflower into the taco shells.
10. Spoon the black beans on top of the cauliflower.
11. Top with diced avocado, pico de gallo and fresh cilantro or your favorite toppings.

INGREDIENTS

4 Tablespoons olive oil, divided

1 Tablespoon minced garlic

1 Tablespoon minced jalapeño

2 cans of black beans, drained

3 Tablespoons EFK Taco Seasoning, divided (page 233)

1 lime cut in half

1 cup diced onion

4 cups riced cauliflower

Taco shells (I like Siete brand, which are grain-free), diced avocado, pico de gallo and chopped cilantro, for serving

WHITE BEAN AND MUSHROOM BURGERS

Dairy-Free, Gluten-Free, Grain-Free, Vegan (Adaptable for SCD)

PREP 12 minutes | COOK 26 minutes | TOTAL 38 minutes | SERVES 4-8

I love bean burgers and make many homemade versions in my kitchen. To get a good consistency that isn't too mushy, I have found that it's helpful to keep the ingredients as dry as possible. After draining and rinsing the beans, I dry them in the oven. I also pat dry any sautéed ingredients I am adding, like the mushrooms and onions. To bind everything together I like to use grain-free cracker crumbs. I blend a box of Simple Mills almond flour crackers in my mini food processor to create the crumbs, but you can use any type of cracker crumbs or breadcrumbs you would like. These burgers are sturdy enough to cook on the grill, but I usually sauté them in olive oil on the stove to brown the sides and give the patties a nice crunch. To adapt for SCD, use SCD-approved beans and crackers.

INGREDIENTS

2 15-ounce cans cannellini or Great Northern beans

2 Tablespoons olive oil, divided

1 pound portobello mushrooms, washed, dried and diced

1 large onion, diced

4 cloves garlic, minced

1 cup of grain-free cracker crumbs or breadcrumbs

2 teaspoons salt

1 1/2 teaspoons chili powder

1 1/2 teaspoons cumin

1 1/2 teaspoons smoked paprika

1/8 teaspoon cayenne pepper

Large lettuce leaves or hamburger buns and your favorite burger toppings, for serving

DIRECTIONS

1. Preheat the oven to 325 degrees.
2. Drain and rinse the beans and pat dry.
3. Spread the beans on a parchment-lined baking sheet and dry in the oven for 15 minutes.
4. In a large sauté pan, heat 1 Tablespoon olive oil over medium-high heat.
5. Add the diced mushrooms and cook for 5 minutes.
6. Reduce heat to medium and add the diced onions and cook for an additional 5 minutes.
7. Add the minced garlic and cook for an additional 3-5 minutes.
8. Drain the mushroom mixture through a strainer and lightly pat dry on a clean kitchen towel.
9. Place the beans in a large bowl and mash with a potato masher or fork.
10. Add the mushroom mixture, cracker crumbs, salt, chili powder, cumin, smoked paprika and cayenne pepper.
11. Mix the ingredients well.

(Continued)

12. Form the mix into 6 burger-sized patties.
13. In a large sauté pan, heat 1 Tablespoon olive oil over medium heat.
14. Place the bean and mushroom burgers in the pan and cook for 2-3 minutes or until golden.
15. Flip the burgers and cook the other side for 2-3 minutes or until golden.
16. Repeat with remaining burgers.
17. Serve on a lettuce leaf or bun with your favorite burger toppings.

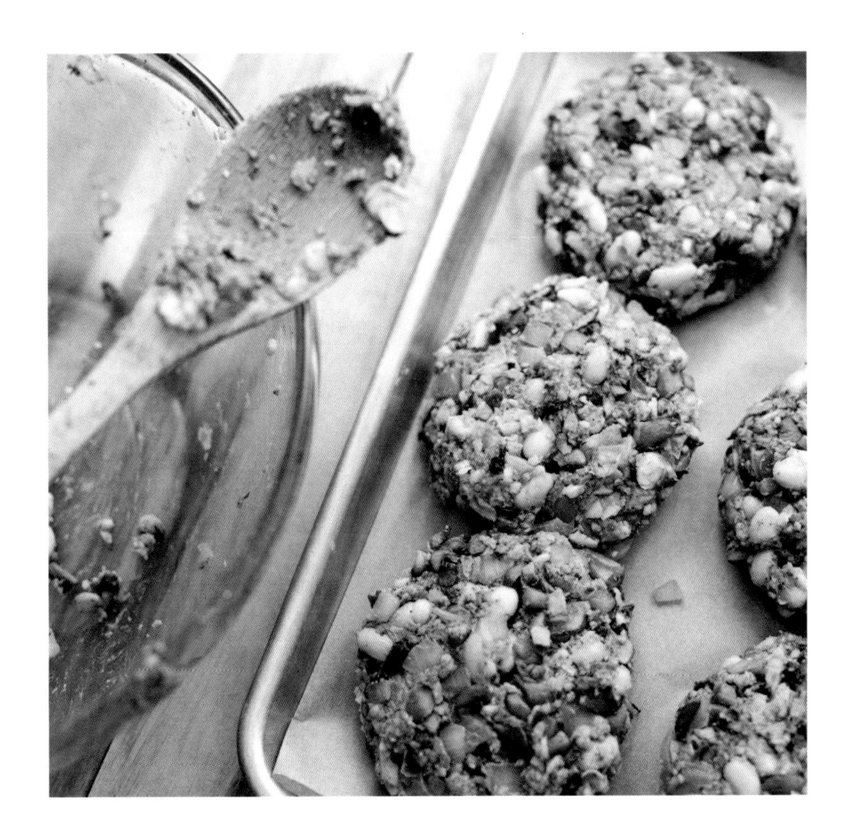

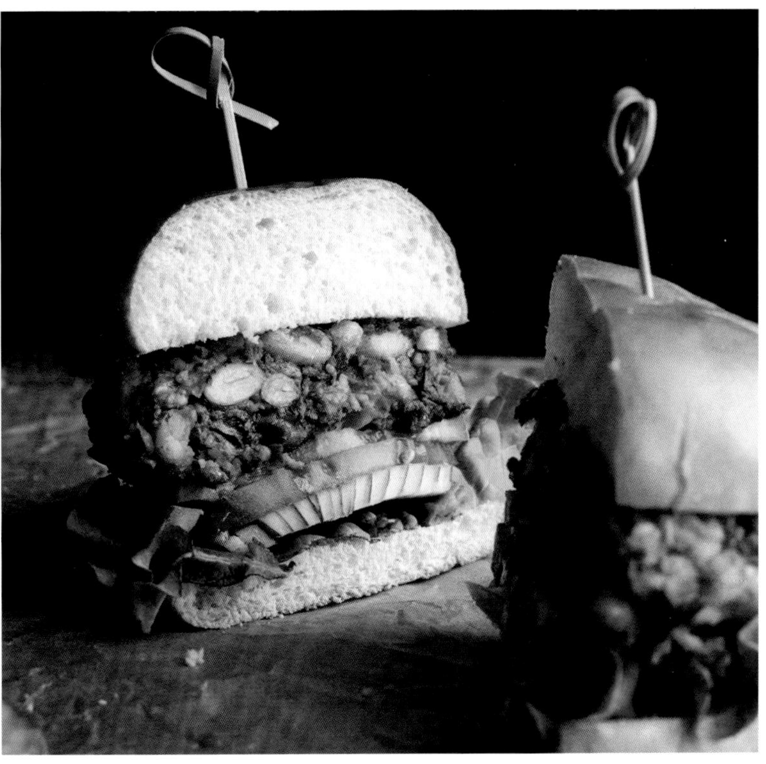

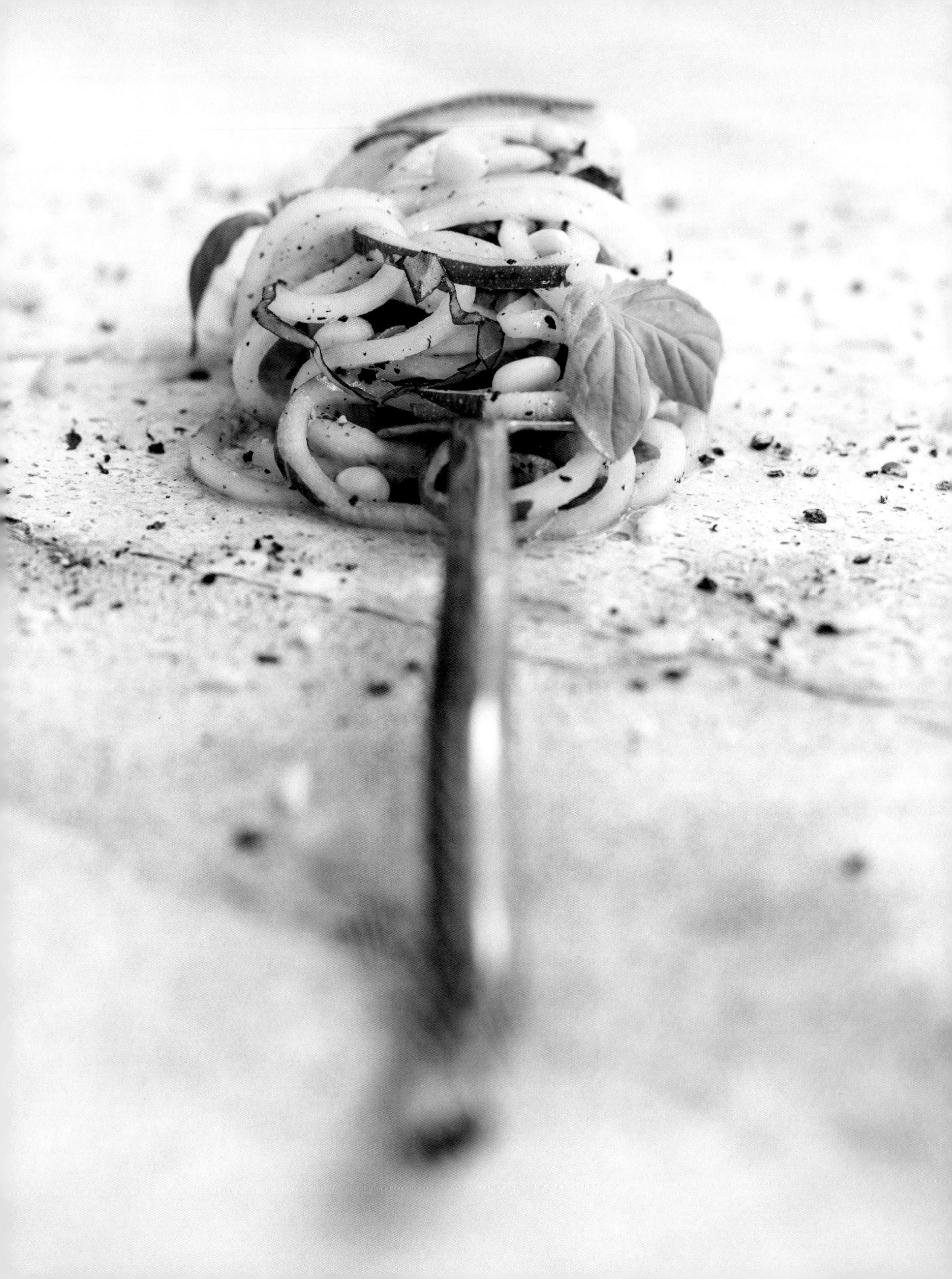

SOUPS AND SIDES

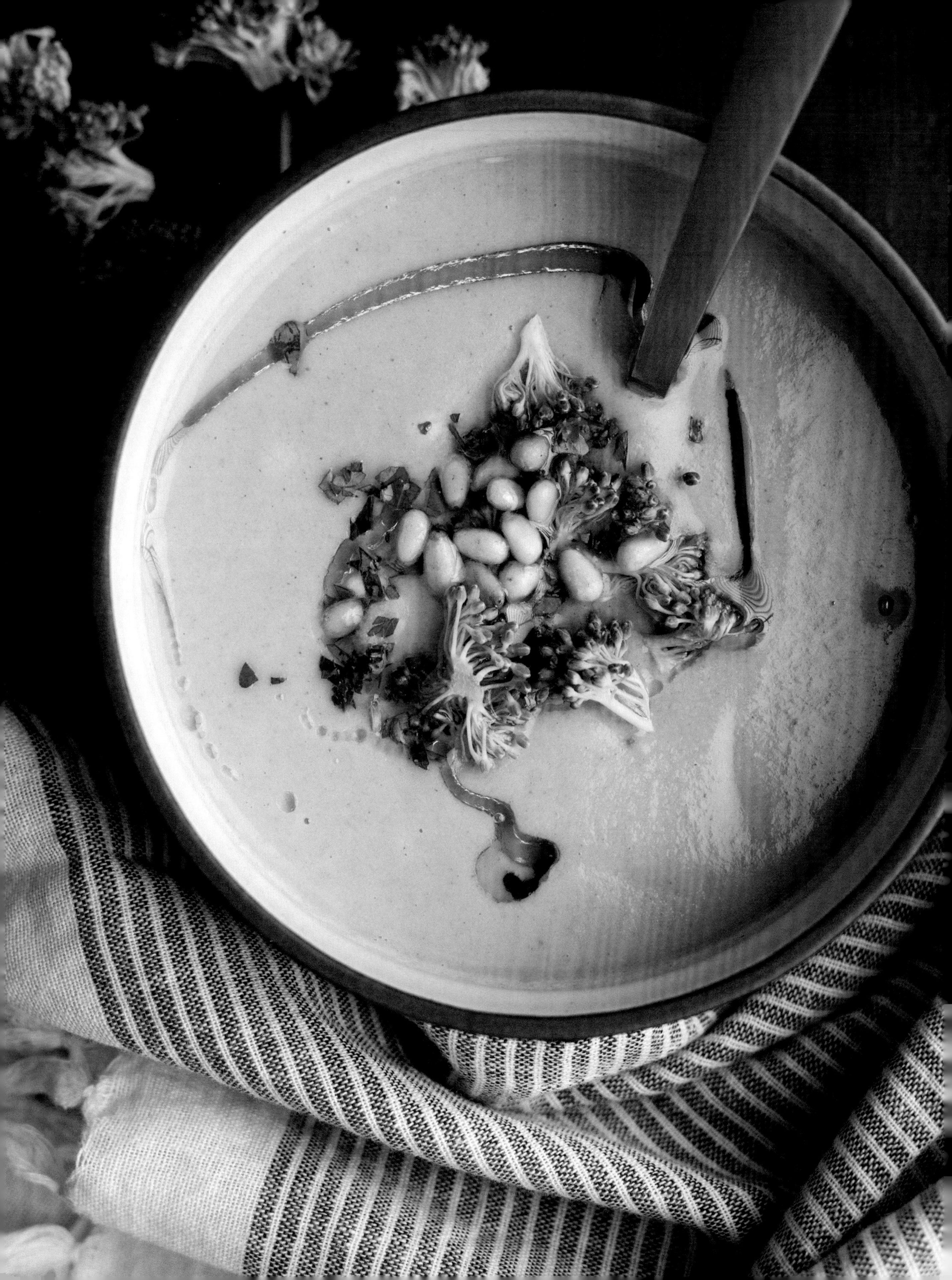

BROCCOLI AND WHITE BEAN SOUP

Gluten-Free, Grain-Free (Adaptable for Dairy-Free, SCD, Vegan)

PREP 5 minutes | COOK 20 minutes | TOTAL 25 minutes | SERVES 3-4

One of my favorite ways to eat vegetables in the winter is in a warm blended soup. Vegetable soups are so easy to make and don't take much time. In this recipe I combine white beans and broccoli. Beans are an inexpensive way to add plant-based protein and fiber to your diet. They're also proven to be helpful in preventing a wide range of diseases.

An important note about digesting beans: Some people have difficulty digesting beans because of the lectins in them. To break down the lectins, you can soak the beans in water overnight, changing the water a few times, and then cook them in a pressure cooker according to the manufacturer's directions. Or you can buy canned beans by Eden Foods. Eden Foods soaks and pressure-cooks its beans before canning, which makes cooking with beans more convenient. To adapt for dairy-free, omit Parmesan cheese. To adapt for SCD, use SCD-approved beans. To adapt for vegan, use vegetable stock and omit Parmesan cheese.

INGREDIENTS

2 Tablespoons olive oil

1 medium onion, diced

3 cloves garlic, minced

15-ounce can of cannellini or other white beans, drained or 1 3/4 cups soaked and cooked beans

12 ounces broccoli florets

3-4 cups chicken or vegetable stock

1 teaspoon salt

1/4 teaspoon white pepper

1 1/2 Tablespoons fresh lemon juice

1/4 cup freshly grated Parmesan cheese

DIRECTIONS

1. In a medium Dutch oven or large pot, heat the olive oil over medium-high heat.
2. Add the onions and sauté for 4 minutes.
3. Add the garlic and sauté an additional 3 minutes.
4. Add the beans, broccoli, 3 cups of stock, salt and white pepper and mix well.
5. Cover and let simmer for 8-10 minutes or until the broccoli is tender.
6. Remove from heat and ladle into a blender.
7. Blend the soup until smooth.
8. Wipe out the Dutch oven or pot and pour in the blended soup. Return the soup over medium heat, adding additional stock to achieve the desired consistency.
9. Add the lemon juice and freshly grated Parmesan cheese.
10. Adjust seasoning if needed and serve.

ROASTED BUTTERNUT WITH SAGE-INFUSED COCONUT CREAM SOUP

Dairy-Free, Gluten-Free, Grain-Free, Paleo, SCD, Vegan

PREP 10 minutes | COOK 1 hour 50 minutes | TOTAL 2 hours | SERVES 4

One of the best ways to warm up after being outside in the crisp fall weather is with a piping-hot bowl of soup. This soup is a favorite in our house. In this simple recipe, the squash is roasted in the oven and then added to sautéed onions with spices and stock and then puréed in a blender until smooth and creamy. You can stop there and be completely satisfied or make it extra special by adding a sage-infused coconut cream and garnishing with crisp fried sage leaves.

INGREDIENTS

1 butternut squash

7 Tablespoons olive oil, divided

Sea salt

Black pepper

1 can full-fat coconut milk, preferably without guar gum

1 bunch fresh sage leaves

2 cups diced yellow onion

1 teaspoon sea salt

1 Tablespoon cumin

1/4 teaspoon white pepper

1 quart vegetable or chicken stock

DIRECTIONS

1. Preheat oven to 450 degrees.
2. Cut the squash in half lengthwise.
3. Using a large spoon, scrape out the seeds and fibrous strands.
4. Place the squash halves cut side up on a baking sheet lined with parchment paper.
5. Lightly coat the tops with 1 Tablespoon of olive oil and sprinkle with salt and black pepper.
6. Roast the squash for 80-90 minutes or until tender.
7. Remove the squash from the oven and let cool.
8. Meanwhile, shake the can of coconut milk well and pour into a small saucepan.
9. Bring to a boil and then reduce the heat to medium low and allow the coconut milk to reduce for 45 minutes.
10. Add 3-4 sage leaves to the coconut milk for the last 15 minutes of reduction and then remove.
11. In a large pot heat 3 Tablespoons of olive oil over medium-high heat.
12. Add the onions and sauté until they are translucent, about 10 minutes.
13. Add 1 teaspoon sea salt, the cumin and white pepper.

(Continued)

14. Scrape the soft flesh out of the butternut squash with a large spoon and add to the onions, mixing well.
15. Add the vegetable or chicken stock and bring to a soft boil.
16. Remove from the heat and let sit for 5 minutes.
17. Purée the soup mixture in a blender until smooth.
18. Return to the pot and reheat if necessary.
19. In a small sauté pan, heat 3 Tablespoons olive oil over medium-high heat until small bubbles form.
20. Fry a few sage leaves at a time until crisp, about 2-3 seconds.
21. Transfer to a paper towel and sprinkle with sea salt and black pepper.
22. To serve, pour the soup into a bowl, swirl in a few large spoonfuls of warm coconut cream and top with fried sage leaves.

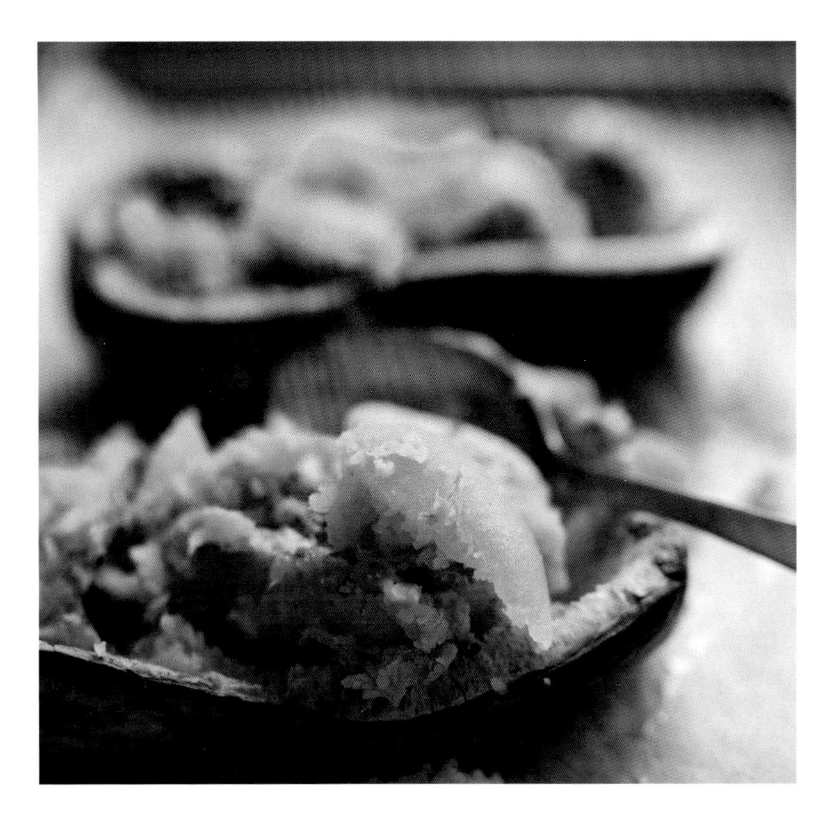

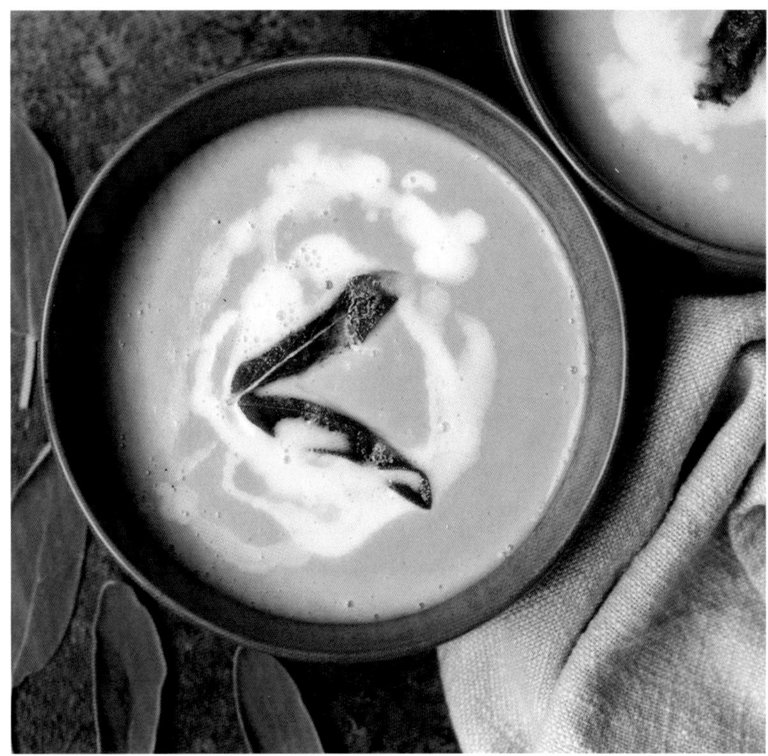

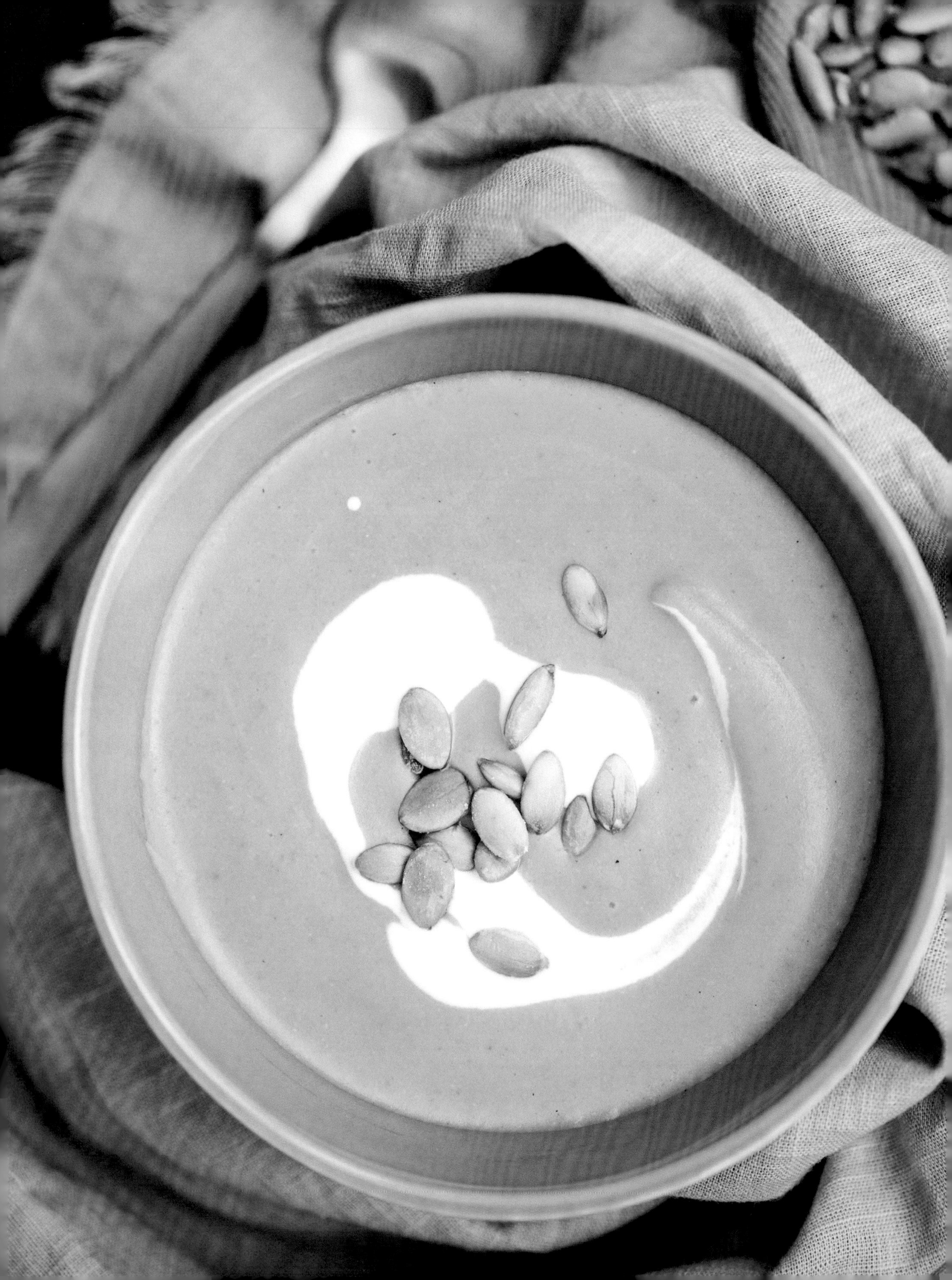

CURRIED RED LENTIL SOUP

Gluten-Free, Grain-Free, SCD (Adaptable for Dairy-Free and Vegan)

PREP 10 minutes | COOK 55 minutes | TOTAL 1 hour and 5 minutes | SERVES 8

Lentils are an excellent source of plant-based protein. They cook quickly and are wonderful for soups. This lentil soup is creamy with a hint of coconut and light curry flavor. If you love curry, feel free to add more curry powder for a stronger flavor. I like to purée most of my soups, but you can skip that step if you like. It tastes great either way. This is a large recipe—I like to go big when I make soup so I can freeze some to have on hand for a quick lunch. If you prefer a smaller batch, the recipe can easily be cut in half.

An important note about digesting lentils: Some people have difficulty digesting lentils because of the lectins in them. To break down the lectins, you can soak the lentils in water for two to four hours before using. To adapt for dairy-free and vegan, use dairy-free plain yogurt.

INGREDIENTS

4 Tablespoons olive oil

4 medium onions, chopped

4 large carrots, peeled and chopped

1 Tablespoon sea salt

2 Tablespoons curry powder

2 teaspoons cumin

1/4 teaspoon cayenne pepper

2 cups red lentils, rinsed

2 quarts vegetable stock

1 15-ounce can of full-fat coconut milk

1 Tablespoon fresh lime juice

Plain yogurt and pepitas, for serving

DIRECTIONS

1. Place the olive oil in a large pot over medium heat.
2. Add the onions and cook for 5 minutes, stirring occasionally.
3. Add the carrots and cook for 10 minutes or until carrots are tender.
4. Add the sea salt, curry, cumin and cayenne pepper. Stir well.
5. Cook for 2 minutes and add the lentils.
6. Add the vegetable stock and bring to a boil.
7. Reduce the soup to a simmer and cook for 25-30 minutes or until the lentils are tender, stirring occasionally.
8. Add the coconut milk and blend well. Return the soup to a boil.
9. Remove from heat and purée with an immersion blender or a stand-up blender in batches.
10. Return to the pot if using a stand-up blender.
11. Add the fresh lime juice and adjust seasoning to taste.
12. Top with your favorite plain yogurt and pepitas.

DAIRY-FREE WHITE CHICKEN CHILI

Dairy-Free, Gluten-Free, Grain-Free (Adaptable for SCD)

PREP 15 minutes | COOK 30 minutes | TOTAL 45 minutes | SERVES 4

White chicken chili makes a delicious meal on a cold day. However, most recipes include a lot of dairy, which can make it heavy and too rich. In this version, I omit the cream and cheese, instead puréeing the ingredients with white beans to give the chili the same creamy consistency as one made with dairy. For the cooked and shredded chicken breasts, I like to use a pressure cooker because it is so quick and easy. I put the chicken breasts in the pressure cooker with a half-cup of chicken stock and turn it on the poultry setting. It only takes 15 minutes. When the chicken is finished cooking, I use a hand mixer to shred it. You can use this method or cook and shred the chicken however you like. The chicken can even be prepared ahead of time for this recipe. To adapt for SCD, use SCD-approved beans.

INGREDIENTS

3 Tablespoons olive oil

2 cups diced onion

1 Tablespoon minced garlic

2 jalapeños, minced

2 teaspoons sea salt

2 Tablespoons cumin

1/2 teaspoon white pepper

1 teaspoon smoked paprika

1 1/2-2 cups chicken stock, divided

2 15-ounce cans of white cannellini or Great Northern beans, drained

2 boneless chicken breasts, cooked and shredded

Avocado, pico de gallo, jalapeño slices, fresh cilantro and tortilla chips, for serving

DIRECTIONS

1. In a medium pot, heat 3 Tablespoons of olive oil over medium-high heat.
2. Add the diced onion and sauté for 8 minutes, stirring occasionally.
3. Add the garlic and jalapeño and sauté for an additional 5 minutes.
4. Add the salt, cumin, white pepper and smoked paprika and mix well. Cook for 2 minutes.
5. Add 1 cup of chicken stock and 1 can of beans; simmer for 10 minutes, stirring occasionally.
6. Remove from heat and purée the mixture with an immersion or stand-up blender.
7. If using a stand-up blender, wipe out the pot with a paper towel and pour the blended soup back into the pot.

(Continued)

8. Return to heat and add the shredded chicken and the other can of beans.
9. Add 1/2 cup of chicken stock and mix well, adding more stock if needed for desired consistency.
10. Return the chili to a simmer and serve.
11. Top with avocado, pico de gallo, jalapeño slices and fresh cilantro and serve with tortilla chips.

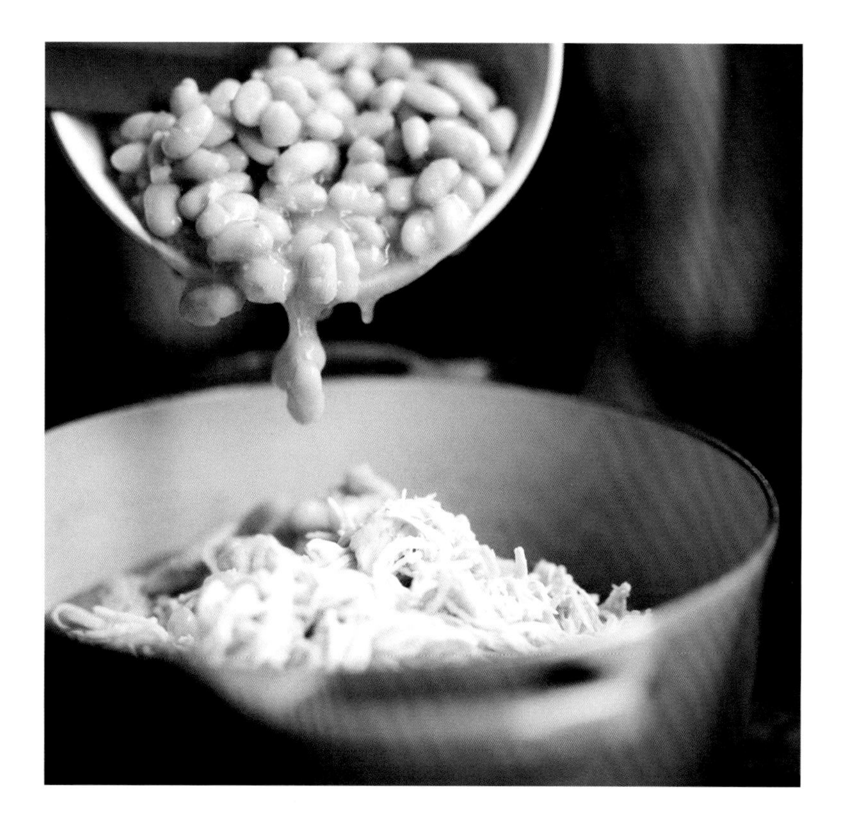

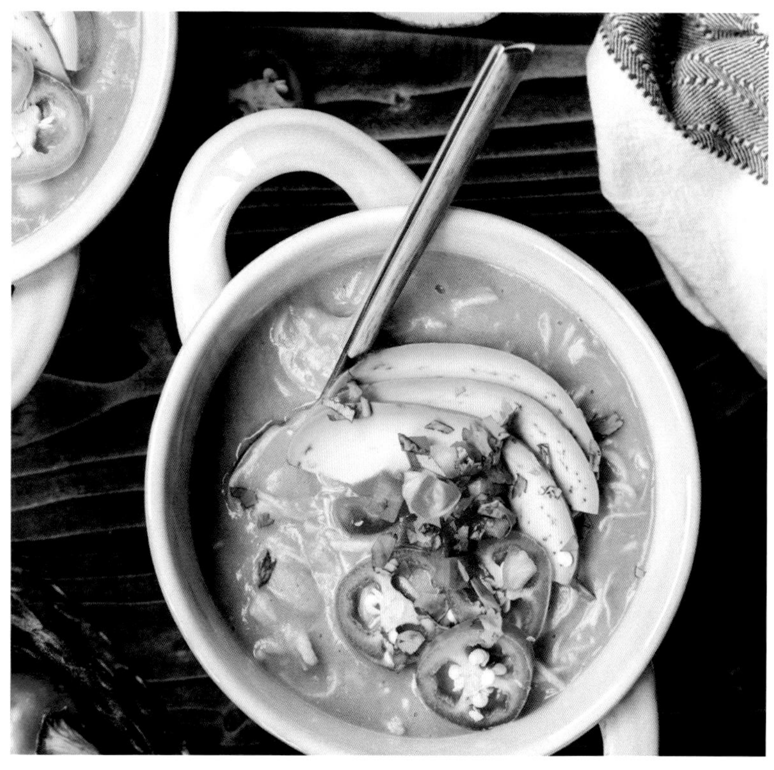

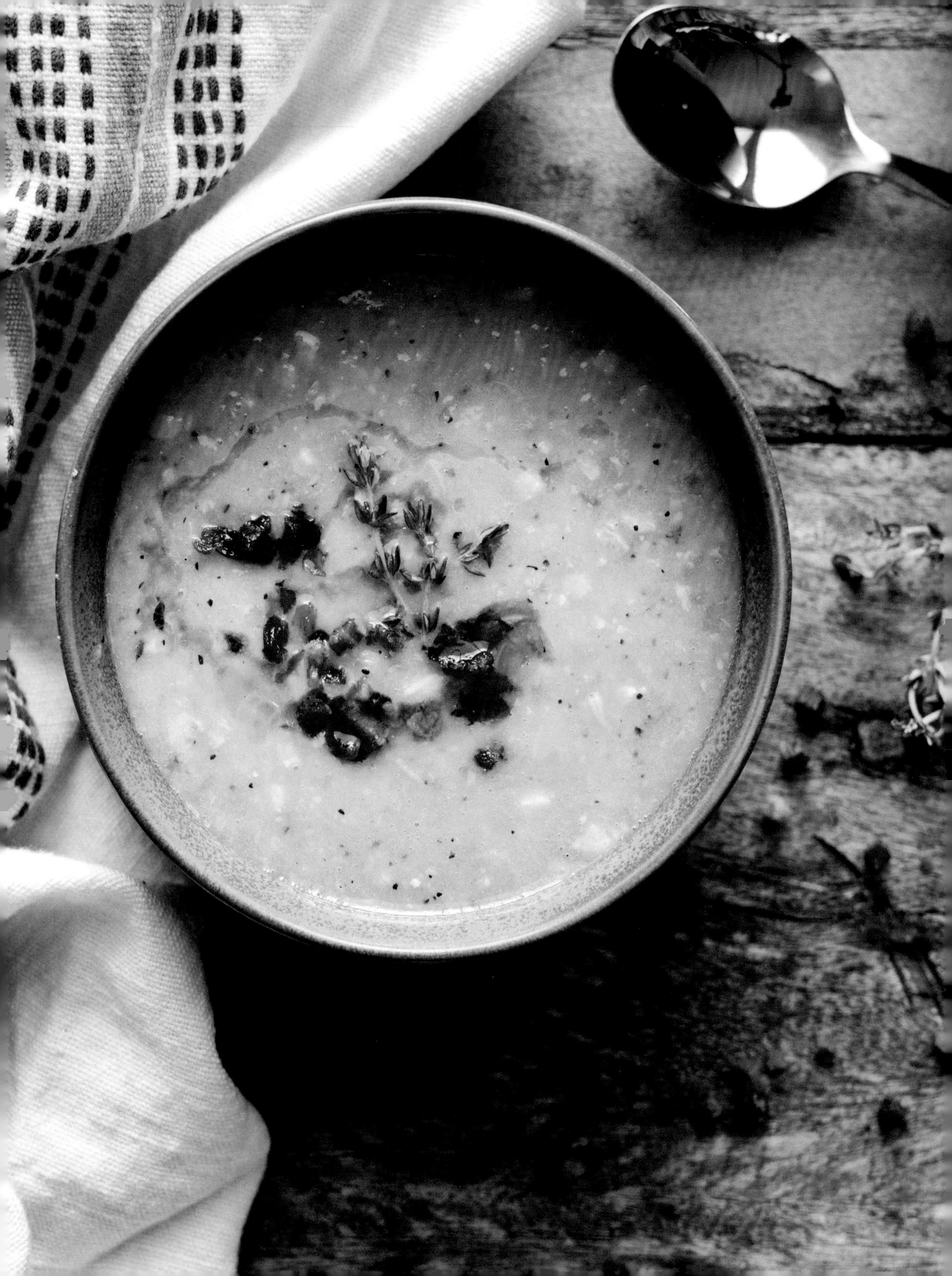

WHITE BEAN AND PANCETTA SOUP

Dairy-Free, Gluten-Free, Grain-Free (Adaptable for SCD)

PREP 8 minutes | COOK 17 minutes | TOTAL 25 minutes | SERVES 4

Nothing is more comforting on a cold or gloomy day than a warm bowl of soup. This white bean and pancetta soup is simple to make and satisfying. Beans are a great source of prebiotic fiber for the microbes in your gut. They also provide ample protein to the diet. This combination of protein and fiber makes beans very filling. The salty pancetta in this recipe gives the mild beans a nice burst of flavor while the fresh thyme and garlic round out the dish splendidly. I like to partially purée this soup so half of the beans are creamy and the other half are left chunky, which gives it a hearty consistency. To adapt for SCD, use SCD-approved beans.

DIRECTIONS

1. Place the olive oil in a large pot over medium heat.
2. Add the onions and cook for 5 minutes, stirring occasionally.
3. Add the pancetta and cook for 3 minutes.
4. Add the garlic, thyme, salt and pepper. Cook for 3 minutes.
5. Add the beans and stock and simmer for 5 minutes.
6. Remove from heat. Using an immersion blender, partially purée. Leave half of the beans chunky and the other half creamy.
7. Return to heat and adjust seasoning.

INGREDIENTS

4 Tablespoons olive oil

2 cups diced onion

8 ounces diced pancetta

1 Tablespoon minced garlic

1 Tablespoon chopped thyme

2 teaspoons sea salt

1 teaspoon black pepper

1 29-ounce can and 1 15-ounce can cannellini or other white beans

2 cups chicken stock

CHICKEN TORTILLA SOUP

Dairy-Free, Gluten-Free, Grain-Free, Paleo

PREP 5 minutes | COOK 40 minutes | TOTAL 45 minutes | SERVES 4

Chicken tortilla soup is easy to make and it's delicious. I love the combination of a flavorful broth with creamy avocado and crunchy tortilla strips. My version has a healthy amount of spice. If you like your tortilla soup on the milder side, you can substitute a can of regular diced tomatoes for one of the fire-roasted ones. For the cooked and shredded chicken breasts, I like to use a pressure cooker because it is so quick and easy. I put the chicken breasts in the pressure cooker with a half-cup of chicken broth and turn it on the poultry setting. It takes 15 minutes. Shred the chicken however you like. For topping the soup, I like to make my own tortilla strips using Siete almond flour tortillas. I stack a few tortillas, slice them into strips, then lightly fry them in avocado oil. You can also skip this step and use your favorite brand of tortilla strips or chips instead.

INGREDIENTS

4 Tablespoons olive oil

1 large onion, diced

1 jalapeño, minced

2 cloves garlic, minced

1 1/2 teaspoons sea salt

1 Tablespoon cumin

2 14-ounce cans fire-roasted diced tomatoes

4 cups chicken broth

2 boneless chicken breasts, cooked and shredded

1 large or 2 small zucchini, diced

2 Tablespoons chopped cilantro

1 lime, juiced

Diced avocado and tortilla strips or chips, for serving

DIRECTIONS

1. Place the olive oil in a large pot over medium heat.
2. Add the onions and jalapeño and cook for 5 minutes.
3. Add the garlic and cook for 3 minutes.
4. Add the salt, cumin and tomatoes. Cook for 5 minutes.
5. Add the chicken broth, shredded chicken and diced zucchini. Simmer for 10 minutes.
6. Add the chopped cilantro and fresh lime juice and stir well.
7. Ladle the soup into bowls and top with avocado and tortilla chips or strips.

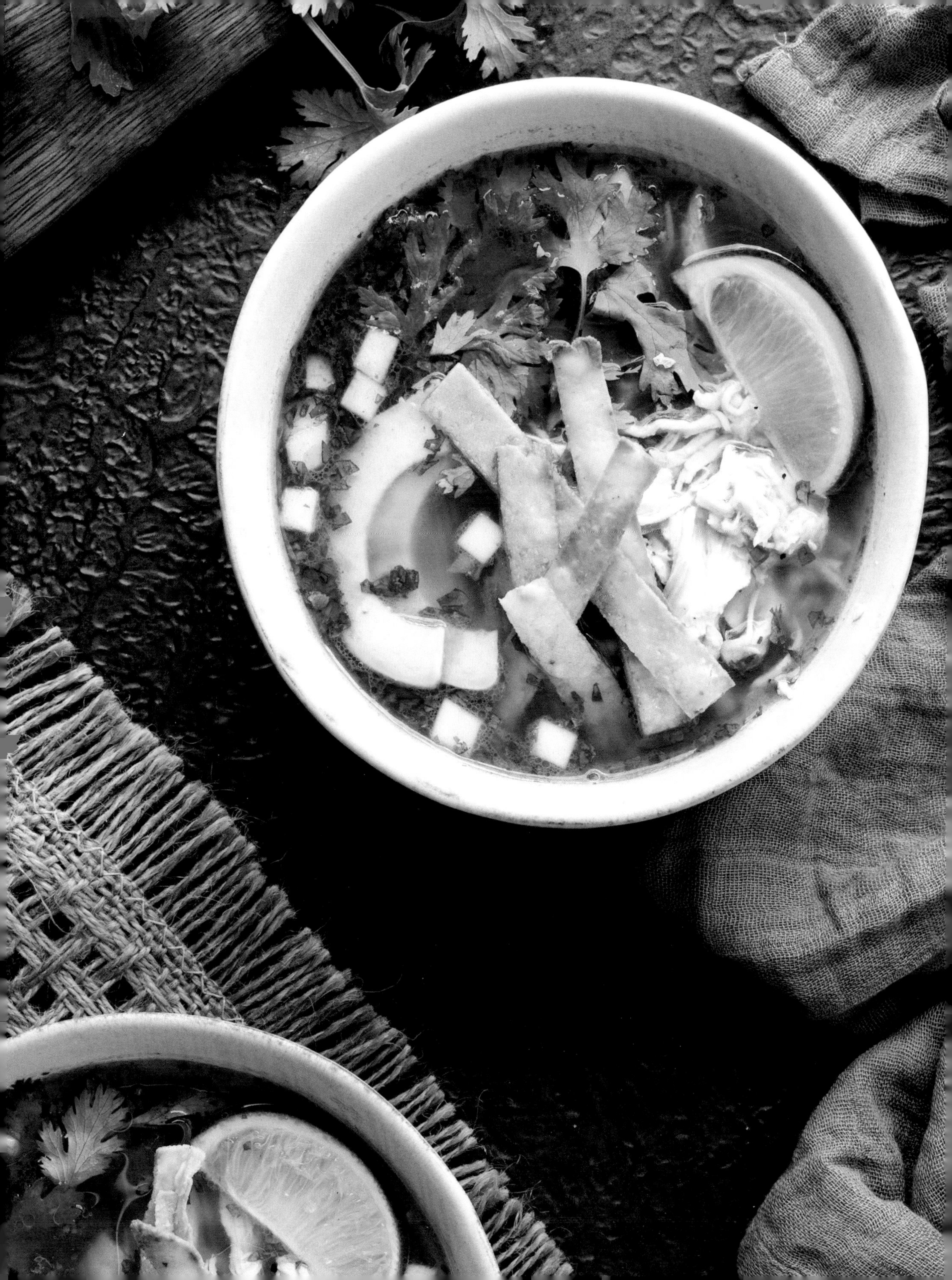

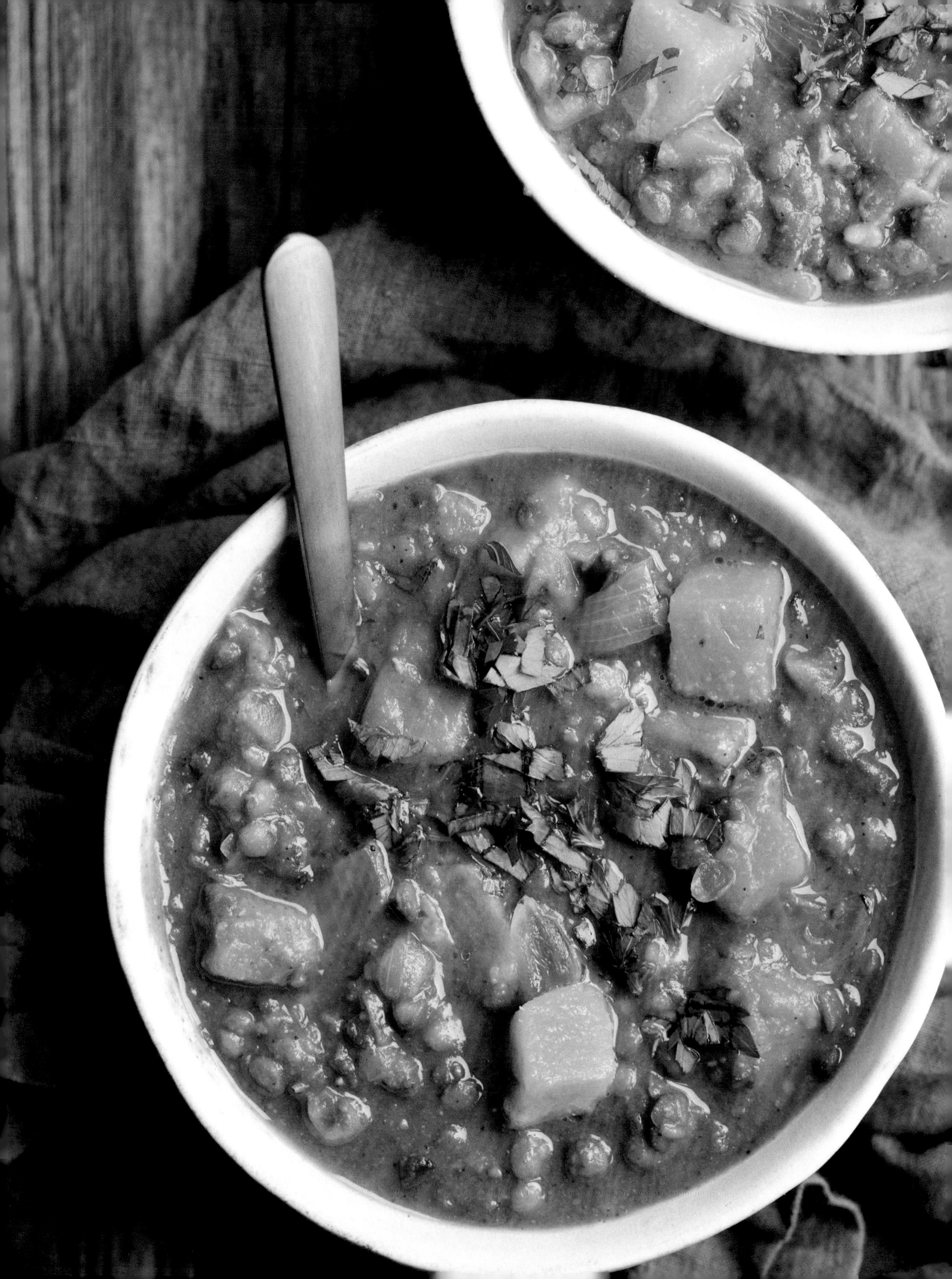

BUTTERNUT SQUASH AND LENTIL STEW

Dairy-Free, Gluten-Free, Grain-Free, SCD, Vegan

PREP 10 minutes | COOK 20 minutes | TOTAL 30 minutes | SERVES 4

This hearty plant-based stew is filled with fiber and is absolutely delicious. The many spices give the stew a rich flavor as well as additional health benefits. The convenience of pre-cut butternut squash and precooked lentils available in stores makes this dish exceptionally easy to prepare. I like to keep those ingredients on hand in the fall and winter so I can quickly whip up a batch for some cold-weather comfort food.

INGREDIENTS

5 Tablespoons olive oil, divided

1 large yellow onion, diced

6 cups of peeled and cubed butternut squash, about 1 1/2 pounds

3 cloves garlic, minced

1 Tablespoon sea salt

1 1/2 teaspoons turmeric

1 1/2 teaspoons cumin

1/2 teaspoon smoked paprika

1 teaspoon coriander

1 teaspoon chili powder

1 1/2 teaspoons ground ginger

1/4 teaspoon cayenne

2 cans or 4 cups of cooked lentils

2-3 cups of vegetable broth

1/2 lime, juiced

DIRECTIONS

1. Add 4 Tablespoons olive oil to a large Dutch oven or large pot over medium-high heat.
2. Add the diced onion and cubed butternut squash.
3. Sauté for 12 minutes stirring frequently.
4. Add 1 Tablespoon olive oil, the minced garlic, sea salt, turmeric, cumin, smoked paprika, coriander, chili powder, ginger, cayenne and lentils and stir well.
5. Cook for 3 minutes, stirring frequently.
6. Add 2 cups of vegetable broth and stir well.
7. Add additional broth to achieve the desired consistency and return to a simmer.
8. Add the fresh lime juice.
9. Adjust seasoning to taste.

ROASTED TOMATO SOUP

Gluten-Free, Grain-Free, SCD (Adaptable for Dairy-Free, Paleo, Vegan)

PREP 15 minutes | COOK 45 minutes | TOTAL 1 hour | SERVES 3-4

Roasted tomato soup is simple to make and tastes much better than the canned versions in the supermarket. I use plum tomatoes, but you can use any kind you like. Or try a variety! This is a great recipe for gardeners looking to use up extra tomatoes. This soup freezes well so you can enjoy the fruit of your garden (or farmers market) year-round. To adapt for dairy-free and paleo, substitute olive oil for butter and omit the Parmesan cheese. To adapt for vegan, substitute olive oil for butter, use vegetable broth and omit the Parmesan cheese.

INGREDIENTS

3 pounds plum tomatoes

1 large yellow onion

6 cloves garlic

1/4 cup olive oil

2 teaspoons sea salt

1 1/2 teaspoons black pepper

2 Tablespoons chopped fresh oregano

1/2-1 1/2 cups chicken or vegetable broth

1-2 Tablespoons grass-fed butter or olive oil

Grated Parmesan cheese, for serving

DIRECTIONS

1. Preheat the oven to 425 degrees.
2. Cut the tomatoes in half lengthwise and place in a single layer on a parchment-lined sheet pan.
3. Peel the onion and cut it in half and then into thick slices.
4. Add the onion and garlic cloves to the pan of tomatoes.
5. Drizzle 1/4 cup of olive oil over the tomatoes, onions and garlic cloves.
6. Sprinkle with salt and pepper.
7. Roast the vegetables for 40-45 minutes.
8. Transfer the tomatoes, onion, garlic and pan juices to a blender.
9. Add the fresh oregano and blend on medium-high for 1 minute.
10. Add 1/2 cup of chicken or vegetable broth and blend for 30 seconds.
11. Check the consistency and add more broth to achieve desired thickness.
12. Adjust salt and pepper to taste.
13. Stir in 1-2 Tablespoons of butter or olive oil for a richer flavor.
14. Top with grated Parmesan cheese.

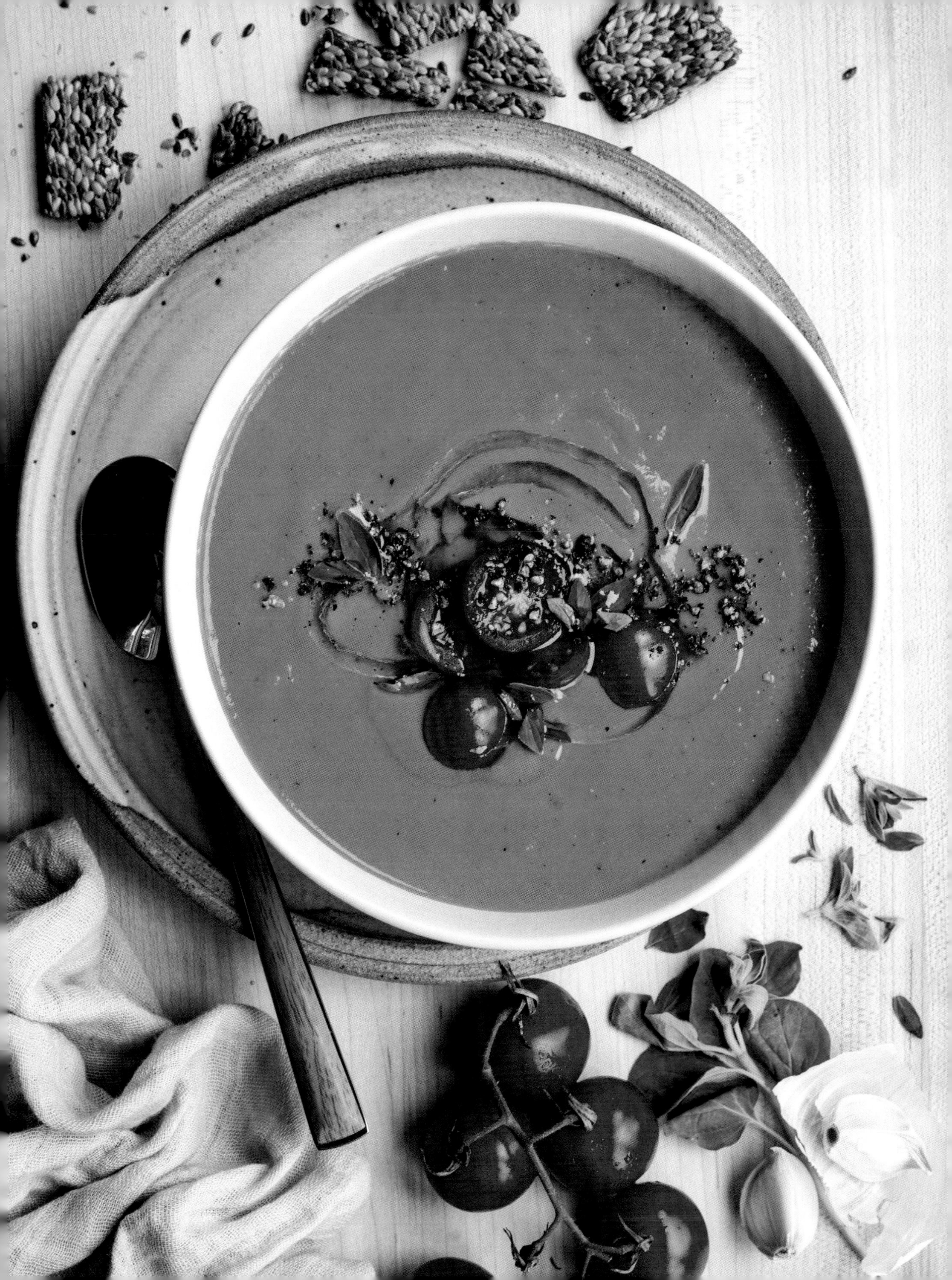

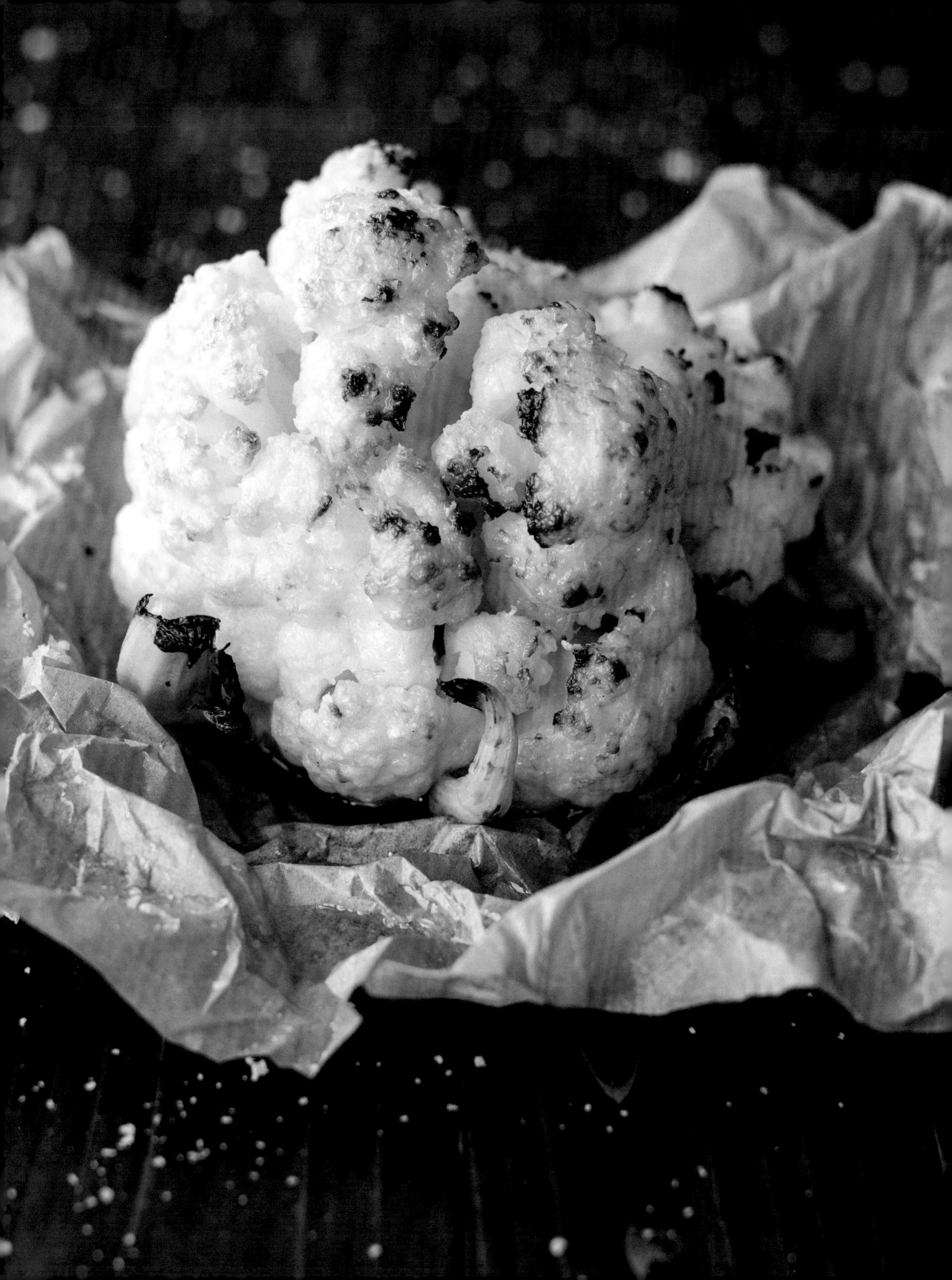

WHOLE ROASTED CAULIFLOWER

Dairy-Free, Gluten-Free, Grain-Free, Paleo, SCD, Vegan

PREP 10 minutes | COOK 50 minutes | TOTAL 1 hour | SERVES 2-4

Roasted cauliflower is so simple and has quickly become one of my favorite side dishes to prepare at home. When I was working on the photo shoot for this recipe with my photographer, Belén, she shared that when she was living in Spain, her house mom always cooked whole heads of cauliflower. It was similar to this version with olive oil and sea salt, but she served it with vinegar. After Belén finished shooting the cauliflower we sat down to enjoy it with a side of vinegar. It was a wonderful addition to an already delicious dish. You can eat the leaves too!

DIRECTIONS

1. Preheat oven to 500 degrees.
2. Bring 6 quarts of water to a boil and add 3 Tablespoons of sea salt; stir to dissolve.
3. Wash the cauliflower and cut the base so it stands upright, keeping the leaves intact.
4. Place the head of cauliflower in the boiling water.
5. Place the lid of a pot or a ceramic plate on top of the cauliflower to keep it submerged.
6. Boil for 7-9 minutes or until a knife inserted in the cauliflower pushes easily through the soft outer layers and meets some resistance in the middle.
7. Place the hot cauliflower on a sheet pan and allow to cool until you no longer see steam coming off of it. This should take about 15-20 minutes.
8. Rub the cauliflower with olive oil and sprinkle with sea salt.
9. Roast the cauliflower in the oven for 15-20 minutes or until browned.
10. Remove from the oven and drizzle with olive oil and sea salt.
11. Serve alone or with your favorite vinegar.

INGREDIENTS

1 small head of cauliflower

Olive oil

Sea salt

Vinegar, for serving

SOUTHWESTERN SWEET POTATO FRIES

Dairy-Free, Gluten-Free, Grain-Free, Paleo (Adaptable for Vegan)

PREP 20 minutes | COOK 50 minutes | TOTAL 1 hour 10 minutes | SERVES 4

Sweet potato fries are on my list of all-time favorite foods. When I order them at a restaurant it takes a tremendous amount of restraint for me to not finish the whole plate. Many restaurants add extra ingredients and use cooking methods that are not necessarily the healthiest. When I make them at home, I don't have to worry about overindulging because they are baked instead of fried, which makes them much healthier. In this recipe, I add Southwestern seasoning to give them a kick and serve them with a simple seasoned fry sauce. The arrowroot is a grain-free starch that helps to make fries crispy. If you are not concerned with the fries being grain-free, you can substitute cornstarch for the arrowroot. To adapt for vegan, use vegan mayonnaise.

INGREDIENTS

2 teaspoons sea salt

1 1/2 teaspoons chili powder

1 1/2 teaspoons cumin

1 1/2 teaspoons smoked paprika

1 teaspoon garlic powder

1/8 teaspoon cayenne

2 Tablespoons arrowroot starch

1/4 cup ketchup

1/4 cup homemade or good-quality mayonnaise

2-3 large sweet potatoes

2 Tablespoons avocado oil

Chopped fresh cilantro and coarse sea salt, for serving

DIRECTIONS

1. Preheat the oven to 425 degrees.
2. In a small bowl combine the sea salt, chili powder, cumin, smoked paprika, garlic powder and cayenne.
3. In another small bowl combine the ketchup and mayonnaise and add 1 1/2 teaspoons of the seasoning mix. Set aside.
4. Add the arrowroot to the remaining seasoning and mix well.
5. Wash and peel the sweet potatoes.
6. Cut the potatoes into 1/4-inch fries, keeping them as close to the same length as possible.
7. Place the fries in a large bowl and toss with the avocado oil.
8. Add the seasoning with the arrowroot and toss to coat the fries well.

(Continued)

9. Spread the fries on an unlined sheet pan without crowding them. If necessary use a second pan for extra fries.
10. Place the sheet pan in the top third of the oven. I find that it works best to bake one sheet pan at a time. If you have a second pan, bake it in another oven or wait until the first batch is done.
11. Bake for 25 minutes and then flip the fries and return to the oven.
12. Bake for an additional 15-25 minutes or until crisp and browned.
13. Place the fries on a serving tray and top with chopped fresh cilantro and coarse sea salt.
14. Serve with the seasoned fry sauce.

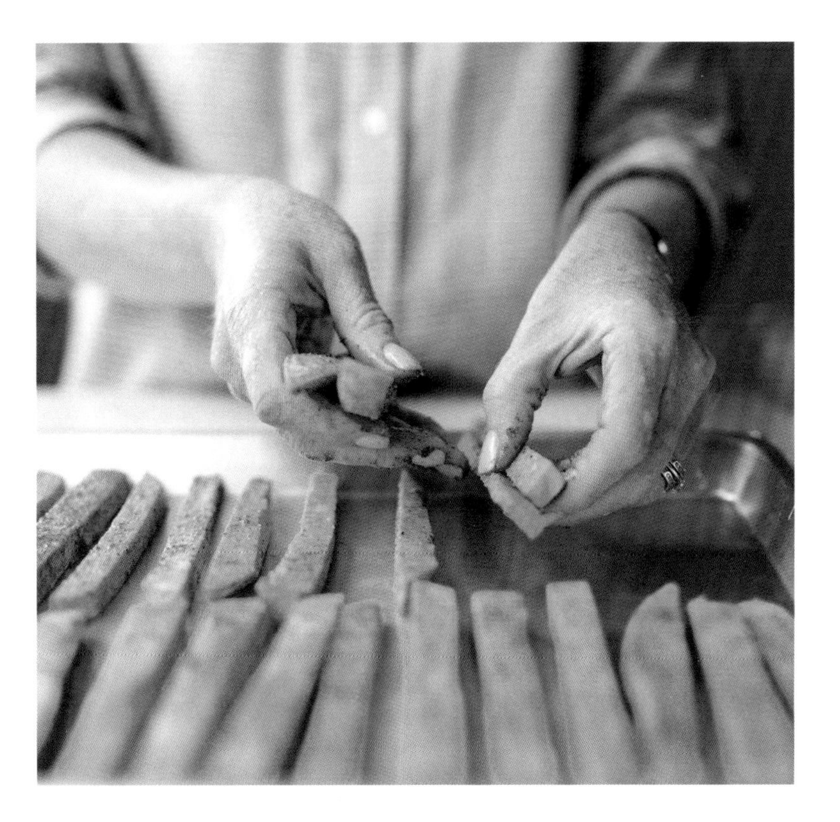

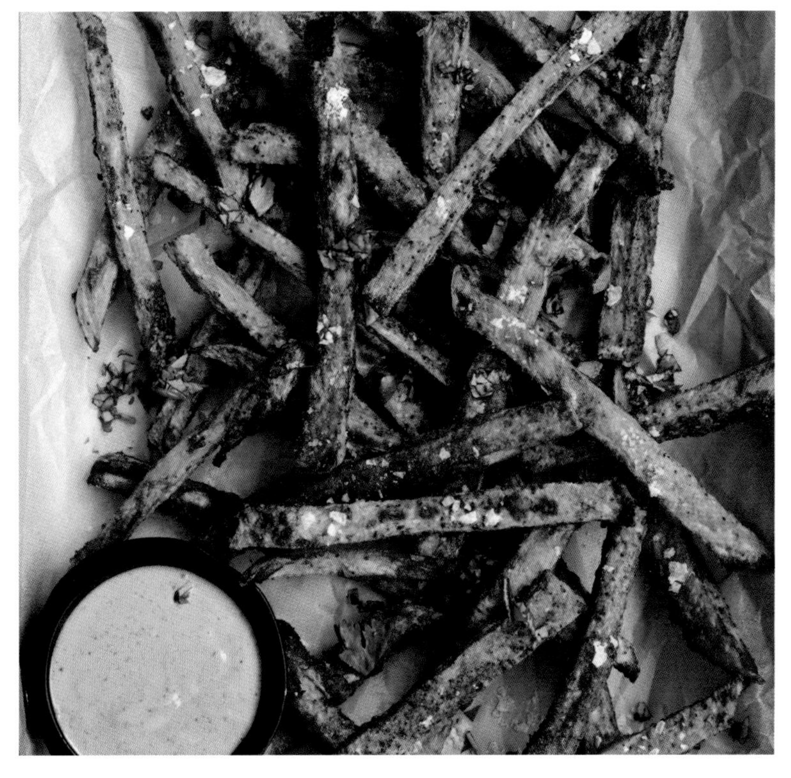

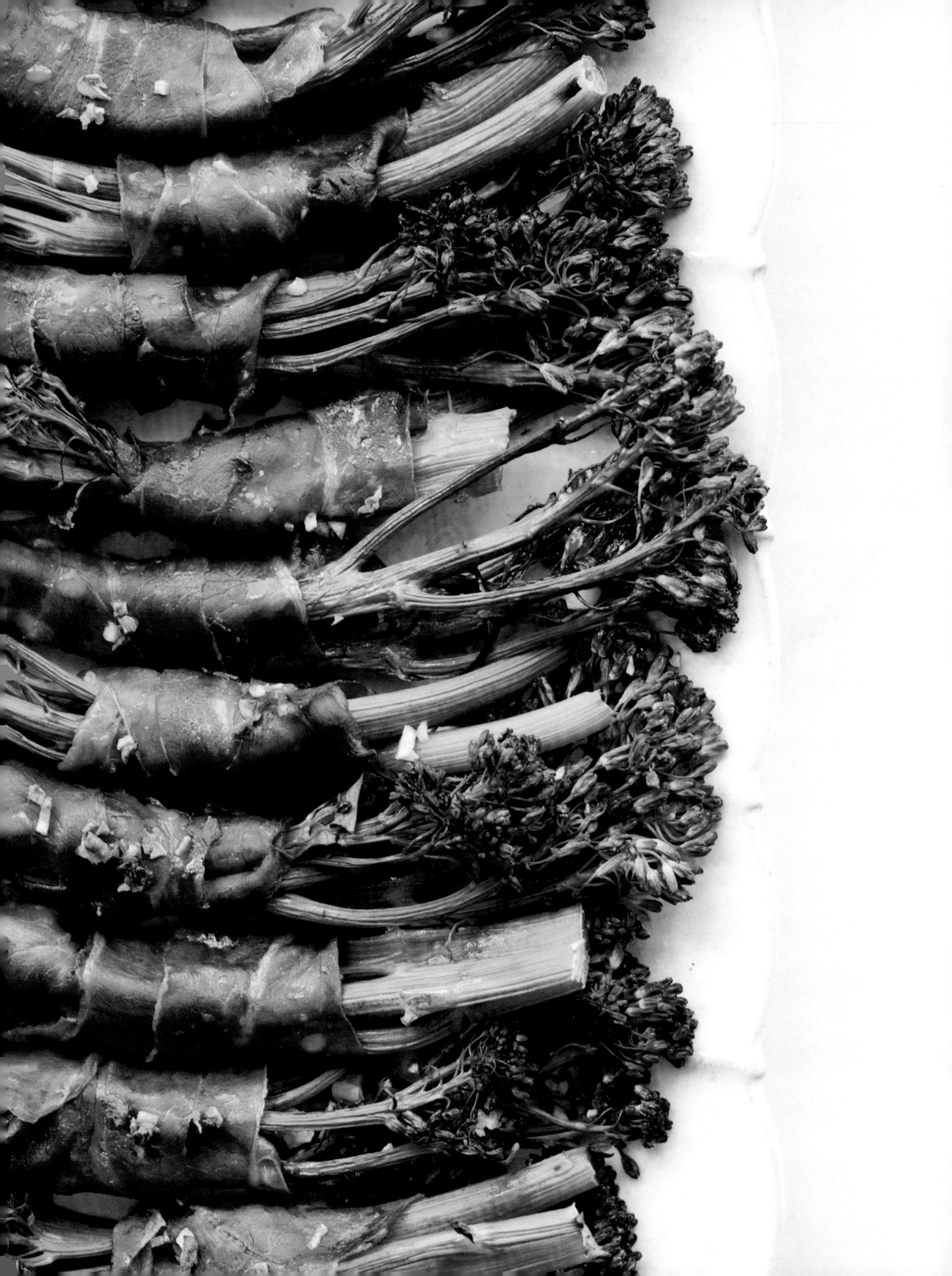

PROSCIUTTO-WRAPPED BROCCOLINI

Dairy-Free, Gluten-Free, Grain-Free, Paleo, SCD

PREP 10 minutes | COOK 20 minutes | TOTAL 30 minutes | SERVES 4

Broccolini is similar to broccoli but with smaller florets and longer, thin stalks. It is milder and more tender than regular broccoli. I like to roast it bundled and wrapped in prosciutto with garlic and lemon. It is so simple and makes a tasty side dish.

INGREDIENTS

1 pound Broccolini

6 slices of prosciutto

Olive oil

2-3 garlic cloves, chopped

1 lemon

DIRECTIONS

1. Preheat the oven to 425 degrees.
2. Rinse and dry the Broccolini.
3. Cut the slices of prosciutto in half lengthwise.
4. Place 2 stalks of Broccolini together and wrap a piece of prosciutto around the stalk to secure.
5. Repeat with remaining Broccolini to make 12 bundles.
6. Place the bundles on a parchment-lined sheet pan.
7. Drizzle olive oil over the Broccolini.
8. Sprinkle the chopped garlic over the olive oil.
9. Roast the Broccolini for 20 minutes or until done.
10. Cut the lemon in half and squeeze the juice over the Broccolini bundles.

FRENCH GREEN BEANS WITH ROASTED HAZELNUTS

Dairy-Free, Gluten-Free, Grain-Free, Paleo, SCD, Vegan

PREP 10 minutes | COOK 20 minutes | TOTAL 30 minutes | SERVES 4

I love green beans and serve them often at my house. They are simple to make and everyone likes them. In this recipe, I toss them in toasted hazelnut oil and add chopped hazelnuts, a squeeze of lemon and coarse sea salt. I roast the hazelnuts myself, but you can use already roasted ones and skip that step if you like.

INGREDIENTS

1/2 cup raw hazelnuts

Maldon or other coarse sea salt

16 ounces French or regular green beans

1 Tablespoon toasted hazelnut oil

1/4 of a lemon

DIRECTIONS

1. Preheat the oven to 350 degrees.
2. Spread hazelnuts on a sheet pan lined with parchment paper.
3. Roast the hazelnuts for 15 minutes or until lightly browned, shaking the pan halfway through roasting.
4. Remove the pan from the oven and transfer the hazelnuts into a clean dish towel.
5. Rub the hazelnuts in the dish towel to remove the bitter skins.
6. Place the hazelnuts on a cutting board and roughly chop.
7. Fill a medium saucepan with 1/2 inch of water and a pinch of sea salt.
8. Add the green beans and bring the water to a simmer.
9. Cook covered until tender, about 5 minutes.
10. Drain the water from the pan.
11. Add the toasted hazelnut oil and chopped hazelnuts to the green beans.
12. Squeeze the juice from the quartered lemon over the beans.
13. Sprinkle with sea salt and toss well.

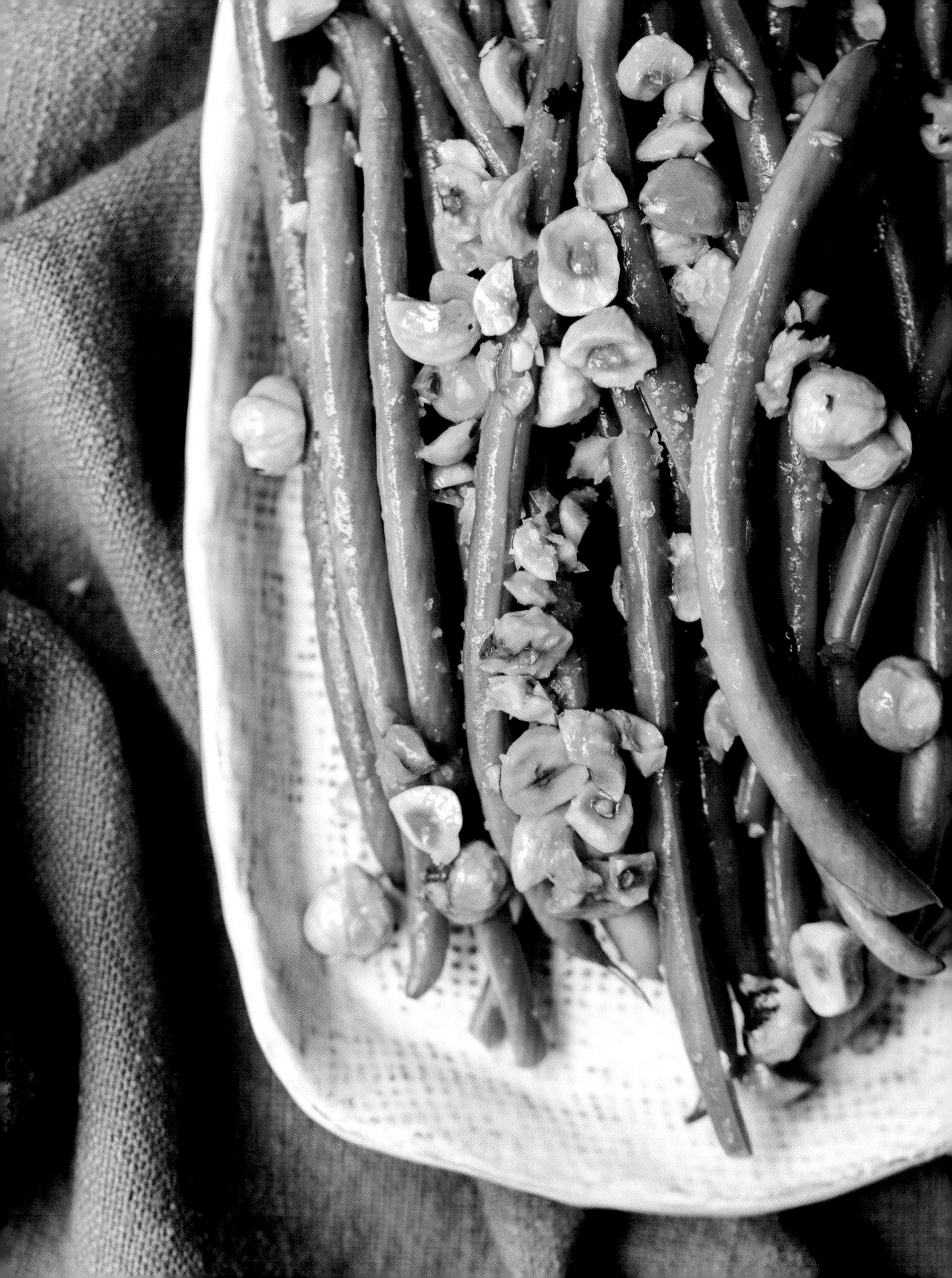

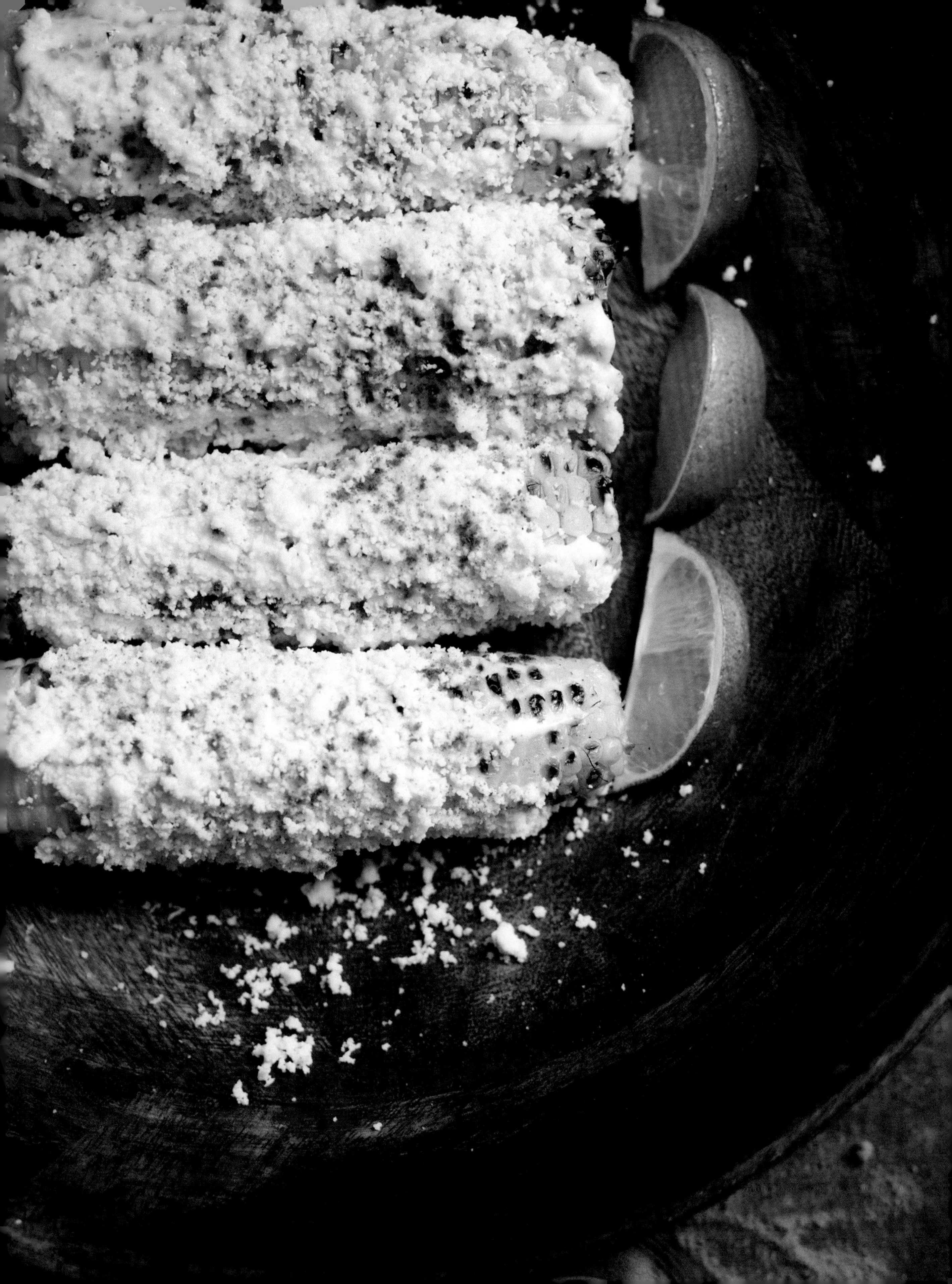

MEXICAN STREET CORN

Gluten-Free

PREP 10 minutes | COOK 12 minutes | TOTAL 22 minutes | SERVES 4

The first time I visited New York City, I went with my sister, Liz. An apparel designer, Liz was traveling there for a trend shopping trip and invited me to join her. She told me, "Since you are the foodie, you can pick where we eat. I only have one place we need to go to, Café Habana for the street corn." Once I tasted the corn there, I understood why this was a must-stop for her. The restaurant's version of this traditional Mexican street food was incredible. After returning home, I set out to duplicate it for my family. I have made it many different ways, and this simple version is the one my family likes the best. I serve it in the summer when sweet corn is in season.

INGREDIENTS

Sea salt

4 ears sweet corn, shucked

1/4 cup homemade or good-quality mayonnaise

1/4 cup Mexican crema or sour cream

4 ounces crumbled cotija cheese

Cayenne pepper

Lime wedges, for serving

DIRECTIONS

1. Fill a large pot with water and add 1/4-1/2 teaspoon of salt.
2. Bring the water to a boil over high heat.
3. Add the corn and cook for 10-12 minutes.
4. If you want to grill the corn, boil it for only 5-6 minutes, then you can brush it lightly with olive oil and grill over high heat until slightly charred. Or you can skip the grilling step.
5. In a small bowl, combine the mayonnaise and Mexican crema or sour cream.
6. Using a spatula, spread the mixture evenly on the hot corn.
7. Roll the corn in the crumbled cotija cheese.
8. Sprinkle with cayenne pepper and sea salt.
9. Serve with lime wedges.

ZUCCHINI NOODLES WITH BASIL AND PINE NUTS

Dairy-Free, Gluten-Free, Grain-Free, Paleo, SCD, Vegan

PREP 10 minutes | COOK 3 minutes | TOTAL 13 minutes | SERVES 3-4

Turning zucchini into noodles is a fun way to enjoy this versatile vegetable. I often use zucchini noodles as a substitute for pasta and they are also delicious as a simple side dish. You can create your own zucchini noodles using a spiralizer or mandoline, or you can purchase them pre-cut at most grocery stores. In this recipe, the fresh basil adds a punch of flavor and the pine nuts add a nice crunch.

INGREDIENTS

3 large or 4 medium zucchini
2/3 cup fresh basil leaves
2 Tablespoons olive oil
2 teaspoons minced garlic
1/3 cup toasted pine nuts
1 teaspoon sea salt
1/2 teaspoon black pepper

DIRECTIONS

1. Trim the zucchini and make noodles using a spiralizer or mandoline.
2. Using a clean kitchen towel, pat the noodles dry.
3. Stack the basil leaves on top of each other and roll them into a cigar shape.
4. Slice the basil roll into thin ribbons (chiffonade) and set aside.
5. Add 2 Tablespoons of olive oil to a large, deep skillet over medium heat.
6. Add the minced garlic and stir.
7. Add the zucchini noodles and sauté for 3 minutes, using tongs to flip and turn the noodles for even cooking.
8. Add the pine nuts, salt and black pepper and cook for an additional minute or until al dente, stirring with the tongs.
9. Remove from heat and add the basil. Stir well.

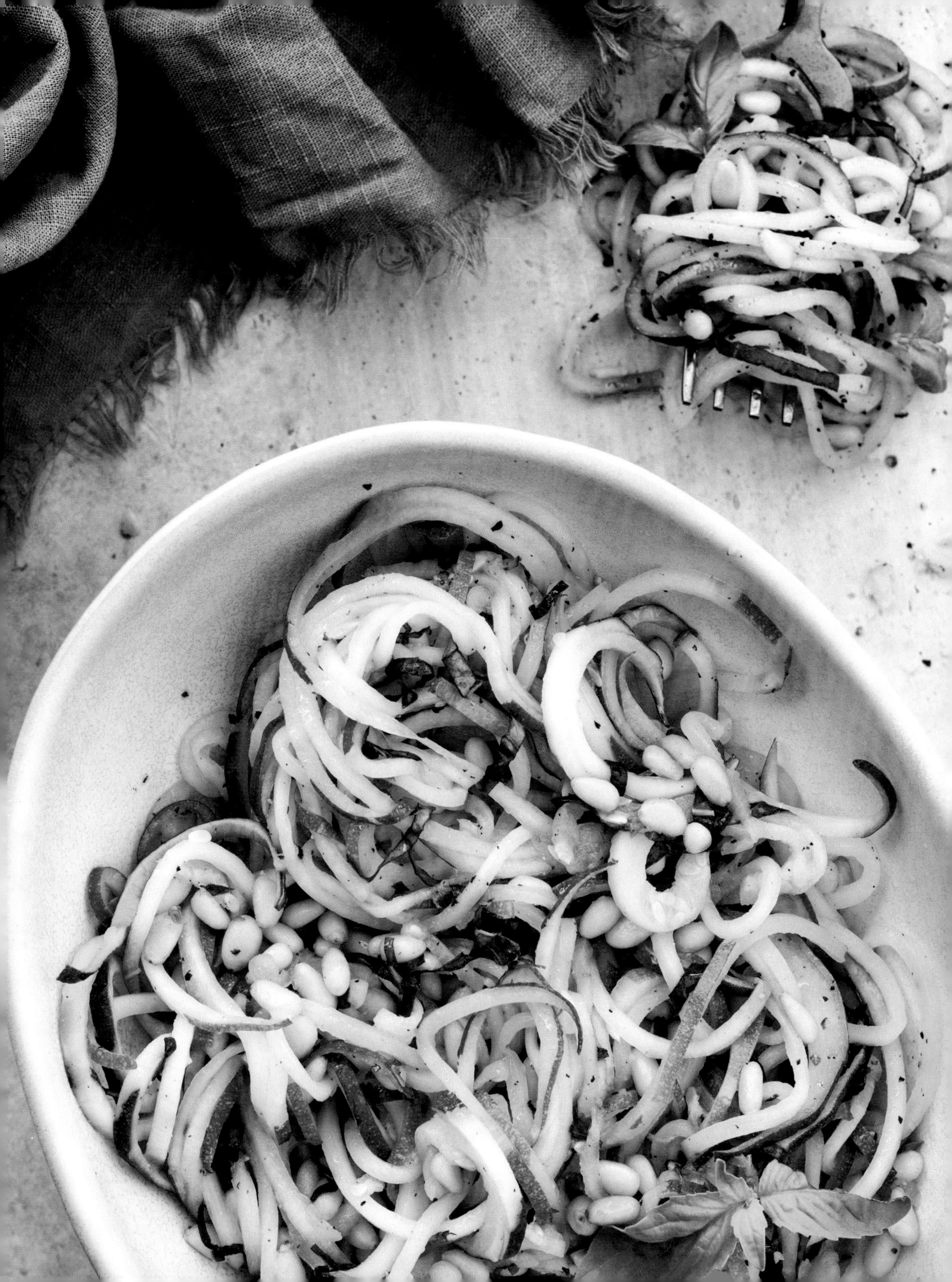

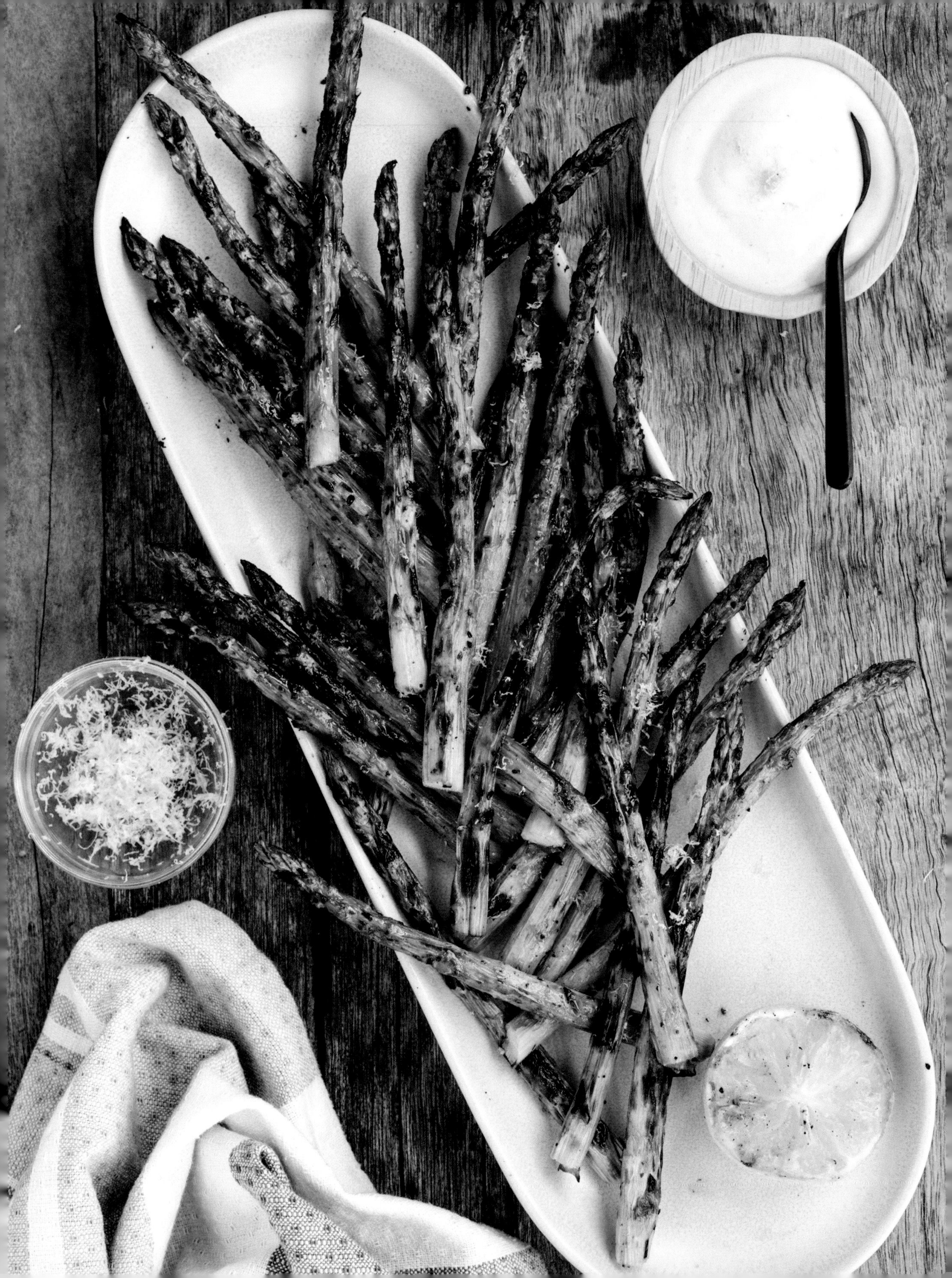

GRILLED ASPARAGUS WITH LEMONY AQUAFABA

Dairy-Free, Gluten-Free, Grain-Free, Vegan

PREP 10 minutes | COOK 20 minutes | TOTAL 30 minutes | SERVES 4

Asparagus is one of my favorite vegetables to grill. I like how the stalks get crispy with a bit of char on the ends. With this recipe, you'll get asparagus that's tender but still has a little crunch and a smoky flavor. Grilling asparagus couldn't be easier and it's delicious with just a simple drizzle of olive oil, a sprinkle of salt and pepper, and a squeeze of lemon juice. To take a platter of grilled asparagus up a notch, I like to serve it with my EFK Lemony Aquafaba on page 217. Aquafaba is the liquid left over from cooked chickpeas and has the consistency of egg whites. My version of the lemony sauce reminds me of hollandaise.

INGREDIENTS

1 pound of asparagus

Olive oil

Sea salt

Black pepper

Lemon half

EFK Lemony Aquafaba (page 217), for serving

DIRECTIONS

1. Preheat the grill to medium-high heat.
2. Rinse the asparagus and pat dry.
3. Snap or cut off the woody ends of the asparagus spears.
4. Lightly coat the asparagus with olive oil and sprinkle with salt and pepper.
5. Using a paper towel or dishcloth, carefully rub a little olive oil on the grill grates.
6. Place the asparagus on the grill perpendicular to the grill bars.
7. Grill for 3-6 minutes depending on thickness.
8. Use tongs to roll them to the other side halfway through grilling.
9. Remove asparagus from the grill and season with salt and pepper and fresh lemon juice.
10. Serve with my EFK Lemony Aquafaba.

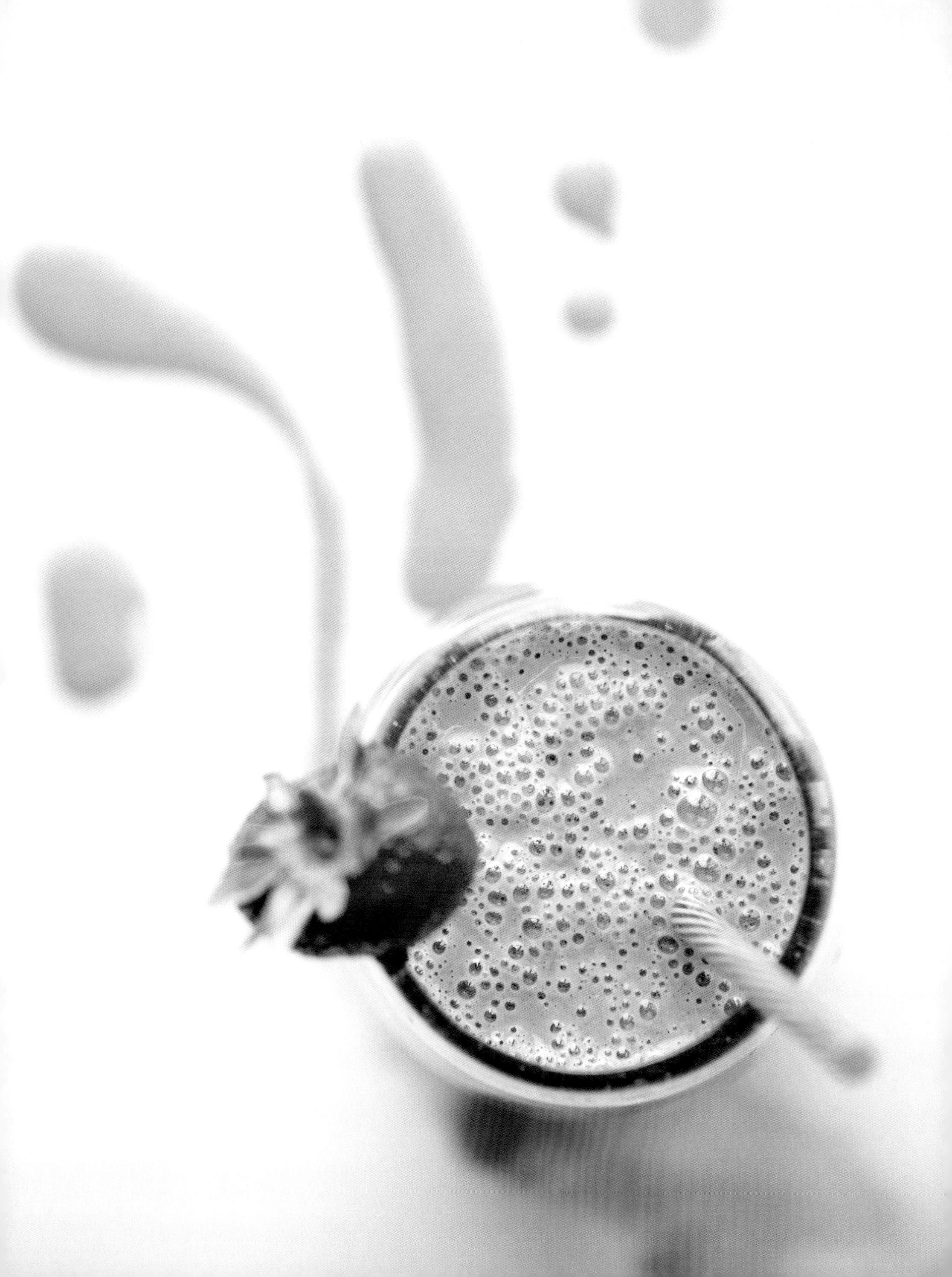

BREAKFAST AND SMOOTHIES

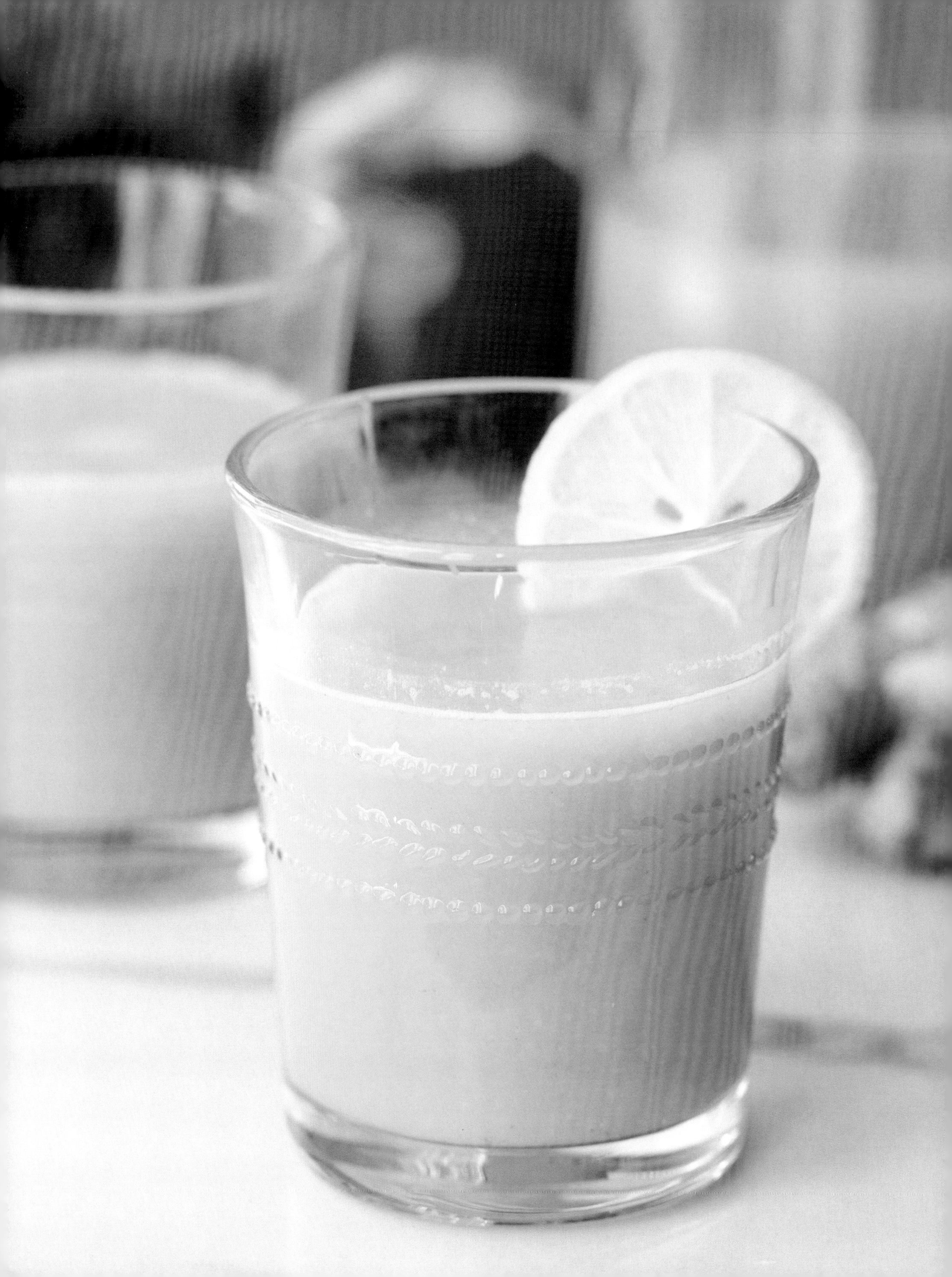

CELERY APPLE GINGER JUICE

Dairy-Free, Gluten-Free, Grain-Free, Paleo, SCD, Vegan

PREP 5 minutes | COOK 0 minutes | TOTAL 5 minutes | MAKES about 5 cups

Enjoying a glass of fresh juice is one of my favorite ways to start the day. This particular juice combines celery, apples, ginger, lemon and mint, making it rich in nutrients and antioxidants. It's like drinking a refreshing glass full of vitamins and minerals. The benefits include reducing inflammation, restoring balance to the gut and improving overall health. Plus it tastes delicious!

DIRECTIONS

1. Rinse the celery and apples and cut into pieces that will fit in your juicer.
2. Peel the ginger and cut in half.
3. Cut the rind off of the lemon and quarter.
4. Rinse the fresh mint.
5. Run all of the ingredients through a juicer.

INGREDIENTS

1 pound fresh celery

3 Honeycrisp apples

1 1/2 inches ginger root

1 lemon

1 bunch of fresh mint

NUT MILK

Dairy-Free, Gluten-Free, Grain-Free, Paleo, SCD, Vegan

PREP 5 minutes | COOK 0 minutes | TOTAL 5 minutes* | MAKES about 5 cups

Nut milks are dairy-free liquids made from ground nuts. They are delicious and make a great substitute for cow's milk. While there is a large variety of packaged nut milks at the grocery store, it is very easy to make them at home. All you need is a high-speed blender and a nut milk bag or cheesecloth and a strainer. The most common nut milk is almond milk, but you can make milk from any nut you choose. Some of my favorites are cashew, macadamia nut, walnut and Brazil nut. This is a basic recipe for nut milk that you can use with any nut. It will keep in the refrigerator for up to four days. You can pour unused milk into an ice cube tray and freeze. Then add to smoothies or iced coffee.

**Does not include soaking time, which is noted in the directions.*

INGREDIENTS

1 cup raw nuts

4 cups filtered water plus more for soaking

Pinch of sea salt

Sweetener of choice, such as pitted dates, pure maple syrup or honey, optional

Vanilla, optional

DIRECTIONS

1. Place the raw nuts in a bowl or large jar and cover with water 2 inches above the top of the nuts.
2. Cover and soak in the refrigerator for 12 hours or overnight.
3. Rinse and drain the nuts and place in a high-speed blender.
4. Add 4 cups of filtered water and a pinch of salt.
5. Add sweetener and vanilla if desired.
6. Blend on high for 2 minutes.
7. Pour the milk through a nut milk bag or a strainer lined with a few layers of cheesecloth.
8. Store in an airtight container in the refrigerator for 3-4 days. If the milk separates, shake or blend it to recombine.

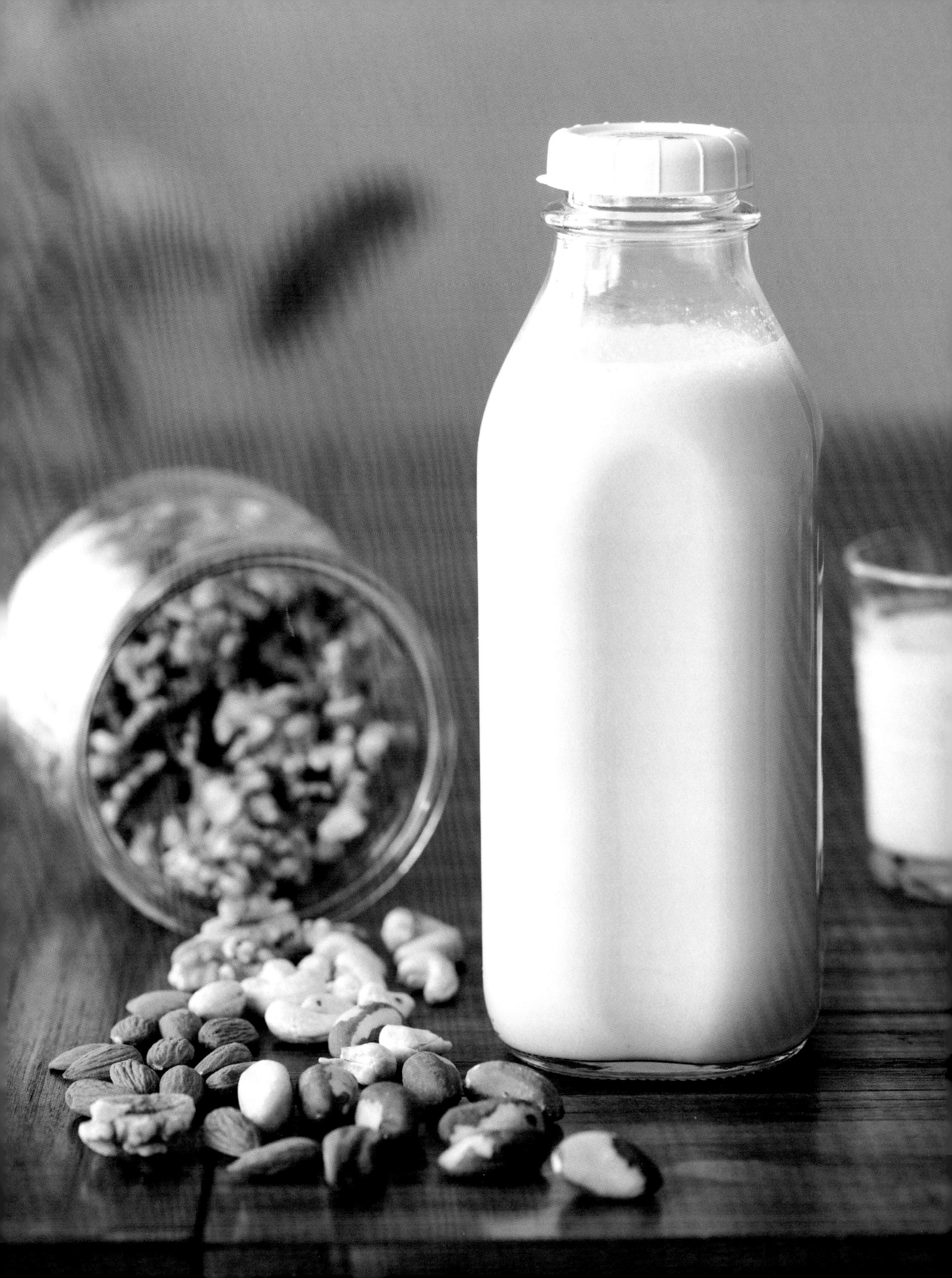

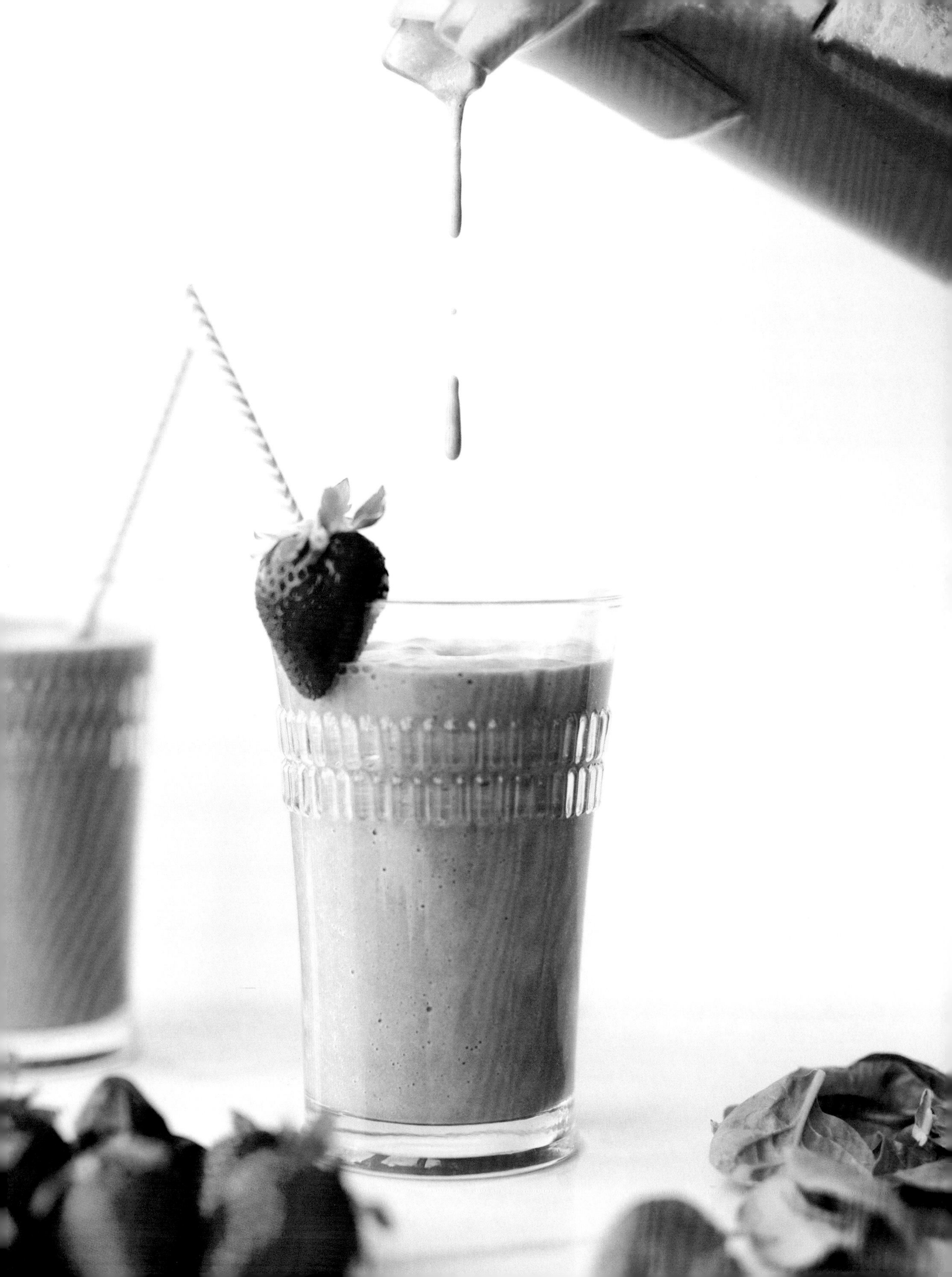

STRAWBERRY BASIL SMOOTHIE

Dairy-Free, Gluten-Free, Grain-Free, Paleo, SCD, Vegan

PREP 5 minutes | COOK 0 minutes | TOTAL 5 minutes | SERVES 2

Strawberries and basil remind me of summer. Combining them gives this green smoothie a unique flavor that is so enjoyable you won't even realize you are drinking two servings of your daily leafy greens. The avocado gives this smoothie the creaminess of a milkshake while adding nearly 20 different vitamins and minerals, dietary fiber and monounsaturated fat—the good fat we all need. The dates add the perfect touch of sweetness.

INGREDIENTS

2 cups unsweetened almond milk

2 cups fresh or frozen strawberries

1/4 avocado

2 dates, pitted

Handful fresh basil, about 10 leaves

4 cups fresh spinach

DIRECTIONS

1. Place all ingredients in a blender.
2. Blend well until smooth.

PEANUT BUTTER AND AÇAÍ SMOOTHIE

Dairy-Free, Gluten-Free, Grain-Free (Adaptable for Vegan)

PREP 5 minutes | COOK 0 minutes | TOTAL 5 minutes | SERVES 2

Açaí is a superfood that originated in the Amazon rainforest of Brazil. These dark purple berries have one of the highest concentrations of antioxidants known to man. Adding them to a smoothie is a great way to incorporate them into your diet. You can find frozen packets of unsweetened açaí in the freezer section of most grocery stores. To add the açaí to a smoothie you can partially thaw a packet in the refrigerator overnight or run a packet under warm water and break up the frozen purée into chunks. Peanut butter and açaí combine together well, creating an almost chocolate flavor. You can make an açaí bowl with this recipe by reducing the amount of almond milk to a few tablespoons for an ice cream-like consistency. Then use your favorite fruits and other toppings to create the bowl that's right for you. To adapt for vegan, substitute two pitted dates for honey.

INGREDIENTS

2 cups unsweetened almond milk

2 packets frozen açaí purée

3 Tablespoons natural peanut butter

2 Tablespoons raw honey

DIRECTIONS

1. Place all the ingredients in a blender.
2. Blend well until smooth.

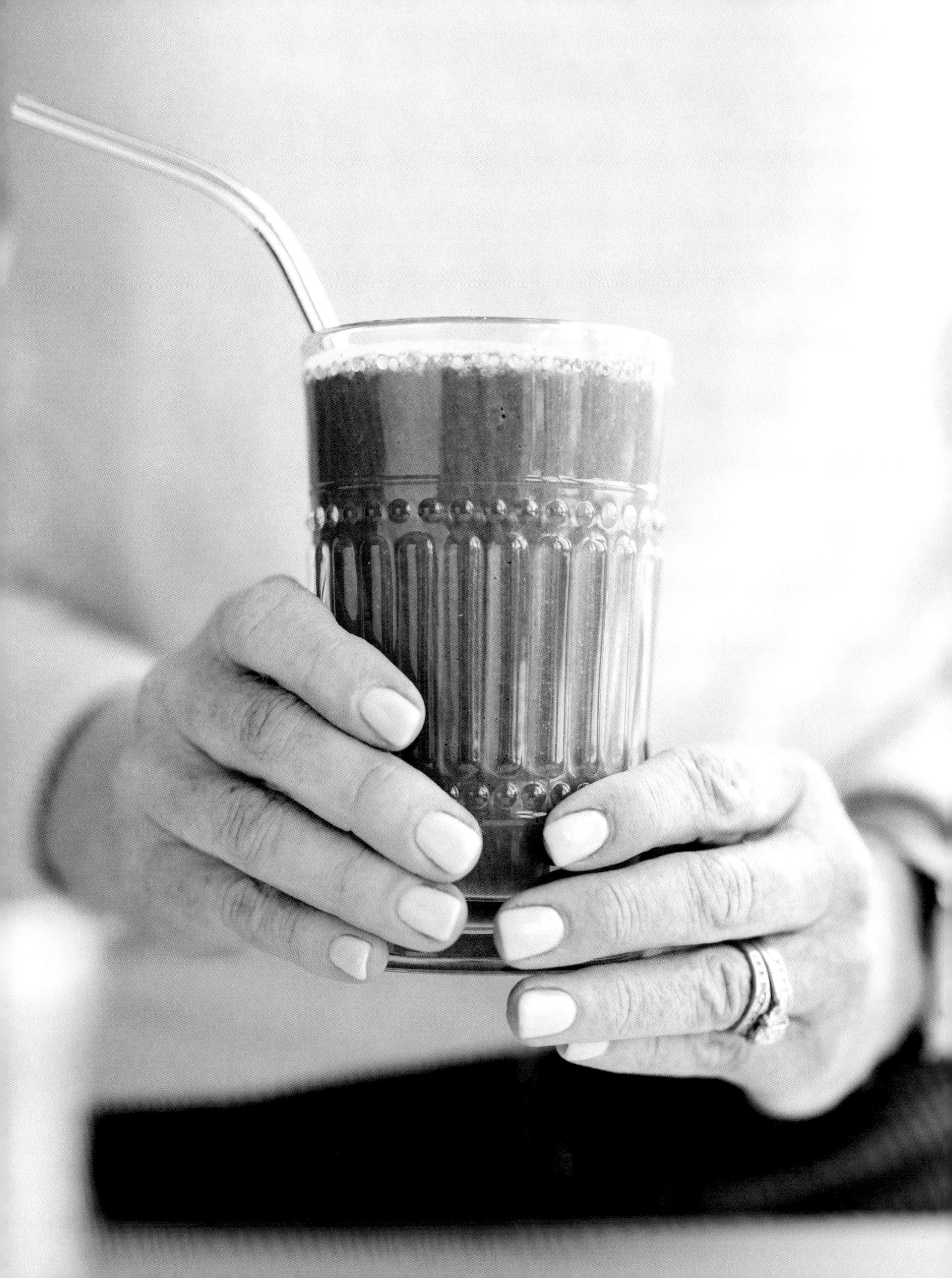

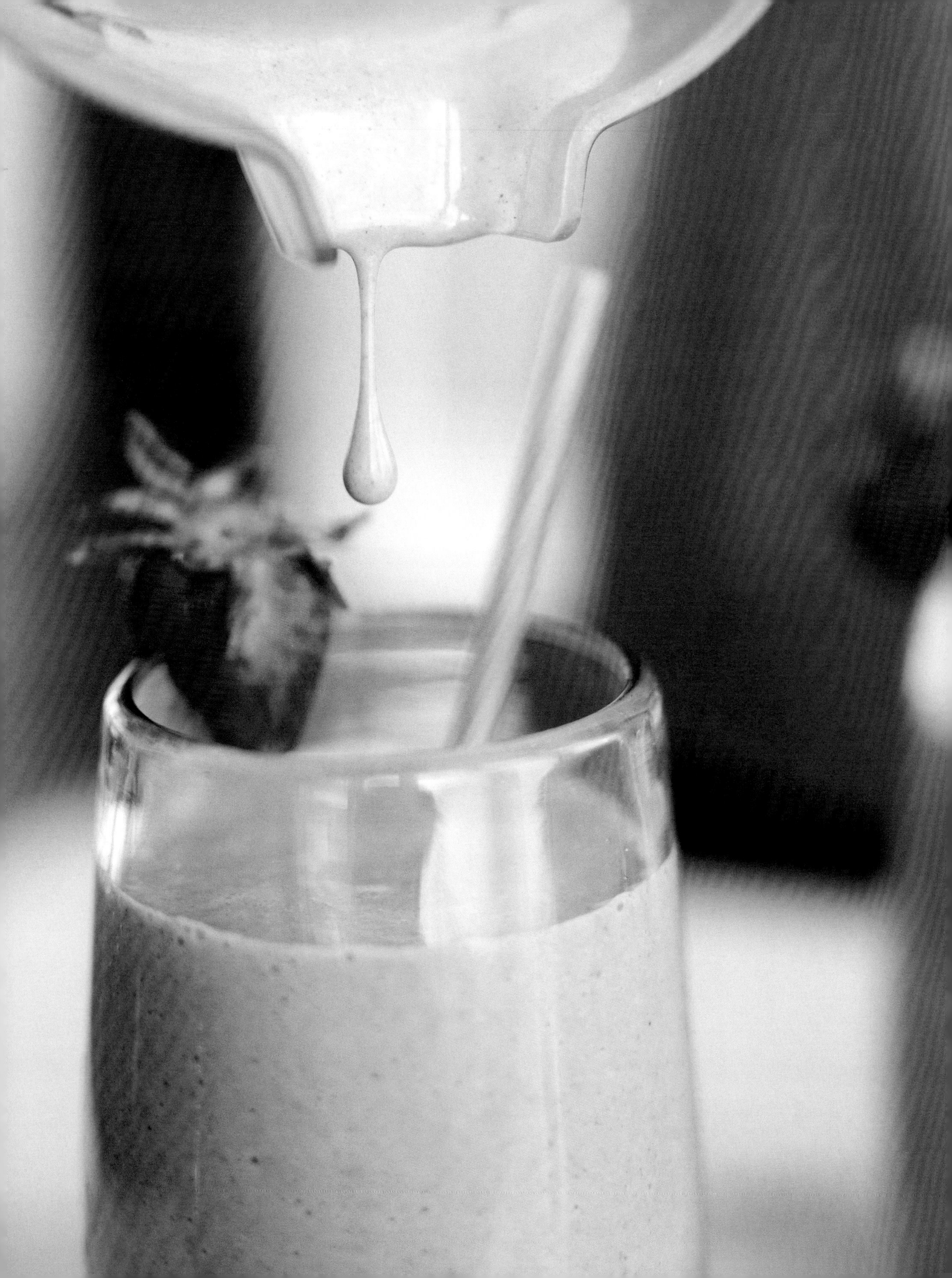

STRAWBERRY MACA CACAO SMOOTHIE

Dairy-Free, Gluten-Free, Grain-Free, Paleo, Vegan

PREP 5 minutes | COOK 0 minutes | TOTAL 5 minutes | SERVES 4

Maca root powder is a supplement with many health benefits. It helps balance hormones, improve libido, increase energy and boost the immune system. Maca has an earthy mesquite-like flavor. When combined with raw cacao, strawberries and bananas, it gives this smoothie the taste of a malted milkshake. I also like to add collagen peptides to this smoothie for skin, hair and joint health benefits.

INGREDIENTS

3 cups almond milk

2 Tablespoons almond butter

4 cups frozen strawberries

2 bananas

1 Tablespoon maca root powder

2 Tablespoons raw cacao powder

3 dates, pitted

2 scoops of collagen peptides

DIRECTIONS

1. Place all ingredients in a blender.
2. Blend well until smooth.

KIWI GREEN SMOOTHIE

Dairy-Free, Gluten-Free, Grain-Free, Paleo, SCD, Vegan

PREP 5 minutes | COOK 0 minutes | TOTAL 5 minutes | SERVES 2-3

This smoothie is clean and refreshing with a sweet and tart flavor. The kiwis are high in fiber and have a large dose of vitamin C as well as other immune-boosting nutrients. Kiwis are also known to aid in digestion. The additional sweetness from the green grapes covers any earthy taste from the greens. Drinking this healthy and delicious smoothie is a delightful way to start the day.

INGREDIENTS

3 cups filtered water

5 kiwis, peeled

3 cups green grapes

1/3 lemon, rind removed

3 ounces spinach

3 ounces kale

DIRECTIONS

1. Place all the ingredients in a blender.
2. Blend well until smooth.

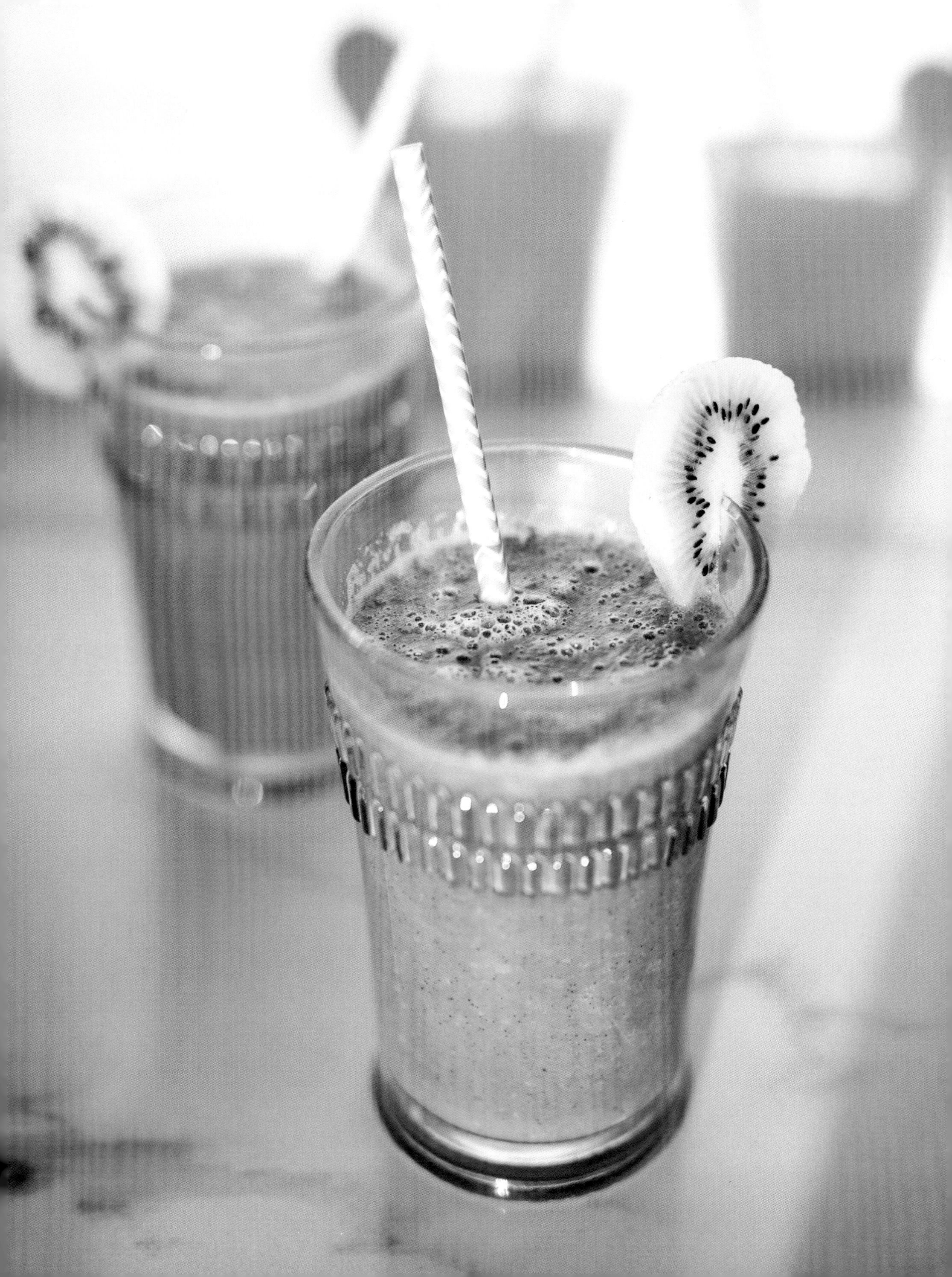

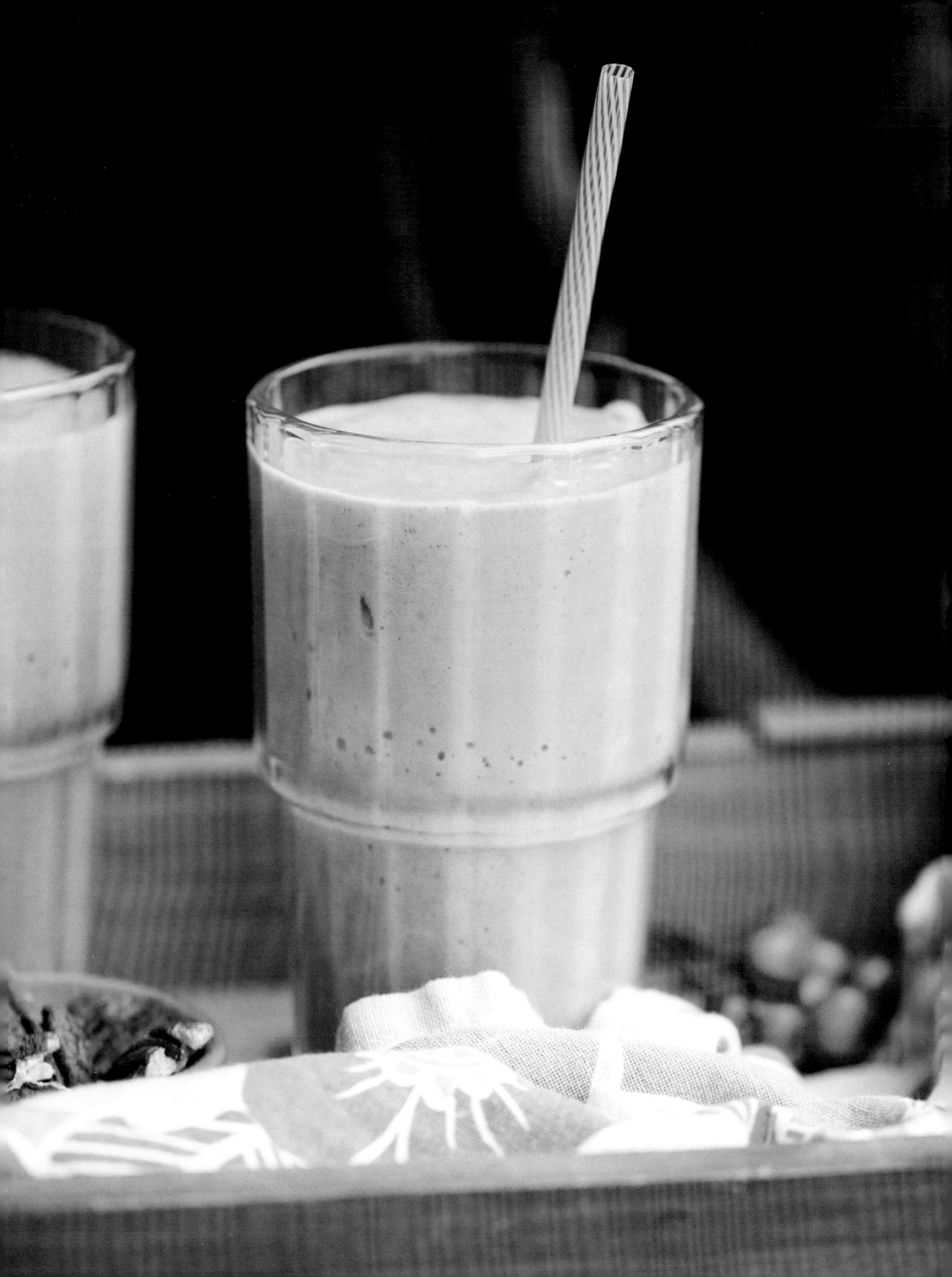

PUMPKIN PIE SMOOTHIE

Dairy-Free, Gluten-Free, Grain-Free, SCD (Adaptable for Vegan)

PREP 5 minutes | COOK 0 minutes | TOTAL 5 minutes | SERVES 2

Pumpkin pie is a popular dessert in November and December. Making a smoothie is a healthful way to enjoy the taste of pumpkin pie without all the extra refined sugar and calories. In a season of holidays when treats and desserts seem to be everywhere, this is a nice option to satisfy your sweet tooth. To adapt for vegan, use dairy-free yogurt and substitute pure maple syrup or one pitted date for honey.

INGREDIENTS

- 1/2 cup almond milk
- 1/2 cup plain yogurt
- 1/2 cup canned pumpkin
- 1 banana, sliced and frozen
- 1 teaspoon honey
- 1/2 teaspoon vanilla
- 1/2 teaspoon pumpkin pie spice
- Handful of ice

DIRECTIONS

1. Place all ingredients in a blender.
2. Blend well until smooth.

POWER SMOOTHIE

Dairy-Free, Gluten-Free, Grain-Free, Paleo, SCD, Vegan

PREP 5 minutes | COOK 0 minutes | TOTAL 5 minutes | SERVES 4

This is my go-to smoothie for after a workout or to drink as a meal on the go. It is full of unprocessed natural plant-based proteins, fats and fiber. The blueberries add a healthy dose of antioxidants without adding too much sugar. I like to make a large batch so I can keep extra in the refrigerator for a few days.

INGREDIENTS

5 cups almond milk
1/2 cup almond butter
1 avocado
2 1/2 cups frozen blueberries
5 ounces spinach
1/4 cup hemp seeds

DIRECTIONS

1. Place all the ingredients in a blender.
2. Blend well until smooth.
3. Store in an airtight container in the refrigerator for up to 3 days.

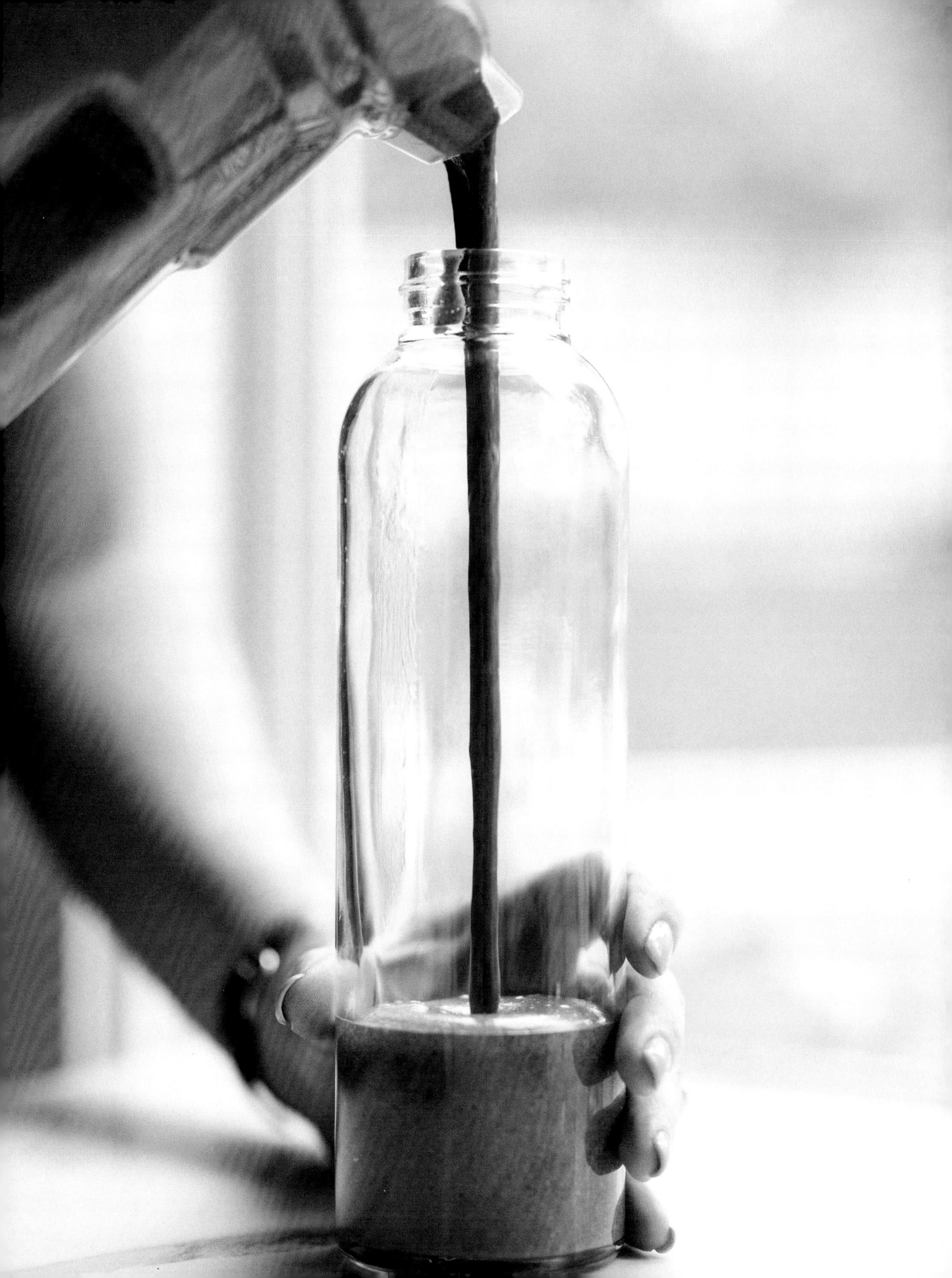

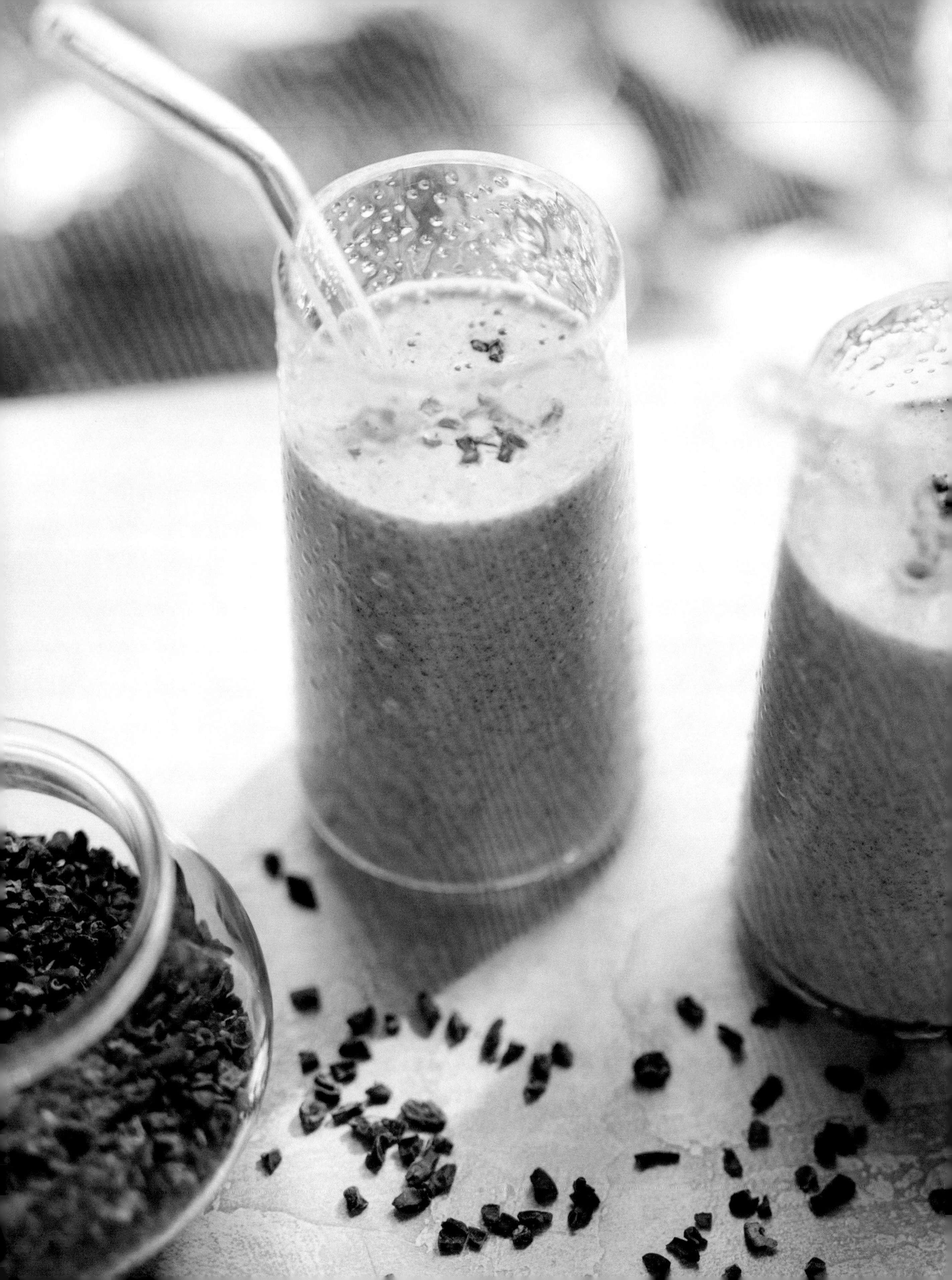

BANANA ALMOND CACAO SMOOTHIE

Dairy-Free, Gluten-Free, Grain-Free, Paleo, Vegan

PREP 5 minutes | COOK 0 minutes | TOTAL 5 minutes | SERVES 3

I had a raw detox business, and I served this smoothie for lunch on day two of the detox. I strategically placed it at that time because it tastes like a milkshake and my clients didn't feel like they were on a detox when drinking it. It was a way of encouraging people that they could keep going and finish the three days. It quickly became a favorite, and after the detox was over, many clients ordered extra Banana Almond Cacao Smoothies to drink when they resumed their regular diet. It is sweetened naturally with bananas and dates, and the almond butter makes it rich and creamy.

INGREDIENTS

3 cups almond milk

3 bananas, cut into chunks and frozen

5 ounces raw almond butter

2 dates, pitted

1/4 cup raw cacao nibs

1/8 teaspoon sea salt

DIRECTIONS

1. Place all ingredients in a blender.
2. Blend well until smooth.

ORANGE CREAMSICLE SMOOTHIE

Gluten-Free, Grain-Free, SCD

PREP 5 minutes | COOK 0 minutes | TOTAL 5 minutes | SERVES 2

This smoothie is reminiscent of a few childhood favorites: the Orange Julius from the mall food court and the Creamsicle from the ice cream truck or grocer's freezer. This is a healthier version made with plain yogurt and sweetened with honey. When my kids were younger, we had this for a treat often and they still enjoy it today.

INGREDIENTS

2 cups freshly squeezed orange juice

1 cup plain homemade or store-bought yogurt

1/4 cup raw honey

1 Tablespoon pure vanilla extract

2 cups ice

DIRECTIONS

1. Place all the ingredients in a blender.
2. Blend well until smooth and creamy.

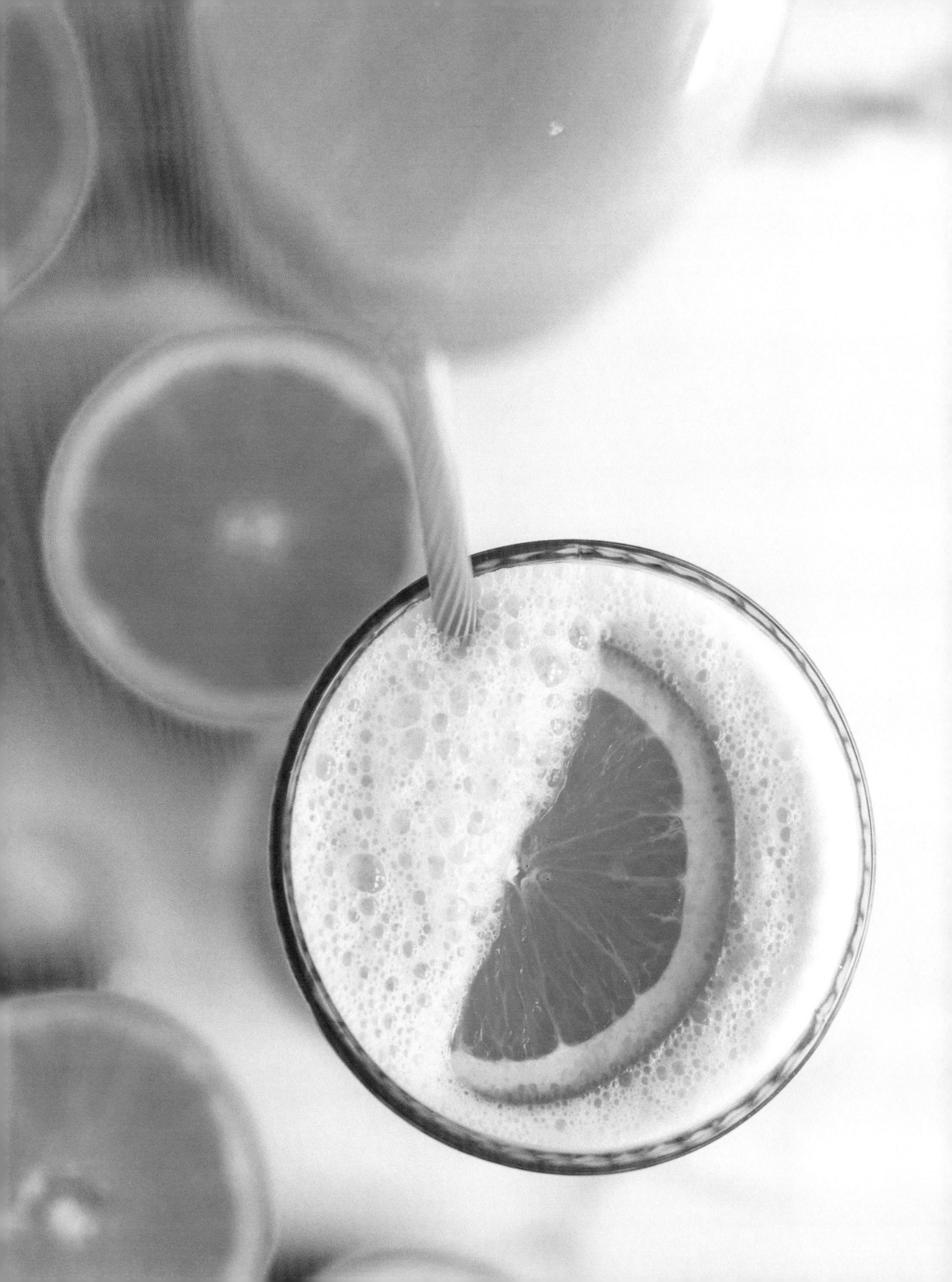

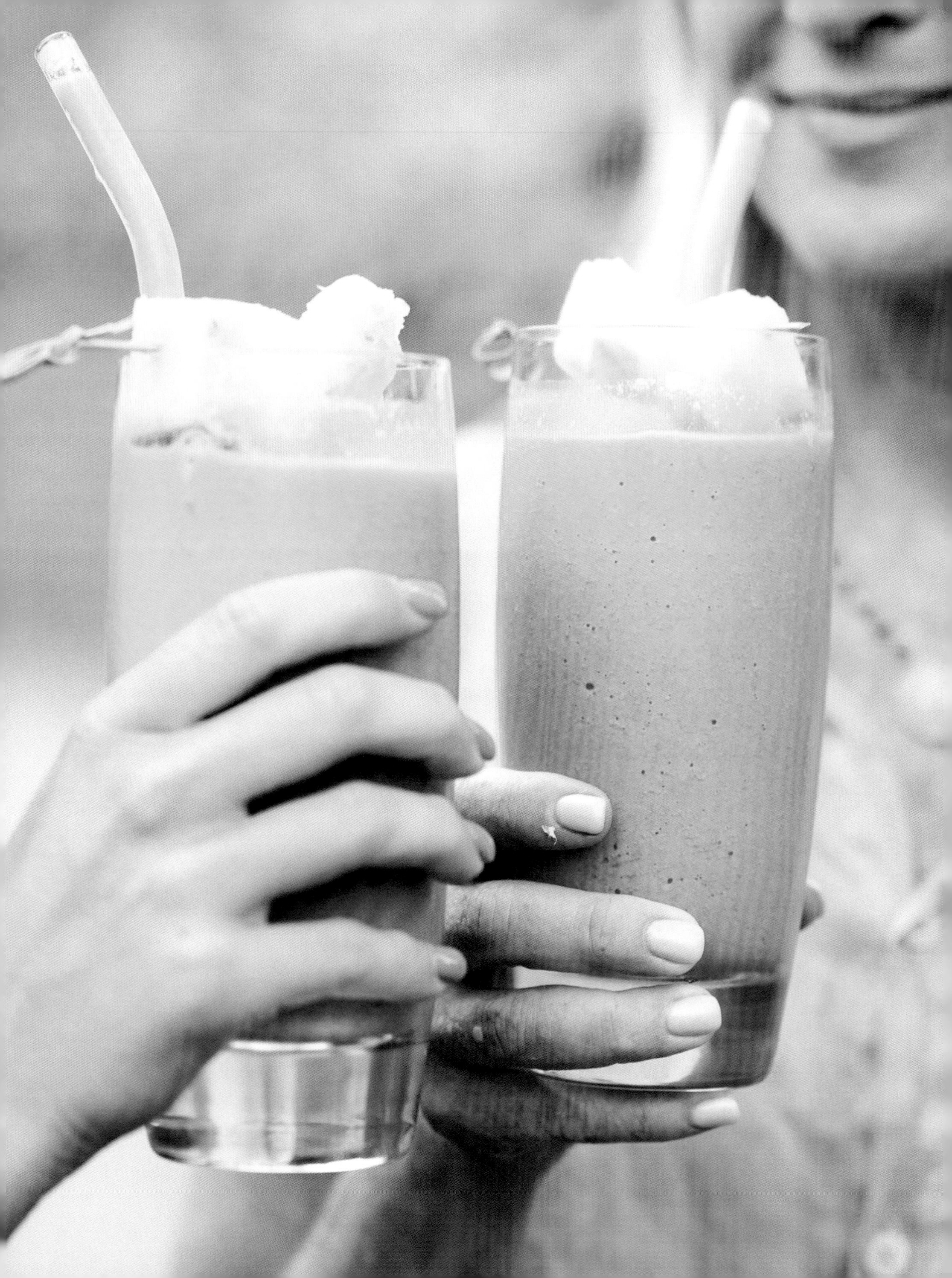

THAI GREEN SMOOTHIE

Dairy-Free, Gluten-Free, Grain-Free, Paleo, SCD, Vegan

PREP 5 minutes | COOK 0 minutes | TOTAL 5 minutes | SERVES 2

Drinking this smoothie is a refreshing way to start the day. It tastes clean and healthy. I like this smoothie because there are so many benefits to each of the ingredients. Enjoying them all in one drink is a huge win. For example, coconut water is full of electrolytes and minerals. Pineapple contains the powerful digestive enzyme bromelain. Cilantro is a great chelator, which means it helps remove toxic heavy metals from the body. Fresh lime is good for the skin and improves digestion. Spinach is a great source of iron, calcium and other nutrients. Avocado is loaded with protein, fiber and good fats.

I love it when I have time to crack open a young Thai coconut and use the water from it. When I do, I also add some of the fresh coconut meat to the smoothie. After pouring out the water, just scrape the soft flesh from the inside of the coconut. You can eat it plain, add it to smoothies or make a fresh coconut pudding. Just blend the coconut meat, coconut water, your sweetener of choice and vanilla.

INGREDIENTS

1 cup fresh or bottled coconut water

3 cups fresh or frozen pineapple

1 lime, rind removed

3 cups fresh spinach

1 cup fresh cilantro

1/2 avocado

Handful of ice

DIRECTIONS

1. Place all the ingredients in a blender.
2. Blend well until smooth.

MATCHA SMOOTHIE BOWL

Dairy-Free, Gluten-Free, Grain-Free, Paleo, Vegan

PREP 7 minutes | COOK 0 minutes | TOTAL 7 minutes | SERVES 2

Lately, my daughter and I have been making a lot of smoothie bowls. We love that we can mix frozen healthy ingredients in a high-speed blender and they come out tasting like an ice cream dessert. This bowl is one of our favorite combinations. We like to top it with unsweetened raw cacao nibs and fresh strawberries, but any fruit, granola or other toppings work well too.

INGREDIENTS

3 dates, pitted

7 ounces (2 packets) frozen coconut purée or frozen coconut meat

1 sliced and frozen banana

1/3 avocado

2 Tablespoons cashew butter

2 teaspoons ceremonial-grade matcha powder

2 Tablespoons almond milk

Raw cacao nibs and fresh strawberries, for serving

DIRECTIONS

1. Place the dates in a small ramekin and cover with hot water.
2. Allow the dates to soak for a few minutes until they get very soft.
3. Drain the dates and chop into small pieces.
4. Break the packets of coconut purée or coconut meat into 2-4 pieces for easier blending.
5. Place the coconut, banana, avocado, dates, cashew butter, matcha powder and almond milk in a high-speed blender.
6. Start blending on low and gradually increase to high speed.
7. The frozen ingredients will be difficult to blend at first so use the tamper stick to help move the ingredients.
8. Blend until the mixture has a smooth, soft serve-like consistency.
9. Using a spatula, scrape the smoothie into a bowl.
10. Top with raw cacao nibs, fresh strawberries and any other toppings you desire.

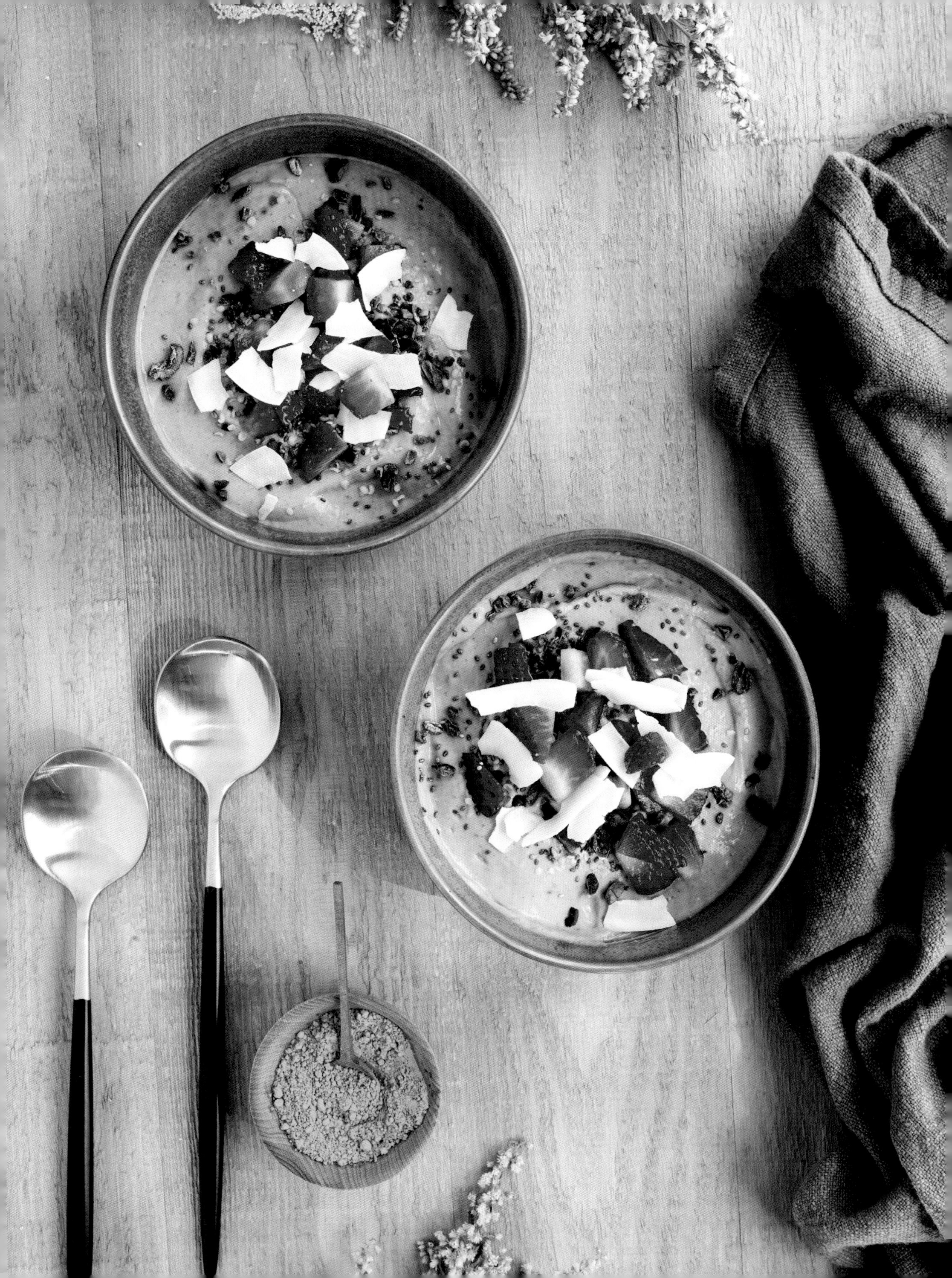

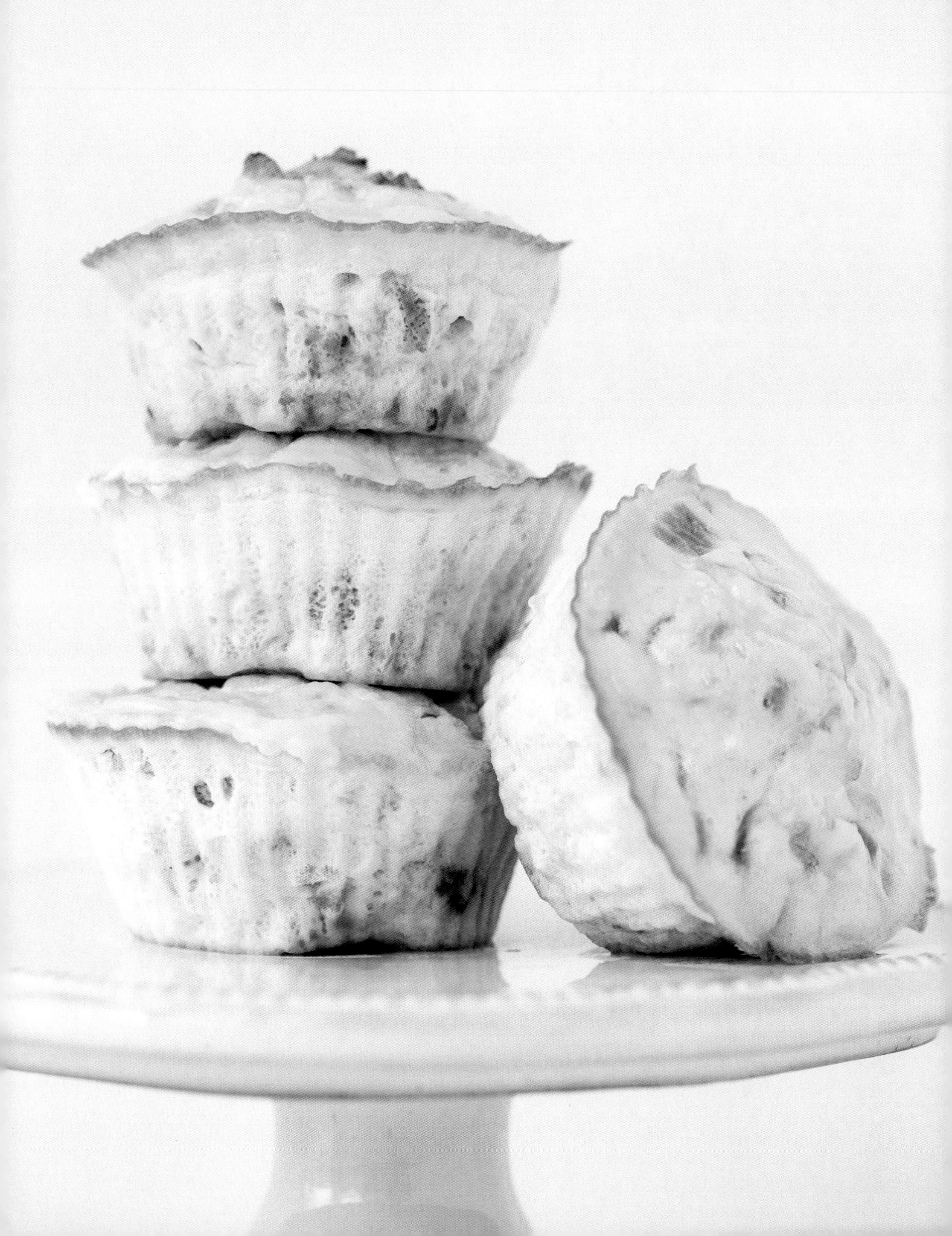

GREEN CHILE AND CHICKEN SAUSAGE EGG CUPS

Dairy-Free, Gluten-Free, Grain-Free, Paleo, SCD

PREP 5 minutes | COOK 35 minutes | TOTAL 40 minutes | MAKES 14 egg cups

These egg cups are the perfect thing to have on hand for a quick breakfast or snack. They can be eaten warm or cold. You would never know they are dairy-free because the coconut milk gives them a creamy consistency. The chicken sausage combined with the green chiles gives them a burst of flavor. This recipe is easy to make, nutritious, delicious, portable and great for busy mornings.

INGREDIENTS

14-16 ounces chicken breakfast sausage

8 eggs

1/2 cup canned full-fat coconut milk, preferably without guar gum

1 4-ounce can diced green chiles

2 teaspoons Dijon mustard

1/2 teaspoon salt

DIRECTIONS

1. Preheat the oven to 375 degrees.
2. Place 14 silicone muffin cups onto a baking sheet or generously grease a muffin pan.
3. In a large sauté pan, cook the sausage over medium heat until browned and set aside.
4. Divide the sausage between the muffin cups.
5. In a large bowl whisk the eggs until well blended.
6. Add the coconut milk and combine.
7. Add the green chiles, mustard and salt.
8. Whisk until well combined.
9. Divide the sausage equally between the muffin cups.
10. Pour the egg mixture over the sausage.
11. Bake for 20-25 minutes or until set.
12. Allow to cool slightly before serving.
13. Store in an airtight container in the refrigerator for up to 1 week and rewarm in the microwave.

GRAIN-FREE APPLE STREUSEL MUFFINS

Dairy-Free, Gluten-Free, Grain-Free, Paleo, SCD

PREP 25 minutes | COOK 20 minutes | TOTAL 45 minutes | MAKES 10-12 muffins

These muffins are moist, delicious and taste like a dessert. But since they are made with almond flour and sweetened with honey, they are actually a healthy breakfast or snack. I like to use Honeycrisp apples, but you can use any baking apple.

INGREDIENTS (STREUSEL)

1 Tablespoon butter or coconut oil, melted

3/4 cup chopped pecans

2 Tablespoons honey

1/4 teaspoon cinnamon

1/2 cup almond flour

INGREDIENTS (MUFFIN)

3 large eggs

2/3 cup honey

2 Tablespoons butter or coconut oil, melted

2 Tablespoons unsweetened applesauce

2 1/2 cups almond flour

2 Tablespoons coconut flour

1/2 teaspoon baking soda

1/4 teaspoon salt

1/2 teaspoon cinnamon

1 cup of diced Honeycrisp or other baking apple

DIRECTIONS

1. Preheat oven to 375 degrees.
2. Line a muffin pan with paper or silicone liners.
3. To make the streusel topping, melt 1 Tablespoon butter or coconut oil in a medium sauté pan.
4. Add the pecans, 2 Tablespoons honey and 1/4 teaspoon cinnamon and cook for 1-2 minutes, stirring.
5. Remove from heat and add 1/2 cup almond flour.
6. Mix well and transfer to a plate or bowl.
7. Crumble and separate the topping with your fingers and set aside to cool.
8. In a large bowl in a stand-up mixer, mix the eggs and 2/3 cup of honey on high for 3 minutes until frothy.
9. Add 2 Tablespoons of melted butter or coconut oil and applesauce.
10. Mix until combined.
11. Add 2 1/2 cups almond flour, coconut flour, baking soda, salt and 1/2 teaspoon cinnamon.
12. Mix on medium for 1 minute, stopping to scrape down the sides of the bowl.
13. Stir in the diced apples by hand.
14. Fill the muffin cups 3/4 full with batter.
15. Top with streusel topping.
16. Bake for 20 minutes until golden brown.
17. Remove from oven and cool.
18. Once cooled, store in an airtight container at room temperature for up to 3 days or in the freezer for up to 1 month.

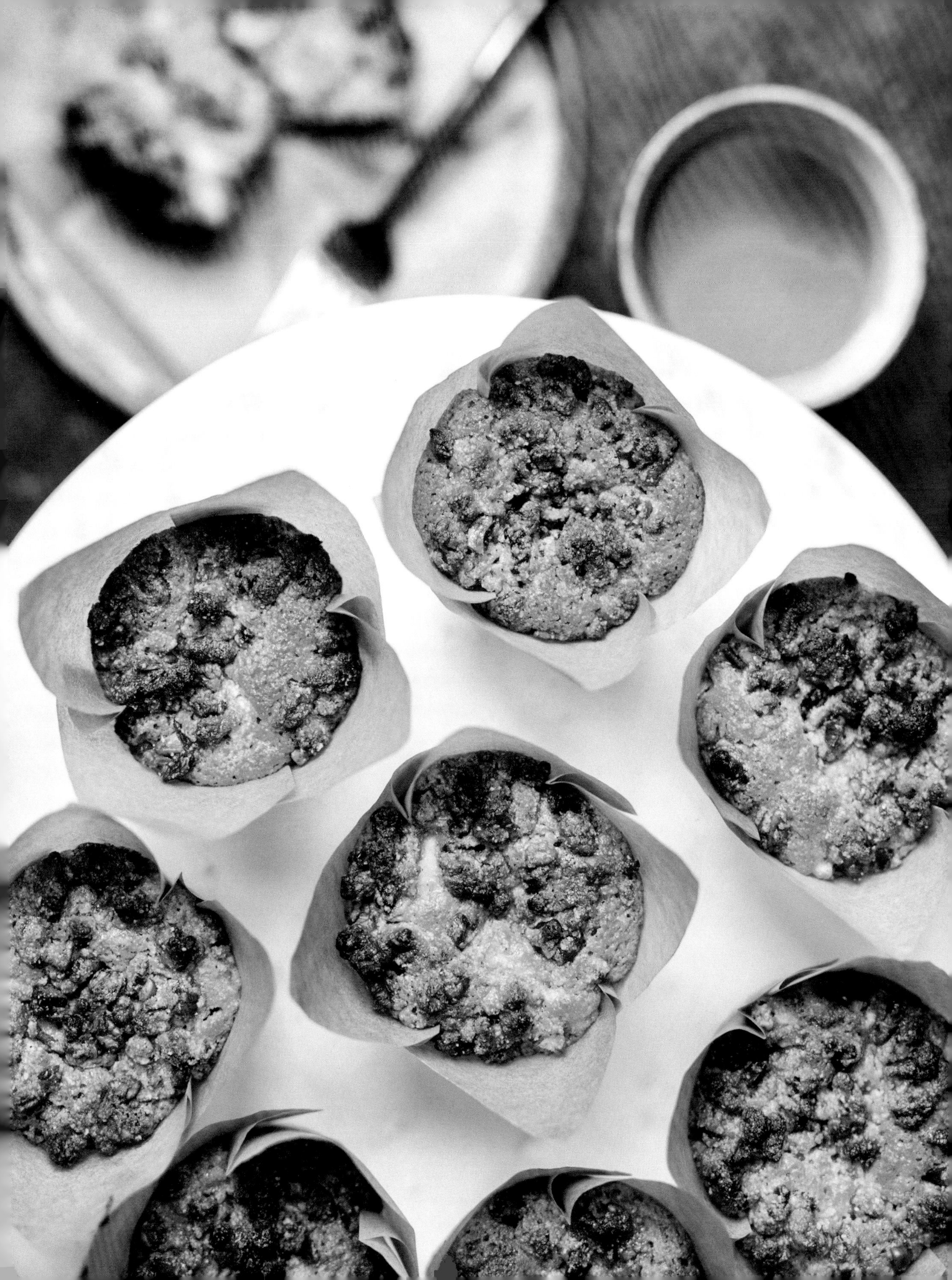

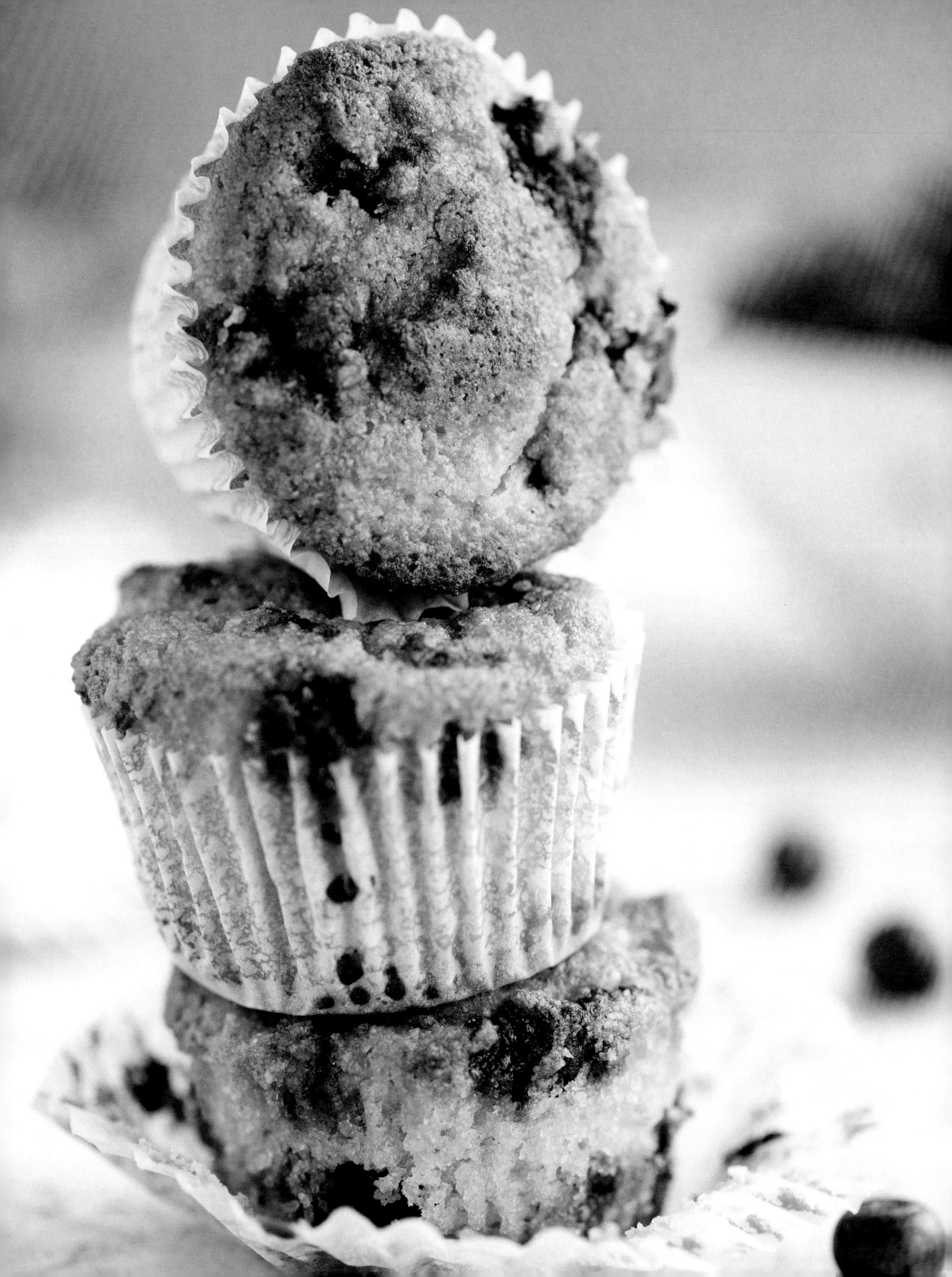

GRAIN-FREE LEMON BLUEBERRY MUFFINS

Dairy-Free, Gluten-Free, Grain-Free, Paleo, SCD

PREP 15 minutes | COOK 20 minutes | TOTAL 35 minutes | MAKES 10-12 muffins

Blueberry muffins are one of my favorite baked treats. Unfortunately, they are often filled with refined flours and sugars, making them less than ideal to enjoy for breakfast. This recipe is a healthier version made with nutrient-rich almond and coconut flours. The muffins are sweetened with honey and applesauce instead of sugar and make a wonderful quick breakfast or snack.

INGREDIENTS

3 large eggs

2/3 cup honey

2 Tablespoons butter or coconut oil, melted

2 Tablespoons unsweetened applesauce

1 1/2 Tablespoons lemon juice

1 Tablespoon lemon zest

1 teaspoon vanilla extract

2 1/2 cups almond flour

2 1/2 Tablespoons coconut flour

1/2 teaspoon baking soda

1/4 teaspoon sea salt

1 cup fresh blueberries

DIRECTIONS

1. Preheat oven to 375 degrees.
2. Line a muffin pan with paper or silicone liners.
3. In a large bowl in a stand-up mixer, mix the eggs and 2/3 cup of honey on high for 3 minutes until frothy.
4. Add the melted butter or coconut oil, applesauce, lemon juice, lemon zest and vanilla.
5. Mix until combined.
6. Add the almond flour, coconut flour, baking soda and salt.
7. Mix on medium for 1 minute, stopping to scrape down the sides of the bowl.
8. Stir in the blueberries by hand.
9. Fill the muffin cups 3/4 full with batter.
10. Bake for 20 minutes or until done.
11. Remove from oven and cool.

SCD YOGURT

Gluten-Free, Grain-Free, SCD

PREP 30 minutes | FERMENT AND COOL 32 hours | TOTAL 32 hours 30 minutes
SERVES 8

Making yogurt from scratch may sound daunting, but it is actually very easy to do if you have a yogurt maker. I started making yogurt years ago when I was on the Specific Carbohydrate Diet. Back then, I purchased a Yogourmet yogurt maker and still use it today. That particular brand can be difficult to find now, but there are many other yogurt makers on the market today.

Homemade probiotic yogurt is the cornerstone of the SCD. When you make it from scratch, you can increase the fermentation time to allow for more beneficial bacteria to be produced and all the lactose from the milk to be digested. This yogurt is fermented for 24 hours whereas commercially produced yogurt is typically only fermented for 8-10 hours. Most store-bought yogurts contain a lot of sugars, artificial sweeteners and colors. Making your own gives you control over sweetening it as well. You pick the sweetener and the amount you want to add. This lactose-free, high-probiotic yogurt is wonderful for helping to restore or maintain balance in the gut.

INGREDIENTS

Half gallon of whole milk

1/2 cup natural full-fat plain commercial yogurt with active cultures or 10 grams of freeze-dried yogurt starter

DIRECTIONS

1. Add milk to a large pot and place over medium-high heat until the milk starts to simmer.
2. Stir constantly to prevent scorching.
3. When the milk reaches 180 degrees, remove from heat.
4. Fill a large bowl with ice water and place the pot of milk in the ice bath to cool.
5. Cool the milk until it reaches 80 degrees.
6. Remove any skin that has formed.

(Continued)

7. Take 1/2 cup of the cooled milk and mix with the yogurt or starter.
8. Add the yogurt mix to the pot of cooled milk and blend well.
9. Pour the mixture into your yogurt maker container and close the top.
10. Place the container into the yogurt maker and fill with warm water to the top.
11. Plug in the yogurt maker and let it run for 24 hours minimum.
12. The yogurt maker should maintain a temperature of 100-110 degrees during this time.
13. Place the yogurt in the refrigerator and allow it to cool for 8 hours.
14. The yogurt is now ready to eat.
15. Store in an airtight container in the refrigerator for up to 2 weeks.

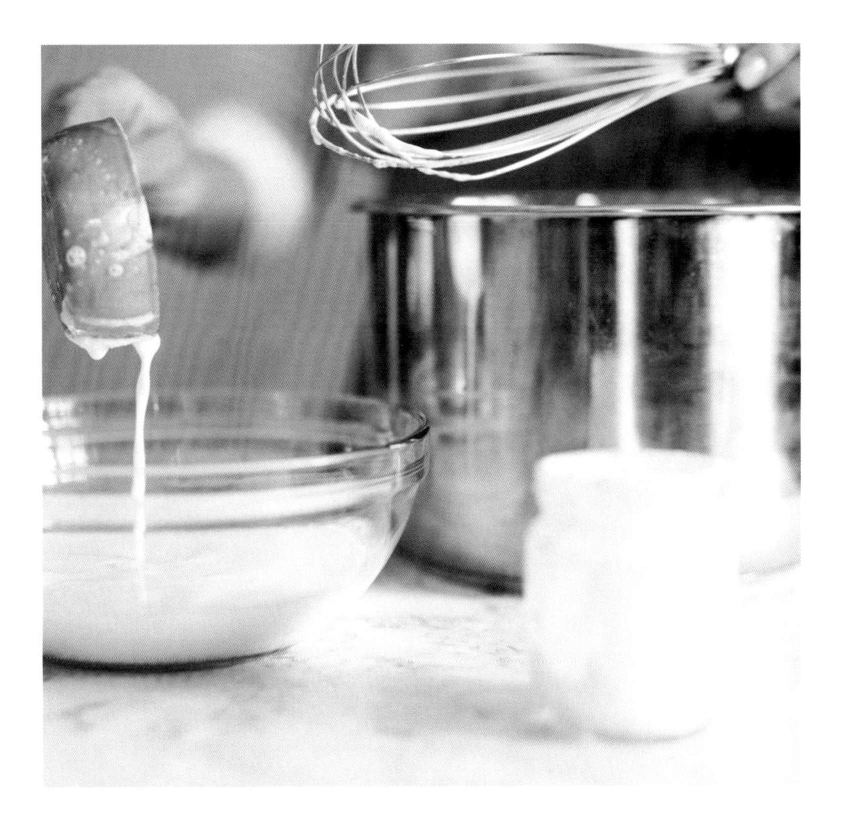

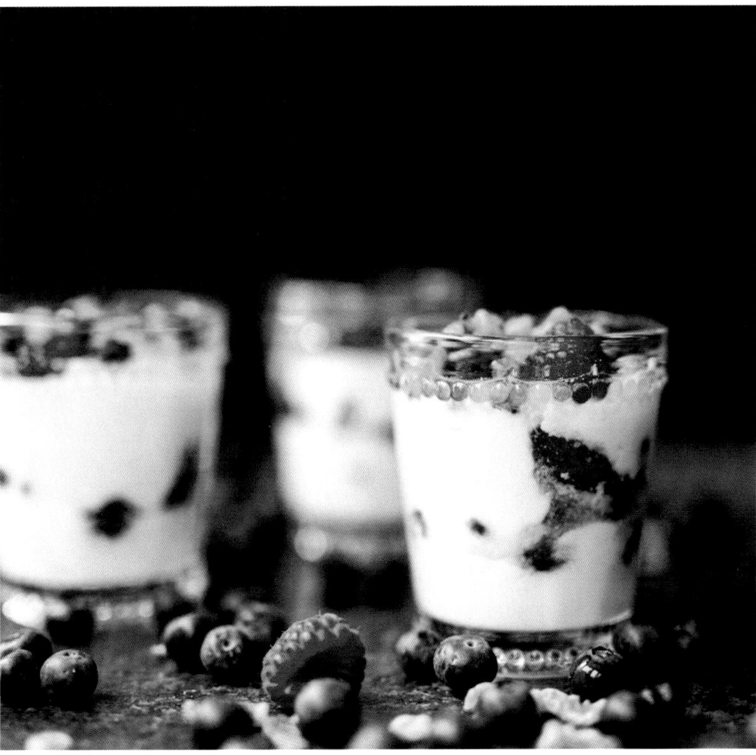

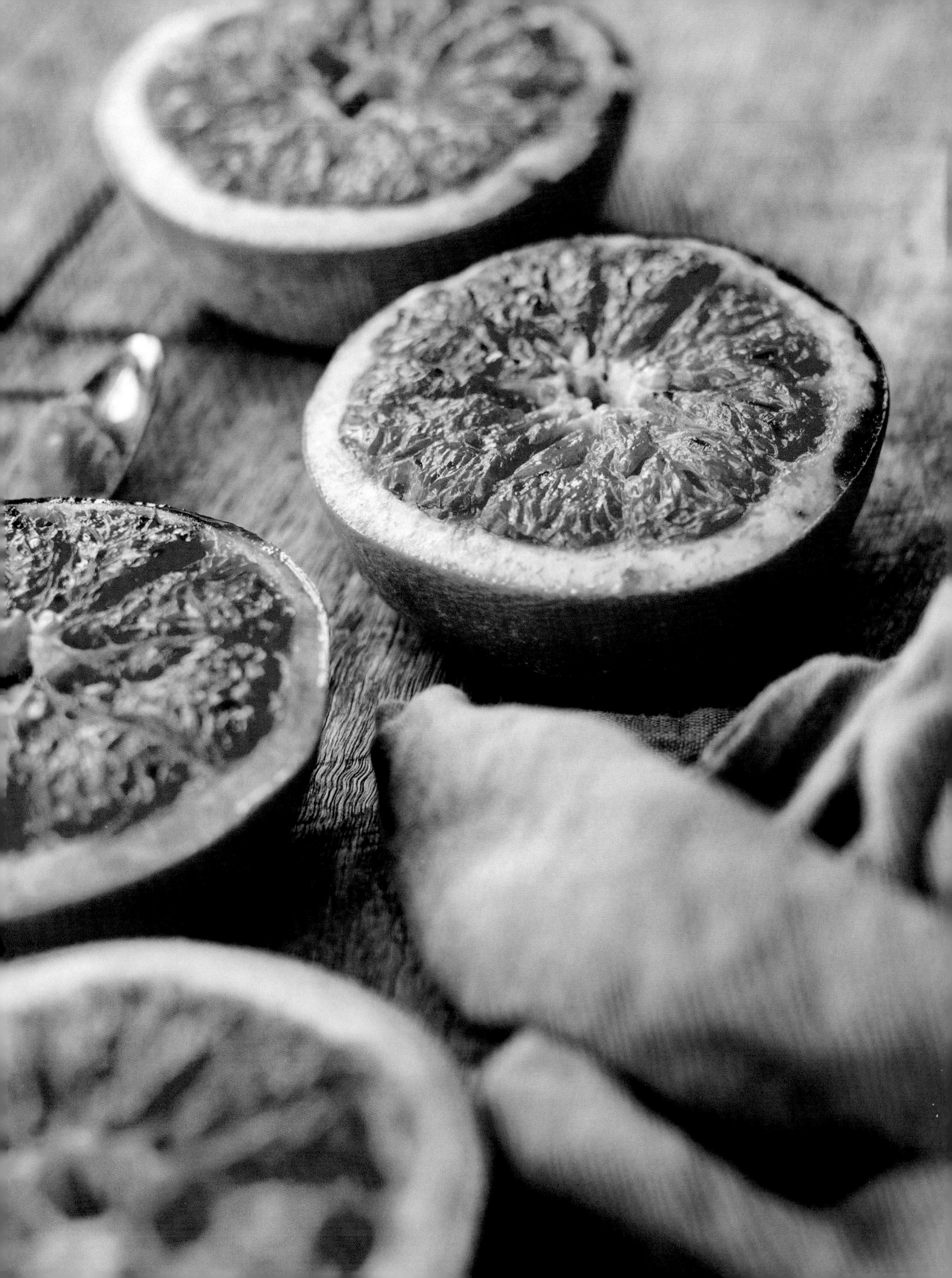

BROILED GRAPEFRUIT

Dairy-Free, Gluten-Free, Grain-Free, Paleo, SCD

PREP 10 minutes | COOK 5 minutes | TOTAL 15 minutes | SERVES 4

I'm delighted to share this four-ingredient recipe! Broiling grapefruit is an easy way to elevate this simple and delicious fruit. I add honey with just a pinch of both cinnamon and sea salt to get the perfect amount of sweetness. Enjoying a warm, bubbly grapefruit half is the perfect way to brighten a dreary winter morning. This recipe can also work as a snack or a dessert.

INGREDIENTS

2 red or ruby grapefruits

2 Tablespoons honey

Pinch of cinnamon

Pinch of sea salt

DIRECTIONS

1. Place the top rack of the oven 4 inches under the broiler.
2. Preheat the oven to broil.
3. Cut the grapefruits in half through the middle.
4. Cut the bottom of each half to keep them securely upright.
5. Slice along the sides of the membranes to separate the segments.
6. Slice around the perimeter of the grapefruit to loosen the sections so they will be easy to remove with a spoon.
7. Place the grapefruit halves on a parchment- or foil-lined sheet pan.
8. In a small bowl, combine the honey, cinnamon and salt.
9. Drizzle the honey mixture over the grapefruit flesh.
10. Broil for 3-5 minutes until lightly browned and bubbly.
11. Let cool for 1 minute and serve warm.

APPLE CINNAMON MILLET PORRIDGE

Dairy-Free, Gluten-Free, Vegan

PREP 5 minutes | COOK 40 minutes | TOTAL 45 minutes* | SERVES 4

A piping-hot bowl of cooked cereal is a great way to start a cold winter day, and this apple millet porridge fits the bill. Millet is a gluten-free grain that is a nutritional powerhouse. It is packed with protein, antioxidants and minerals. It is also high in fiber, which helps make you feel full longer. The apples, cinnamon and maple syrup make this a delicious, satisfying and aromatic breakfast.

**Does not include soaking time, which is noted in the directions.*

INGREDIENTS

1 cup of millet, soaked overnight

2 cups water

2 cups almond milk

1/4 cup pure maple syrup

2 apples, cored and diced

2 teaspoons cinnamon

1/2 teaspoon ground ginger

1/4 teaspoon salt

Diced apples, walnuts, pure maple syrup, almond milk and cinnamon, for serving

DIRECTIONS

1. Rinse and drain the soaked millet.
2. Combine millet, water, almond milk, maple syrup, diced apples, cinnamon, ginger and salt in a large saucepan and bring to a boil.
3. Reduce the heat, cover and simmer for 30 minutes or until all the liquid is absorbed.
4. Serve the porridge in bowls and top with diced apples, walnuts, maple syrup, almond milk and a sprinkle of cinnamon.

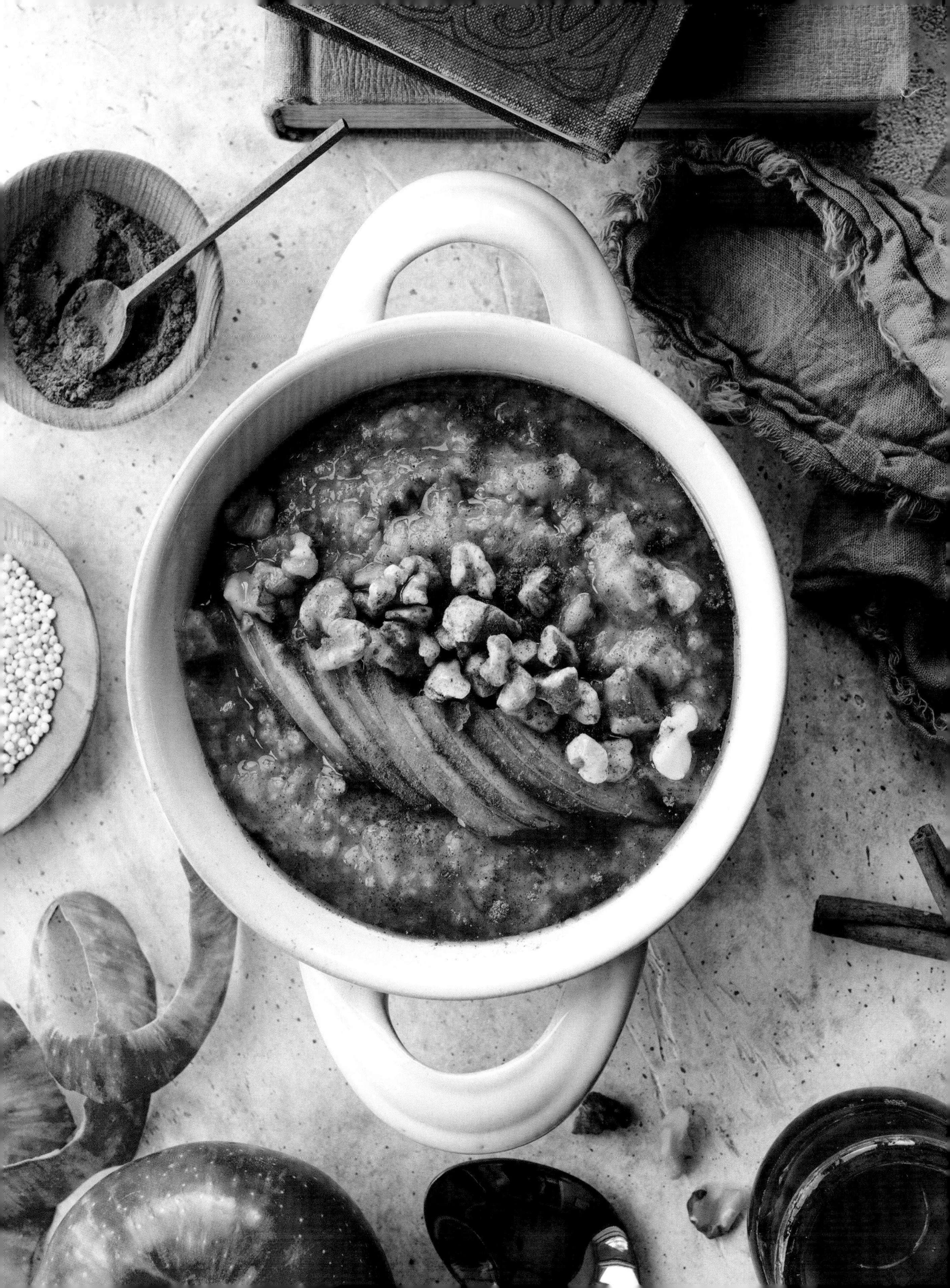

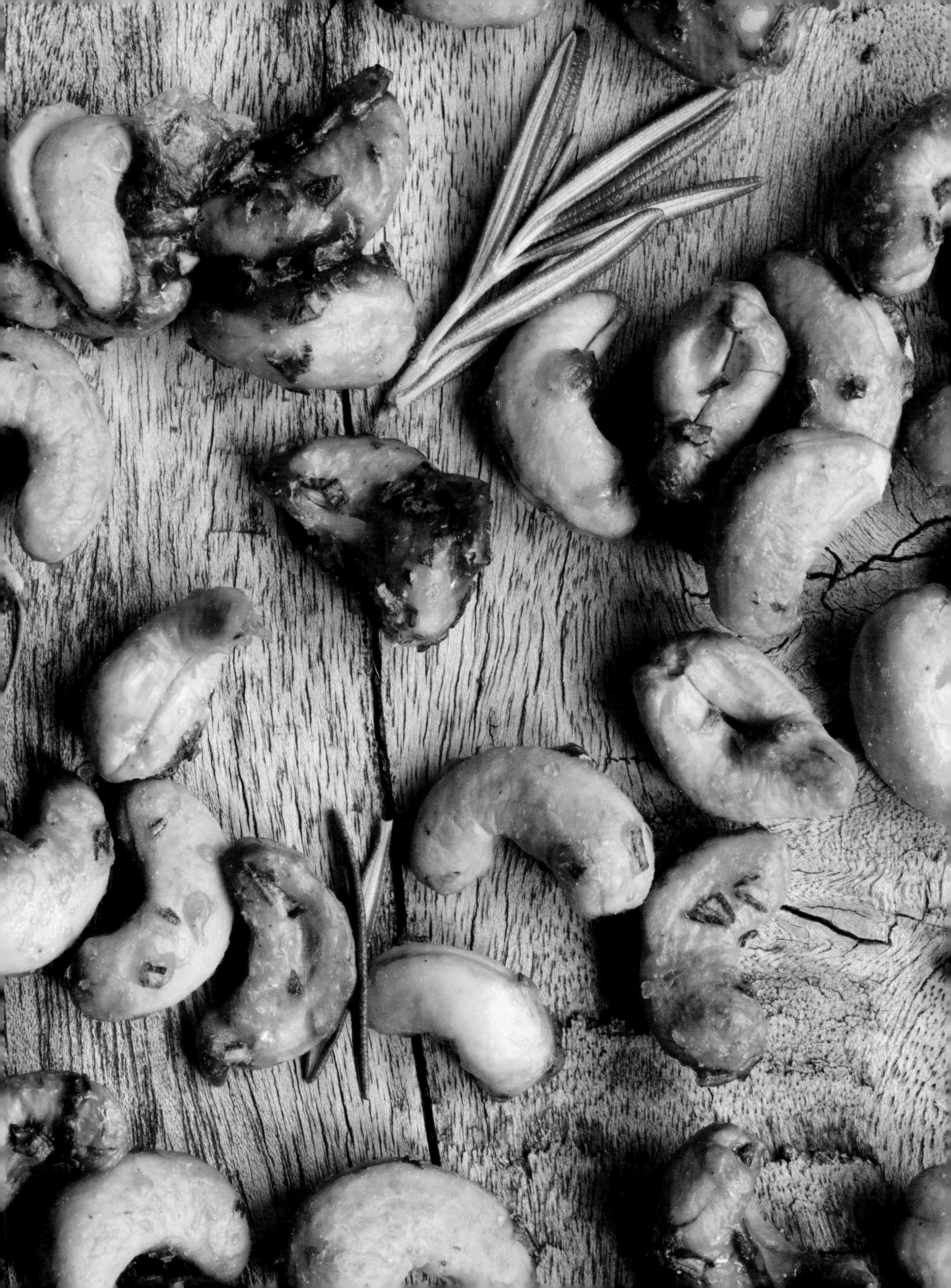

APPETIZERS AND SAVORY SNACKS

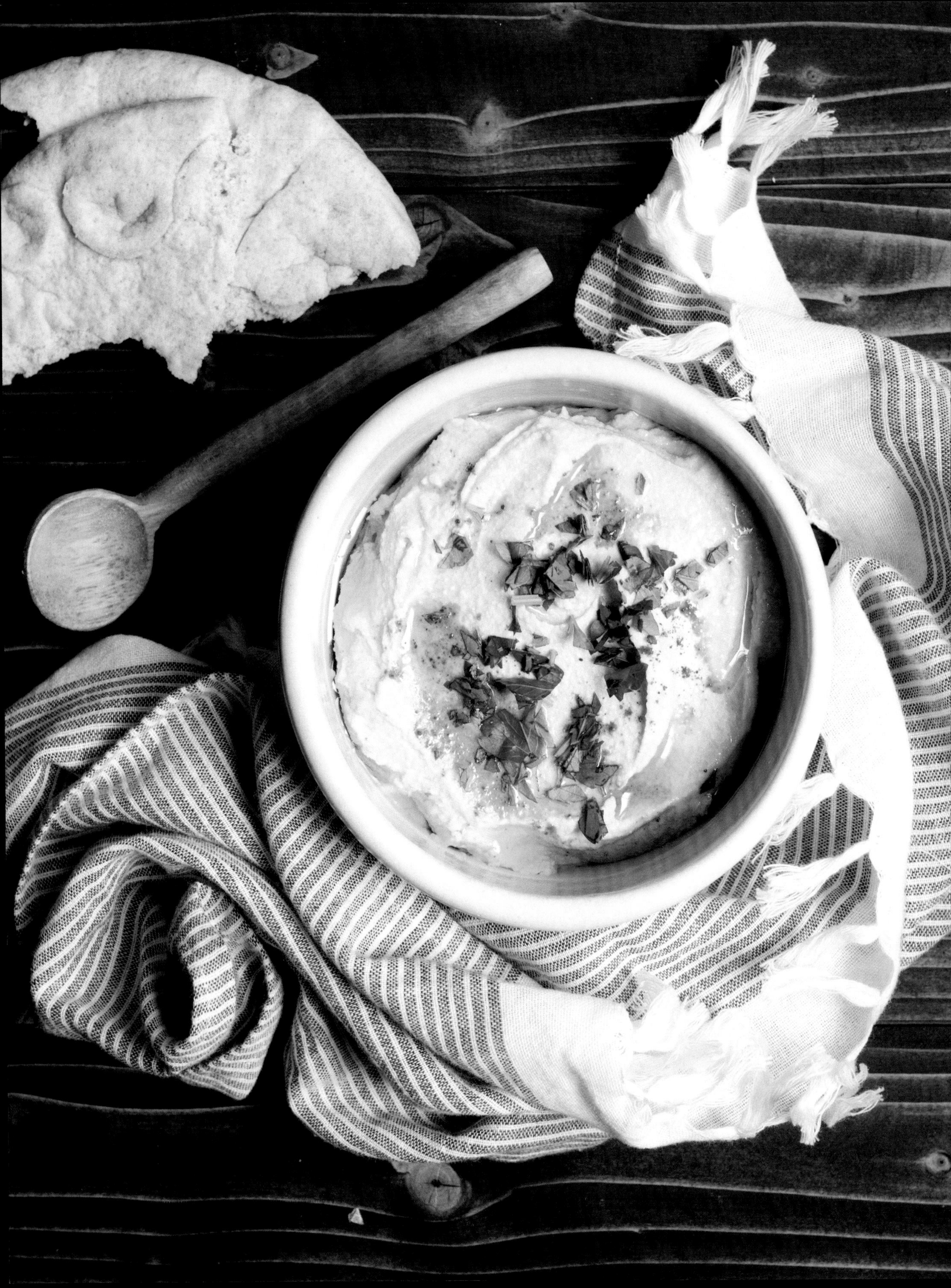

HUMMUS

Dairy-Free, Gluten-Free, Grain-Free, Vegan

PREP 10 minutes | COOK 0 minutes | TOTAL 10 minutes | SERVES 12

Hummus is a delicious nutrient-packed spread or dip that originated in the Middle East and quickly became popular throughout the world. This simple, classic hummus recipe is easy to make and tastes much better than the store-bought versions. I blend the ingredients in the food processor for a few extra minutes to achieve an extra-creamy consistency.

INGREDIENTS

2 cans chickpeas, drained

6 Tablespoons tahini

6 Tablespoons fresh lemon juice

1/2 cup olive oil

4 garlic cloves, minced

1 Tablespoon salt

4 teaspoons cumin

Olive oil, smoked paprika and chopped parsley, for serving

DIRECTIONS

1. Place the chickpeas, tahini, lemon juice, olive oil, garlic, salt and cumin in a food processor.
2. Blend for 1 minute, then stop and scrape down the sides of the processor bowl.
3. Blend for an additional 3-5 minutes or until smooth and creamy.
4. Transfer to a dish for serving and garnish with drizzle of olive oil, a sprinkle of smoked paprika and chopped parsley.
5. Store in an airtight container in the refrigerator for up to 5 days.

GREEK LAYER DIP

Gluten-Free, Grain-Free (Adaptable for Dairy-Free and Vegan)

PREP 20 minutes | COOK 0 minutes | TOTAL 20 minutes | SERVES 12-16

This dip is a fun and flavorful appetizer to serve at a party or bring to a potluck. I like to serve it with home-baked pita chips and cucumber slices. Making your own hummus and pita chips is easy. My EFK Hummus recipe is on page 159. The recipe for my EFK Baked Pita Chips is on page 164. But if you are in a hurry, you can pick up your favorite brands at the grocery store. To adapt for dairy-free and vegan, omit the feta cheese. It still tastes fantastic!

INGREDIENTS

2 cans chickpeas, drained

6 Tablespoons tahini

6 Tablespoons fresh lemon juice

1/2 cup olive oil

4 garlic cloves, minced

1 Tablespoon salt

4 teaspoons cumin

1 cup chopped peeled seedless cucumber

1 cup sliced cherry tomatoes

1 cup chopped pitted Kalamata olives

1/2 cup crumbled feta cheese, optional

1/2 cup chopped flat leaf parsley

Olive oil, cucumber slices and pita chips, for serving

DIRECTIONS

1. Place the chickpeas, tahini, lemon juice, olive oil, garlic, salt and cumin in a food processor.
2. Blend for 1 minute, then stop and scrape down the sides of the processor bowl.
3. Blend for an additional 3-4 minutes or until smooth and creamy.
4. Spread the hummus on a large platter.
5. Sprinkle the chopped cucumber over the hummus.
6. Continue by sprinkling the tomatoes, Kalamata olives, feta cheese and parsley.
7. Drizzle with olive oil and serve with cucumber slices and pita chips.

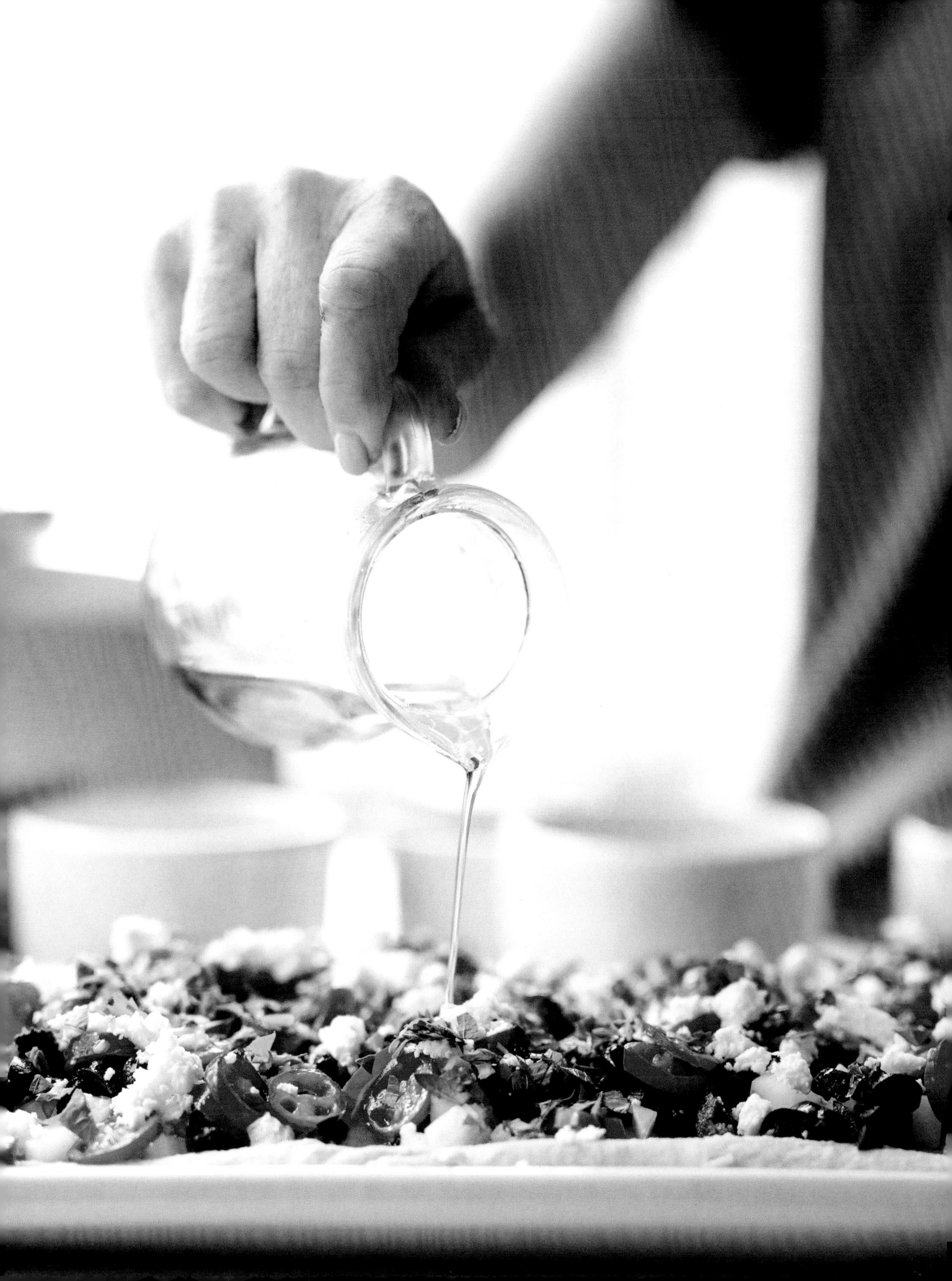

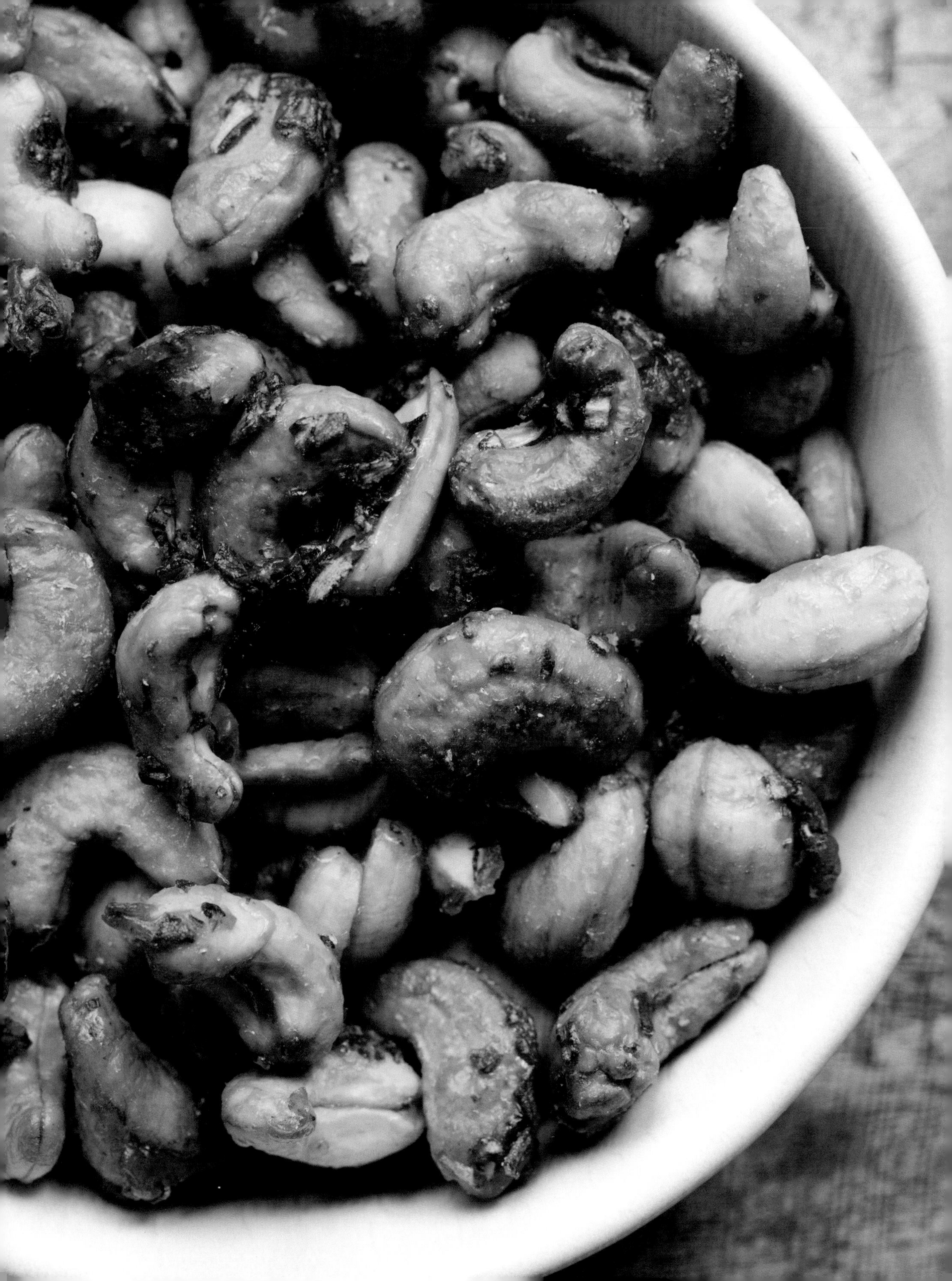

ROSEMARY CASHEWS

Dairy-Free, Gluten-Free, Grain-Free, Paleo, Vegan

PREP 2 minutes | COOK 35 minutes | TOTAL 37 minutes | SERVES 8

When I'm entertaining, I like having something ready for guests to nibble on when they arrive. These roasted cashews are easy to throw together and are guaranteed to elevate a cocktail hour or afternoon snack. They are sweet and salty with a subtle kick of heat. Packaged in a cute container, they also make a thoughtful hostess or holiday gift. There are many flavored nuts available for purchase, but making your own is healthier and less expensive.

INGREDIENTS

2 cups of whole raw cashews

1/4 cup pure maple syrup

1 Tablespoon coconut oil

2 Tablespoons chopped rosemary

1 1/2 teaspoons sea salt

1/4 teaspoon cayenne pepper

DIRECTIONS

1. Preheat the oven to 300 degrees.
2. Spread the cashews on a dry sheet pan.
3. Roast the cashews in the oven for 10 minutes.
4. In a saucepan combine the maple syrup, coconut oil, rosemary, sea salt and cayenne pepper.
5. Warm over medium heat and stir until well combined.
6. Add the cashews to the maple syrup mixture and cook over medium-high heat for 3 minutes, stirring continuously.
7. Line the sheet pan with parchment paper.
8. Spread the cashew mixture on the sheet pan and return to the oven.
9. Roast for 5 minutes and then stir the cashews.
10. Roast for an additional 5 minutes and then stir the cashews again.
11. Continue to roast for an additional 5 minutes or until browned.
12. Remove from the oven and allow to cool, breaking apart clusters as needed.
13. Once cooled to room temperature, serve or store in an airtight container.

BAKED PITA CHIPS

Dairy-Free, Vegan (Adaptable for Gluten-Free)

PREP 10 minutes | COOK 15 minutes | TOTAL 25 minutes | SERVES 8

Baking your own pita chips is simple to do and worth the extra effort. They are so fresh and crisp, making it difficult to go back to eating the store-bought ones. I like to use the 365 brand whole-wheat pita rounds from Whole Foods. They split easily and have great flavor. To adapt for gluten-free, use gluten-free pita bread.

INGREDIENTS

2/3 cup olive oil

1 teaspoon smoked paprika

1 teaspoon cumin

3/4 teaspoon salt

4 pita bread rounds

DIRECTIONS

1. Preheat oven to 350 degrees.
2. In a small bowl combine the olive oil, paprika, cumin and salt.
3. Using scissors, cut the edges off the pitas and separate into 2 pieces.
4. Brush the rough side of the pita with the seasoned olive oil, stirring occasionally to keep the seasonings evenly distributed.
5. Stack the pita halves, rough side up, and cut into 8 triangles.
6. Place the triangles on a parchment-lined sheet pan.
7. Bake for 10-15 minutes until browned.
8. The chips will bake unevenly, so after about 10-12 minutes, remove the chips that are done while leaving the others to continue baking.
9. Once cooled to room temperature, serve or store in an airtight container for up to 3 days.

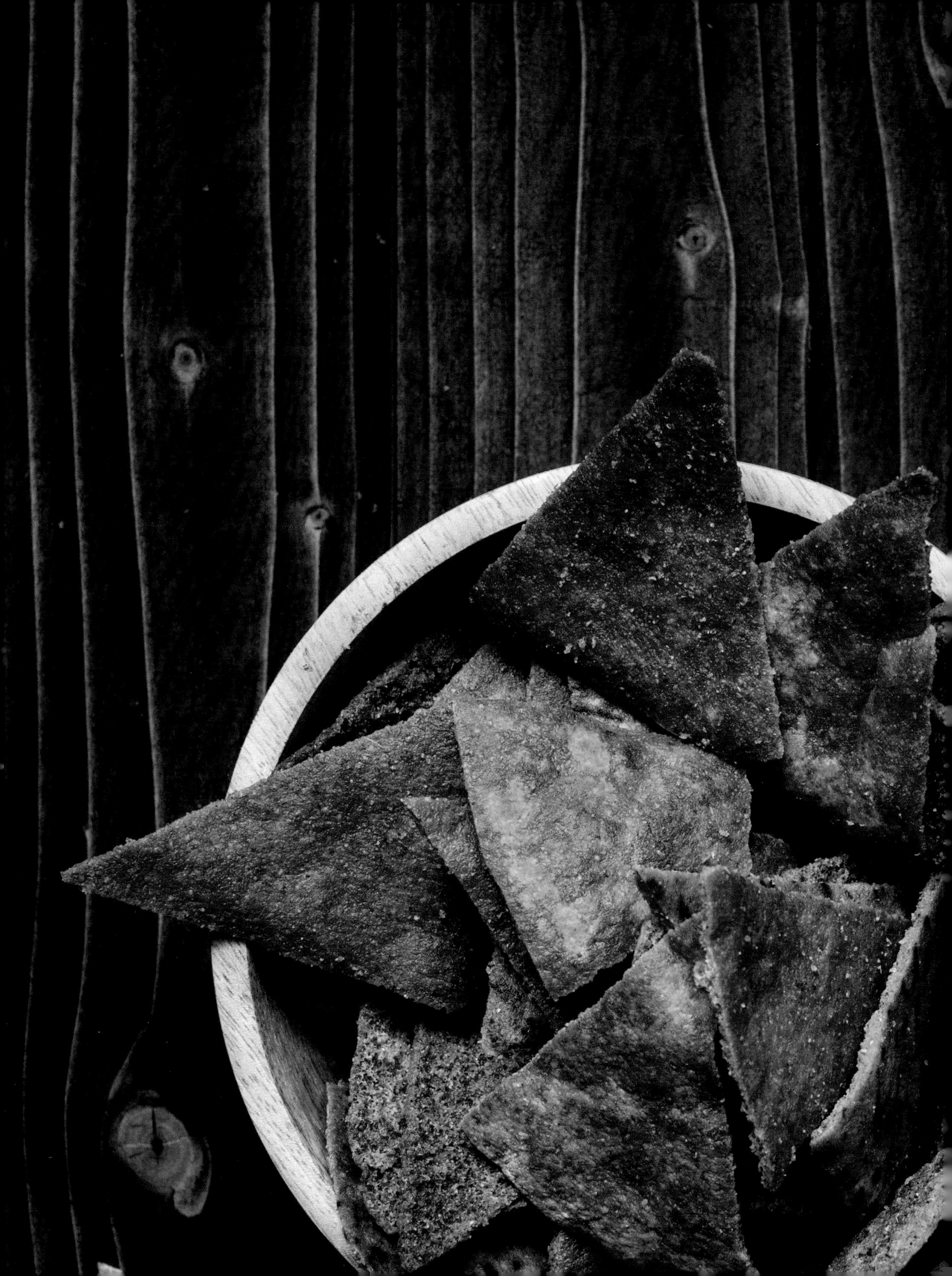

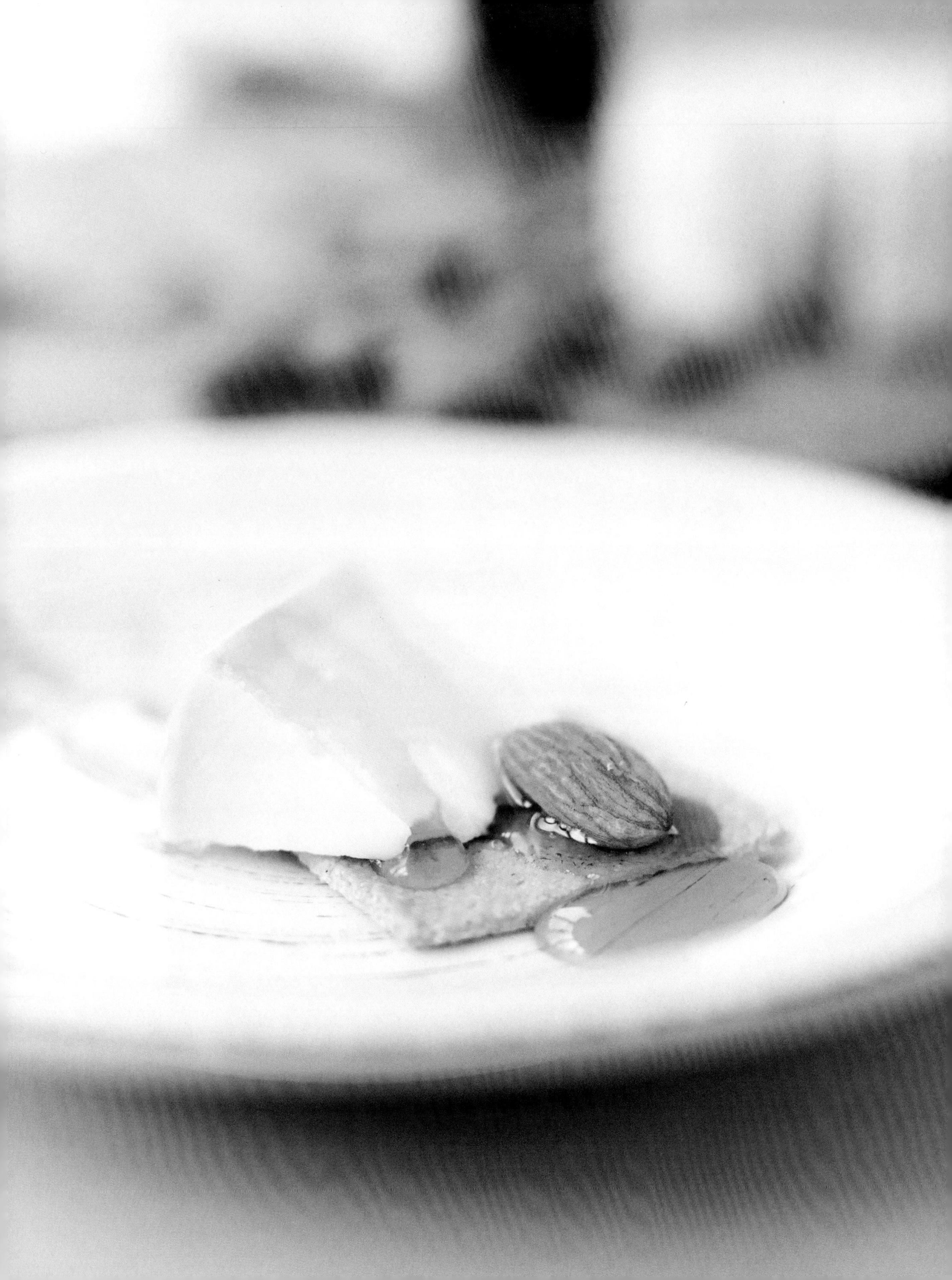

GRAIN-FREE OLIVE OIL CRACKERS

Dairy-Free, Gluten-Free, Grain-Free, Paleo, SCD, Vegan

PREP 8 minutes | COOK 15 minutes | TOTAL 23 minutes | SERVES 6

These grain-free, vegan crackers are incredibly easy to make. They are a delicious substitute for regular crackers or chips if you are following a grain-free or low-carb diet. Top these crisp crackers with your favorite toppings, cheeses or spreads. You can also add a tablespoon of your favorite chopped fresh herbs for a stronger flavor.

INGREDIENTS

1 1/2 cups blanched almond flour

1/2 teaspoon sea salt

1/2 teaspoon fresh ground pepper

2 1/2 Tablespoons olive oil

2 Tablespoons water

DIRECTIONS

1. Preheat the oven to 325 degrees.
2. Combine almond flour, salt and pepper in a medium bowl.
3. Add olive oil and water and then mix well.
4. Knead with your hands to form a ball.
5. Place on a sheet of parchment paper and cover with another sheet of parchment paper.
6. Roll out the dough into a large rectangle to 1/8-inch thickness.
7. Score the crackers with a sharp paring knife or use a multi-wheel dough cutter.
8. Bake for 12-15 minutes or until golden brown.
9. Once cooled to room temperature, serve or store in an airtight container.

GUACAMOLE

Dairy-Free, Gluten-Free, Grain-Free, Paleo, SCD, Vegan

PREP 5 minutes | COOK 0 minutes | TOTAL 5 minutes | SERVES 6

If I could eat one thing for the rest of my life, I think it would be guacamole. I don't even need the chips. I would eat it with a spoon. Nothing beats homemade guacamole. I like it with everything—eggs, wraps, fish, steak, veggies, chips. Everyone has different preferences so feel free to adjust the amount of jalapeño, garlic, lime juice and salt to your taste.

INGREDIENTS

4 ripe avocados

1 tomato, seeded and diced

1 sweet onion, diced

1/2 cup fresh cilantro, chopped

3 limes, juiced

3 cloves garlic, minced

1 jalapeño, seeded and minced

1 1/2 teaspoons sea salt

DIRECTIONS

1. Cut the avocados in half, remove the pit and scoop the flesh into a medium bowl.
2. Lightly mash the avocados with a potato masher or fork.
3. Add the remaining ingredients and stir well.
4. Adjust salt, lime juice, jalapeño and garlic to taste.
5. Serve immediately or store in the refrigerator in an airtight container. To prevent browning, press plastic wrap to the surface of the guacamole before your place the lid on the container.

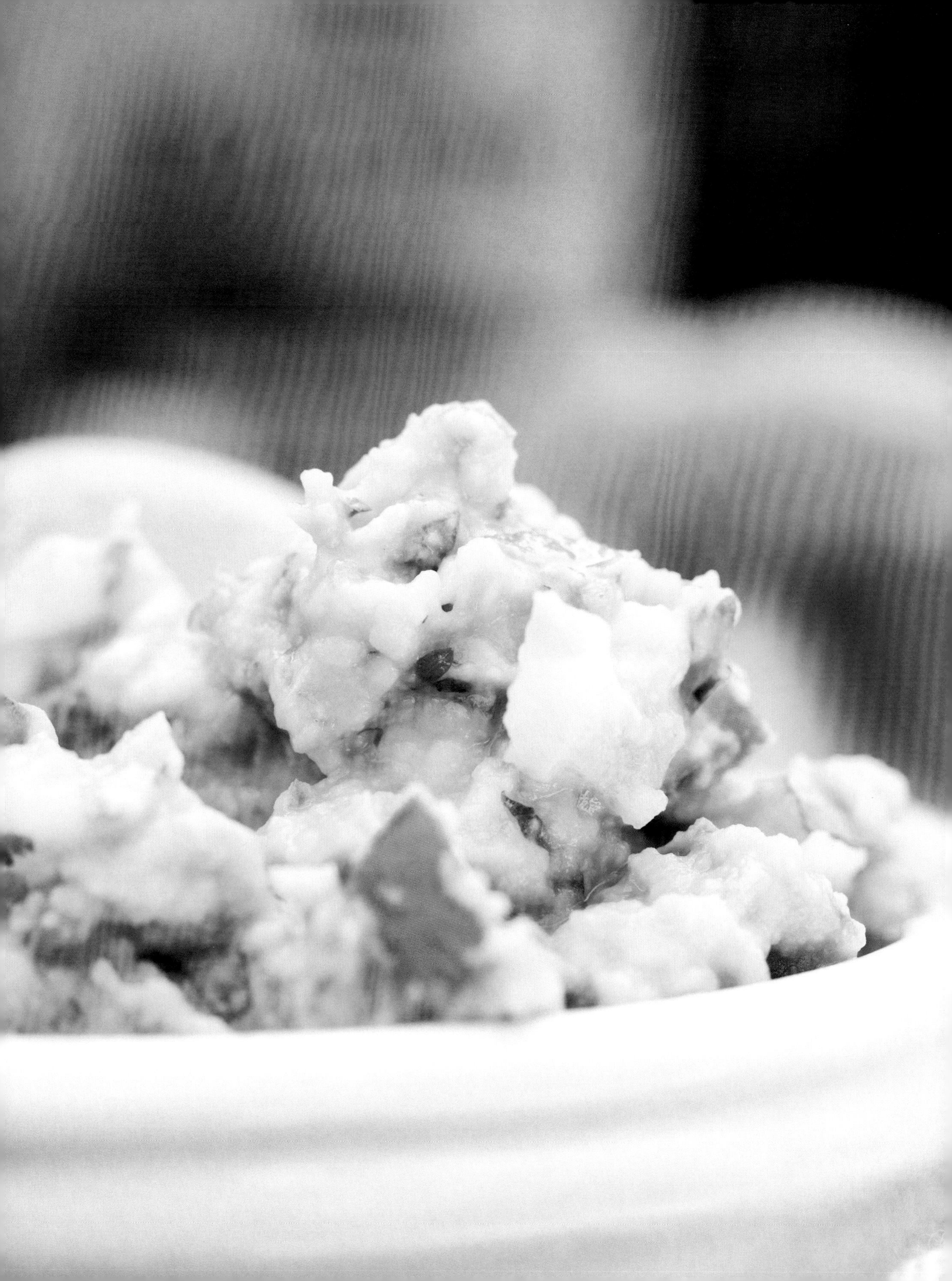

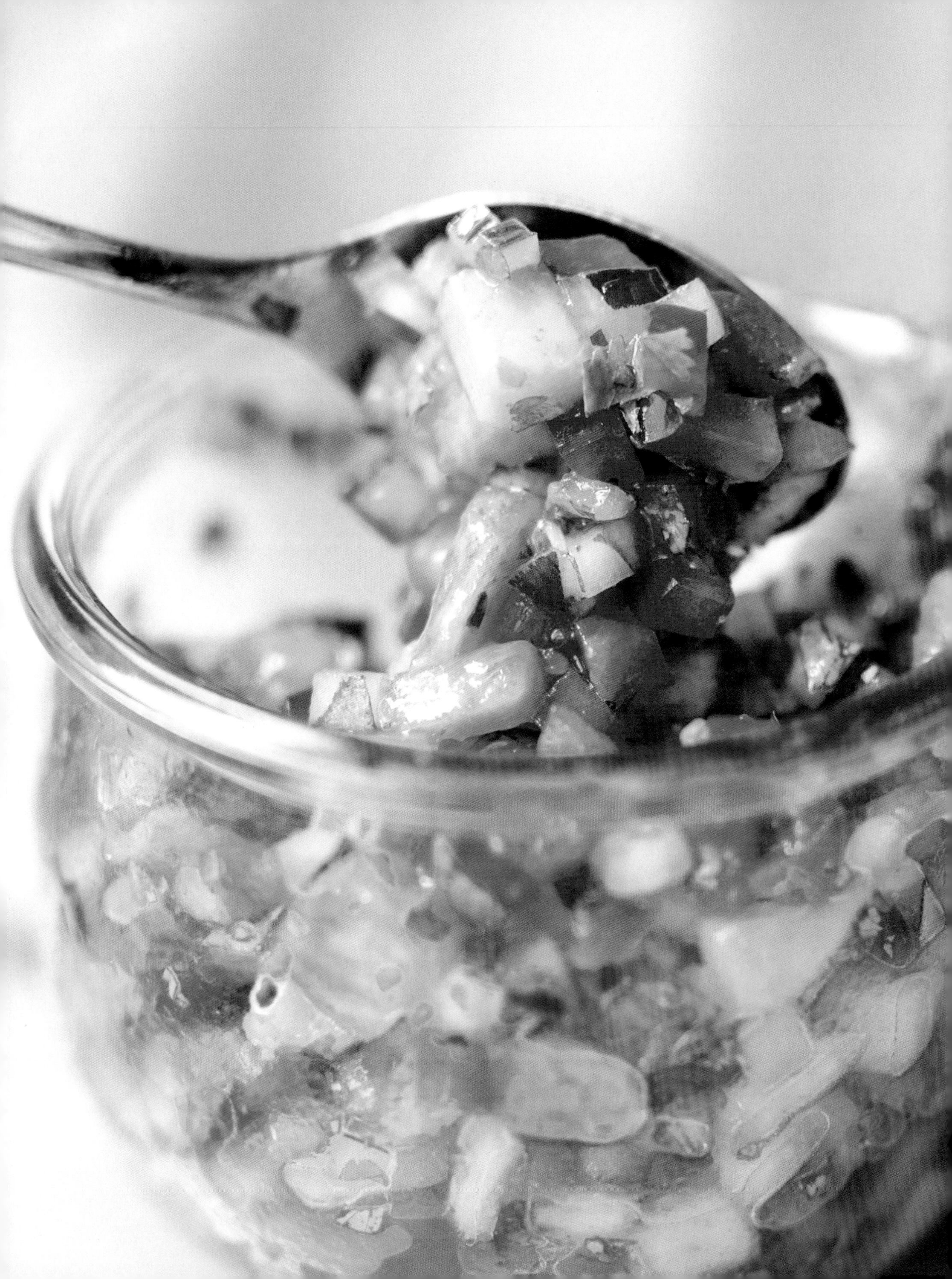

PEACH SALSA

Dairy-Free, Gluten-Free, Grain-Free, Paleo, SCD, Vegan

PREP 10 minutes | COOK 0 minutes | TOTAL 10 minutes | SERVES 6

This fresh peach salsa is delicious served with chips and tacos. It also makes a wonderful condiment for grilled pork and fish. It's light and flavorful, and it will brighten any meal.

INGREDIENTS

2 peaches, skin removed and diced

1/3 cup diced red pepper

1/4 cup diced red onion

1 Tablespoon chopped cilantro

1 teaspoon olive oil

1 teaspoon fresh lemon juice

1/8 teaspoon crushed red pepper

Pinch of sea salt

DIRECTIONS

1. Place all of the ingredients in a bowl and gently mix to combine.
2. Cover and refrigerate until serving.
3. The salsa is best served the same day but can be stored in an airtight container in the refrigerator for up to 3 days.

CHEDDAR PECAN CRACKERS

Gluten-Free, Grain-Free, SCD

PREP 10 minutes | COOK 20 minutes | TOTAL 30 minutes | SERVES 10

These grain-free crackers make a great snack or cheese board accompaniment. They are light, nutty and crunchy, with a little kick from the cayenne. If the dough feels too sticky, put it in the refrigerator for 15-30 minutes. It will firm up and be easier to work with.

INGREDIENTS

1 cup almond flour

1 cup shredded sharp cheddar cheese

1/2 teaspoon baking soda

3/4 teaspoon sea salt

1/4 teaspoon smoked paprika

1/4 teaspoon cayenne pepper

1/4 cup chopped pecans

1/4 cup cold water

DIRECTIONS

1. Preheat the oven to 350 degrees.
2. Place the almond flour, shredded cheddar cheese, baking soda, salt, paprika, cayenne and pecans in a medium bowl.
3. Using a fork, mix the ingredients well.
4. Add the cold water and mix well with the fork until a dough forms.
5. Line a sheet pan with parchment paper.
6. Take one teaspoon of dough and roll into a ball. Place on the sheet pan.
7. Repeat with the remaining dough.
8. Press down on the balls of dough with the bottom of a glass. Cover the glass with a piece of parchment paper to keep from sticking.
9. Bake for 13 minutes and then flip the crackers.
10. Return to the oven and bake for an additional 5-7 minutes or until done.
11. Once cooled to room temperature, serve or store in an airtight container.

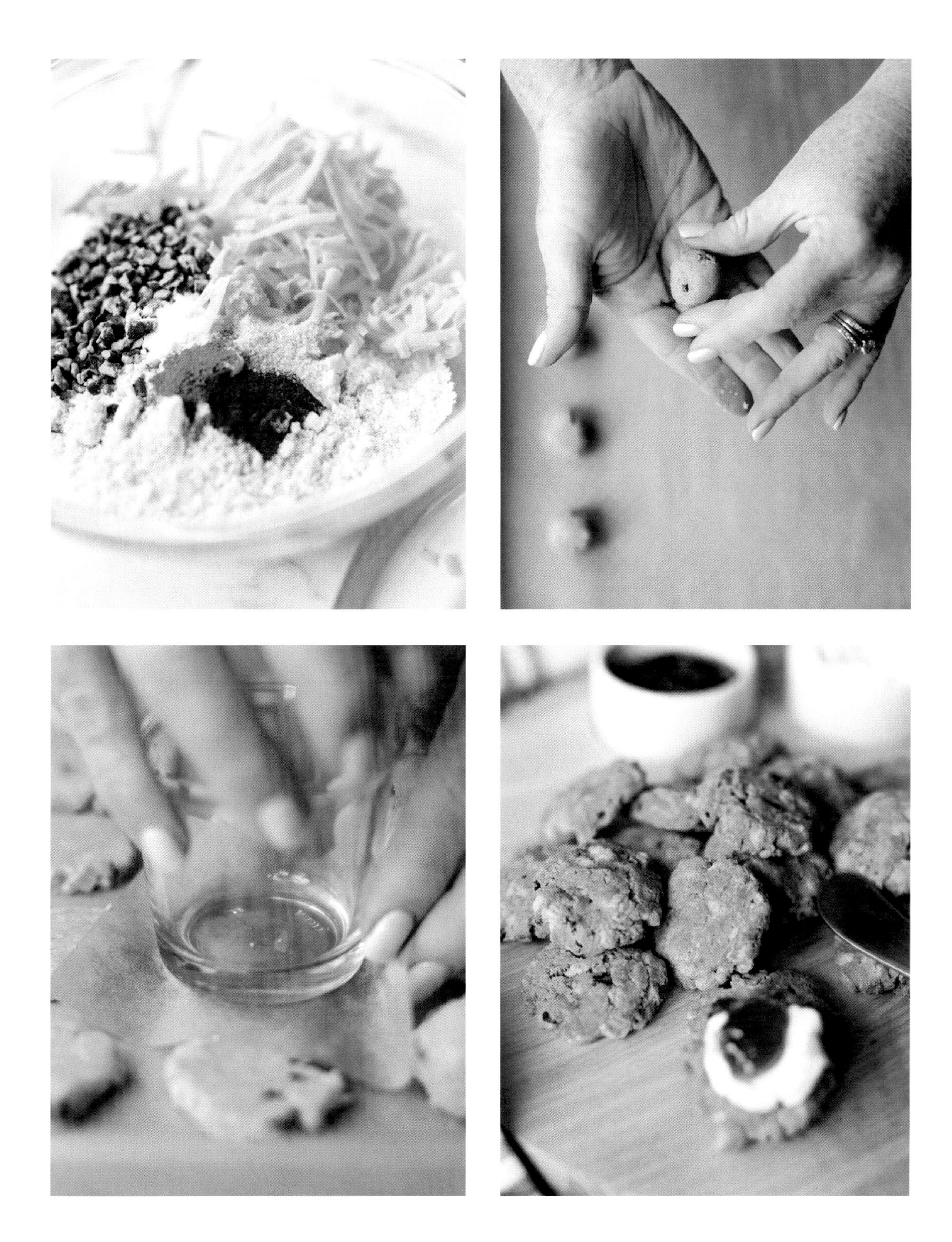

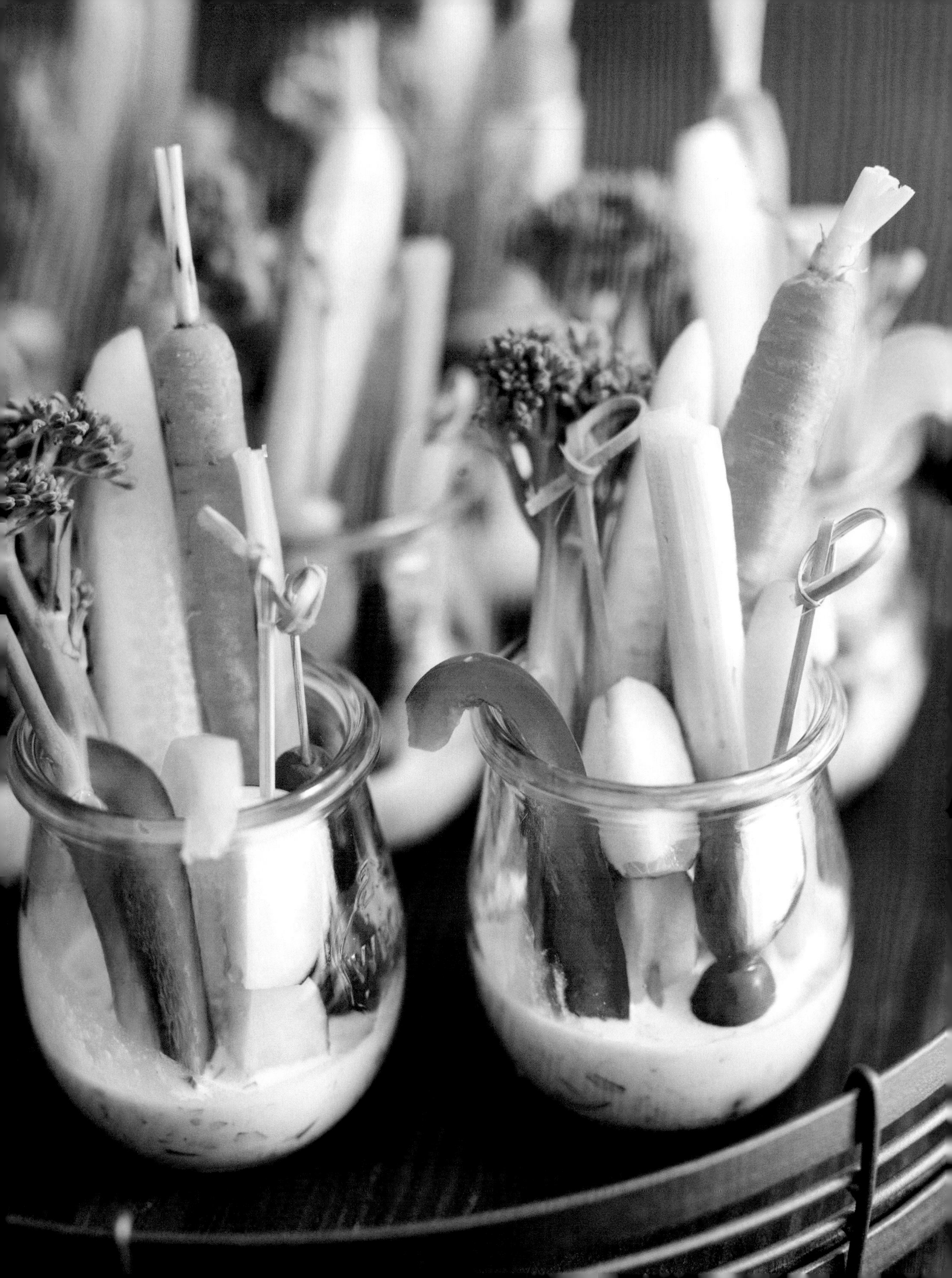

INDIVIDUAL VEGGIES AND DIP

Dairy-Free, Gluten-Free, Grain-Free, Paleo, SCD, Vegan

PREP 10 minutes | COOK 0 minutes | TOTAL 10 minutes

When I am entertaining, I like to serve fresh vegetables and dip on the buffet or offer them with appetizers. A fun way to serve veggies and dips is in individual portions. They look beautiful arranged in small glass jars with a delicious dip at the bottom. This also makes it easier for guests to help themselves. I have listed the vegetables I often serve, but you can use any variety you choose. For dipping, I like to use my EFK Dairy-Free Cilantro Ranch on page 226 or EFK Hummus on page 159, but you can use any dressing or dip you like.

INGREDIENTS

Carrots

Cucumbers

Celery

Broccolini

Peppers

Radishes

Cherry tomatoes

Bamboo cocktail picks

Small glass jars

EFK Dairy-Free Cilantro Ranch (page 226) or EFK Hummus (page 159)

DIRECTIONS

1. Cut long vegetables into sticks with enough height to peek out of the glass jars by an inch or two.
2. Skewer cherry tomatoes, radishes and other small vegetables on bamboo picks.
3. Fill the bottom of the glass jars with dip 1/4 to 1/2 inch deep.
4. Arrange vegetables in the glass jars.
5. Place jars on a serving tray.

GRILLED BRIE WITH BERRIES AND HONEY

Gluten-Free, Grain-Free, SCD

PREP 10 minutes | COOK 6 minutes | TOTAL 16 minutes | SERVES 6

When following the Specific Carbohydrate Diet, you are allowed to have a few low-lactose cheeses. Fortunately, brie made that list, so when I was following the SCD, I was able to eat it occasionally. For a special treat, I would grill a wheel of brie and serve it with fresh berries and a drizzle of honey and eat it with my grain-free olive oil crackers. Today this recipe is my go-to when entertaining in the summer because it's easy to make and everyone loves it. I like to serve it with grilled slices of baguette and grain-free crackers. For the berries, I usually use a combination of whatever I have on hand. Sliced strawberries, blueberries, raspberries and blackberries all work well.

INGREDIENTS

1 cup of fresh berries

1 baguette

Olive oil

Sea salt

1 8-ounce wheel of brie

Honey

DIRECTIONS

1. Preheat the grill to medium-high heat.
2. Rinse and slice (if needed) your berries and set aside.
3. Using a serrated knife, slice the baguette on the bias.
4. Place about 1/3 cup of olive oil in a small bowl and add 1/2 teaspoon of salt.
5. Using a basting brush, swirl the oil and salt together and brush both sides of each of the baguette slices.
6. Unwrap the brie and brush both sides with olive oil.
7. Place the brie on one side of the grill and fill the remaining space with the baguette slices.
8. The bread will brown quickly so check frequently and flip the pieces when they are crisp and brown on the underside.
9. Set the baguette slices aside when they finish browning.

(Continued)

10. Grill the brie for 2 minutes and then carefully flip it over with a large spatula.
11. Grill for an additional 2-4 minutes and transfer to a serving plate when done.
12. Top the brie with the berries and drizzle honey over the top. (Be sure to add extra berries in you use a larger wheel of brie.)
13. Serve with the grilled baguette and grain-free crackers.

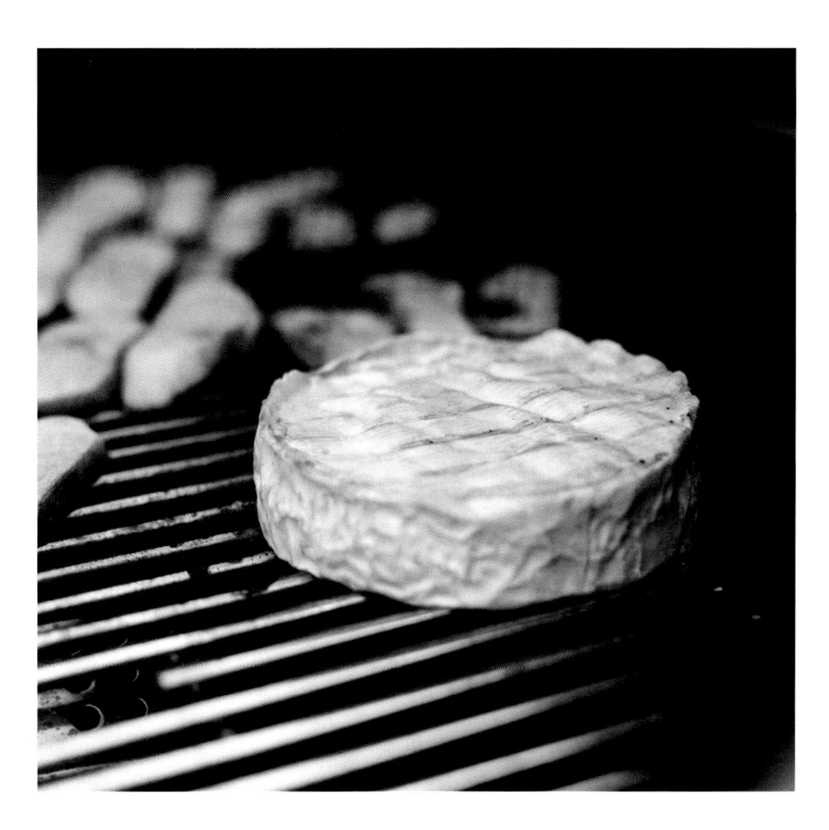

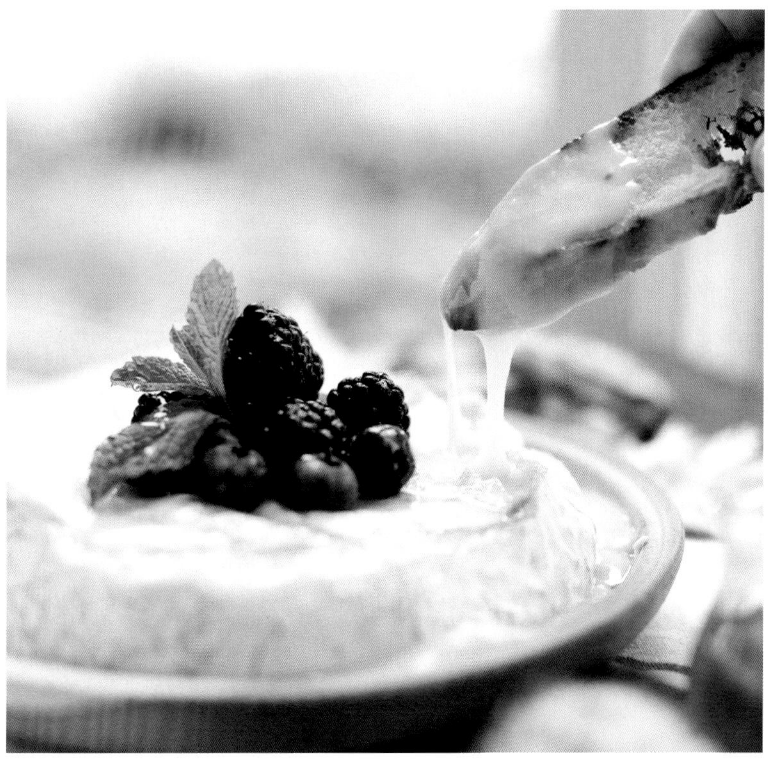

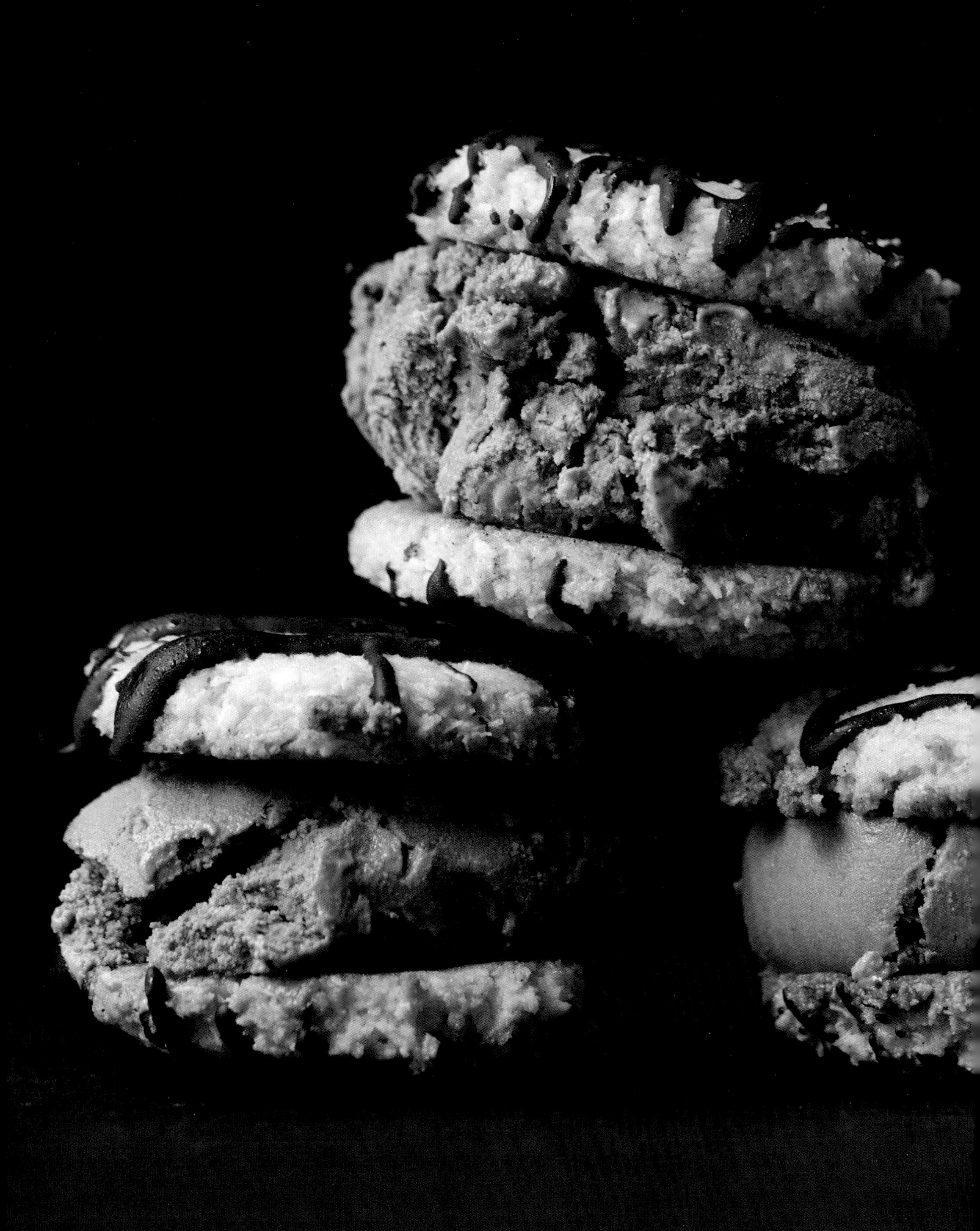

SWEETS AND TREATS

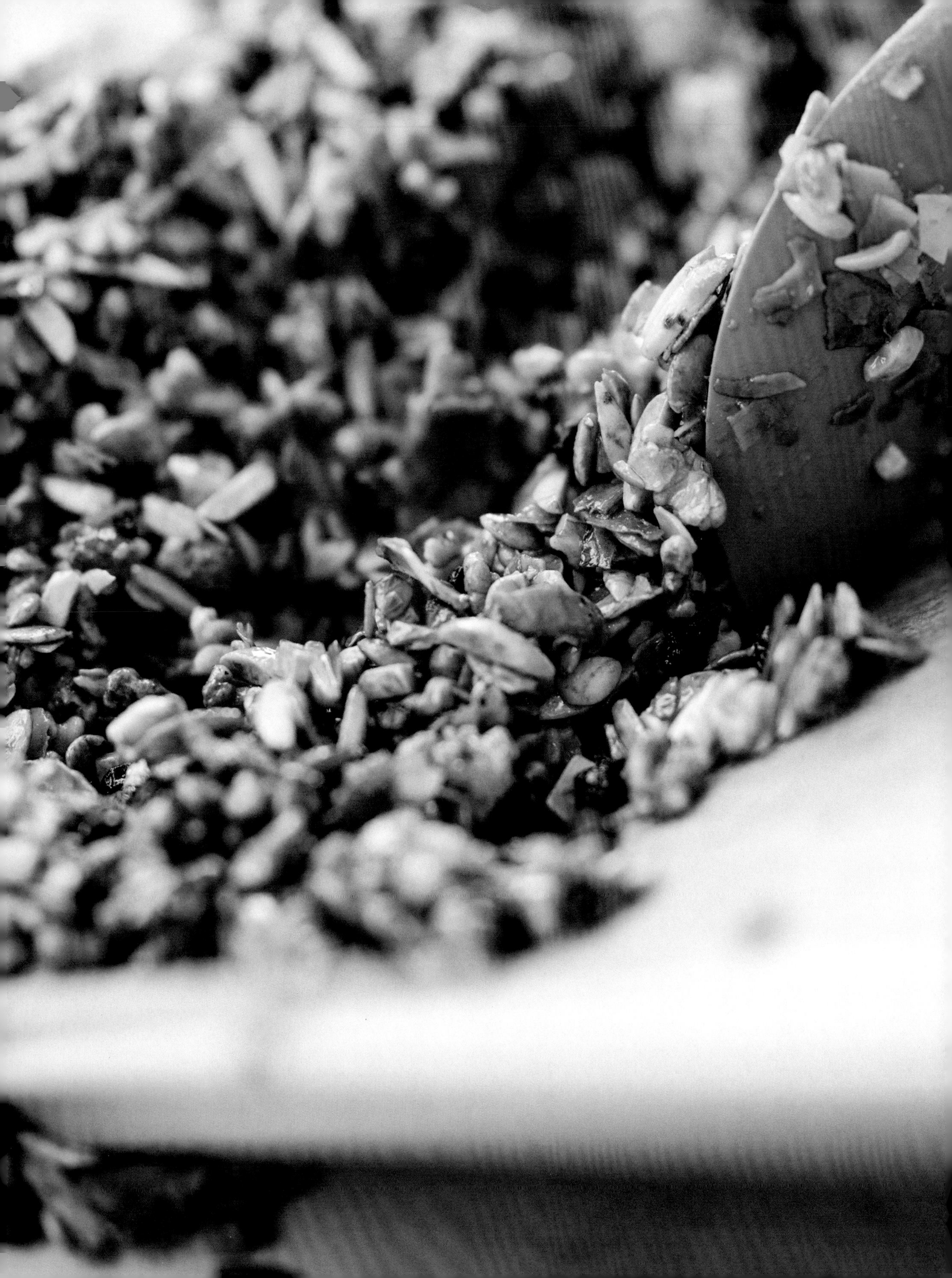

GRAIN-FREE GRANOLA

Gluten-Free, Grain-Free, SCD (Adaptable for Dairy-Free, Paleo, Vegan)

PREP 3 minutes | COOK 32 minutes | TOTAL 35 minutes | MAKES 6 cups

When I was following the Specific Carbohydrate Diet, I couldn't eat grains of any kind. I really missed granola, and back then I couldn't find any grain-free varieties in stores so I created this recipe using nuts, seeds and coconut flakes. Even though I can tolerate most grains again, and there are now many grain-free granola options in stores, I still prefer this homemade version. It makes a wonderful snack, cereal or topping for yogurt and açaí bowls. To adapt for dairy-free and paleo, substitute coconut oil for butter. To adapt for vegan, substitute pure maple syrup for honey and coconut oil for butter.

INGREDIENTS

1 1/2 cups walnut pieces

1 1/2 cups raw slivered almonds

1 1/2 cups unsweetened coconut flakes

3/4 cup pumpkin seeds

1/2 cup honey or pure maple syrup

2 Tablespoons butter or coconut oil

1/2 teaspoon real vanilla extract

1 cup dried blueberries, unsweetened or sweetened with just fruit juice

DIRECTIONS

1. Preheat oven to 350 degrees.
2. In a large bowl combine walnuts, almonds, coconut and pumpkin seeds and set aside.
3. In a small saucepan combine honey or maple syrup with the butter or coconut oil.
4. Bring to a simmer and cook for 2 minutes.
5. Remove from heat and stir in the vanilla extract.
6. Pour the warm liquid over the nut mixture in the bowl and stir well.
7. Spread the granola mixture on a sheet pan lined with parchment paper or silicone liner.
8. Bake for 20-25 minutes or until golden brown, stirring every 4-5 minutes.
9. Stir in the blueberries for the last 4-5 minutes of cooking.
10. Spread granola onto sheets of parchment paper or silicone liners and cool.
11. Once cooled, store in an airtight container.

GRAIN-FREE TOASTED COCONUT COOKIES

Dairy-Free, Gluten-Free, Grain-Free, Paleo, Vegan

PREP 10 minutes | COOK 22 minutes | TOTAL 32 minutes | MAKES 20 cookies

These tasty, chewy cookies are vegan and grain-free. The toasted coconut and maple syrup complement each other's natural sweetness. They are wonderful on their own or drizzled with dark chocolate. My husband loves them without the chocolate, so when I make them I only use the chocolate over half of them.

INGREDIENTS

1 cup unsweetened shredded coconut

1 1/2 cups blanched almond flour

2/3 cup pure maple syrup

1/2 teaspoon grain-free baking powder (I like Hain brand)

1/4 teaspoon sea salt

1 1/2 teaspoons real vanilla extract

1 3-ounce bar dairy-free dark chocolate

DIRECTIONS

1. Preheat the oven to 350 degrees.
2. Sprinkle the coconut on a dry cookie sheet.
3. Toast in the oven for 5 minutes or until golden, shaking the pan every minute or so.
4. Set the toasted coconut aside.
5. In a medium bowl place the coconut, almond flour, maple syrup, baking powder, salt and vanilla and stir well.
6. Scoop tablespoons of dough on a parchment-lined cookie sheet.
7. Press down slightly with the bottom of a glass covered with a piece of parchment paper to keep from sticking.
8. Bake for 15 minutes or until golden.
9. Cool on a baking rack.
10. Break the chocolate bar into pieces and melt in the microwave or in a double boiler.
11. Stir well and drizzle the chocolate with a spoon over the cooled cookies.
12. Set in the freezer until chocolate is set.
13. Store in an airtight container for up to 3 days or in the freezer for up to 2 weeks.

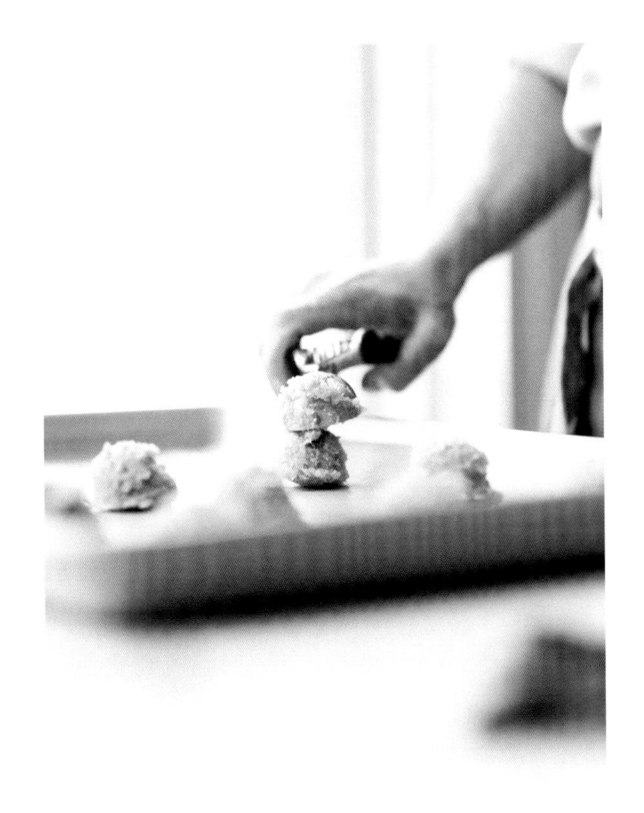

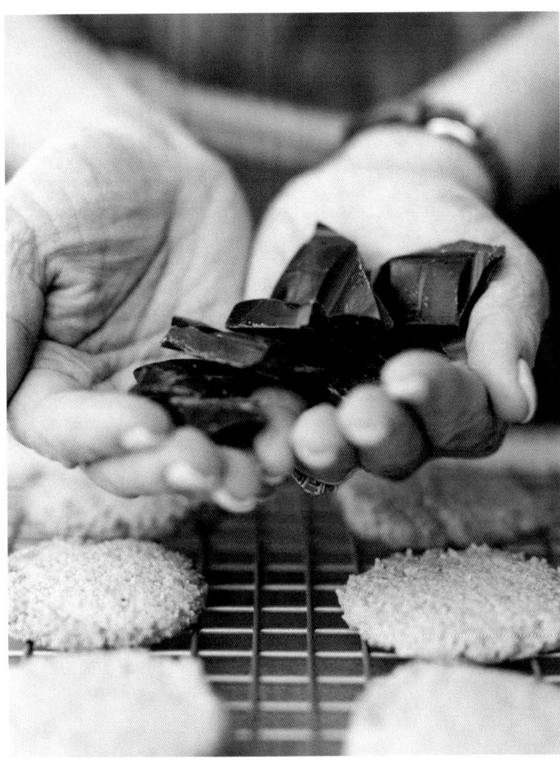

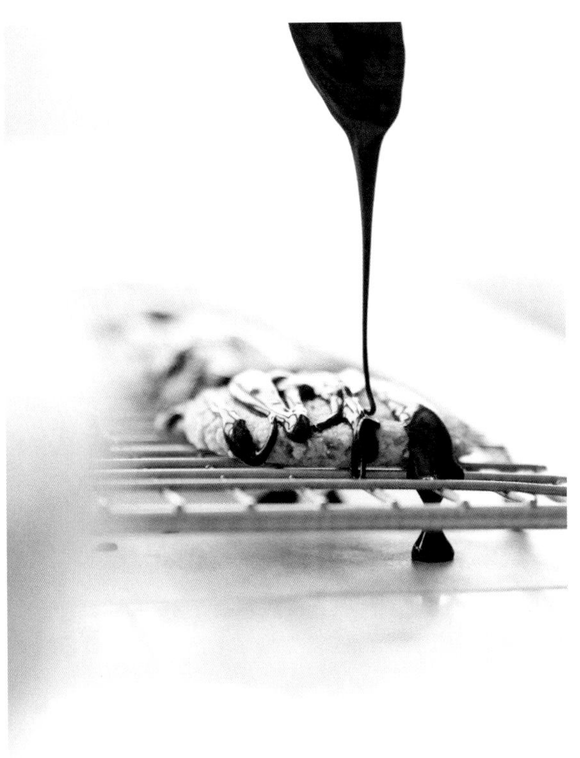

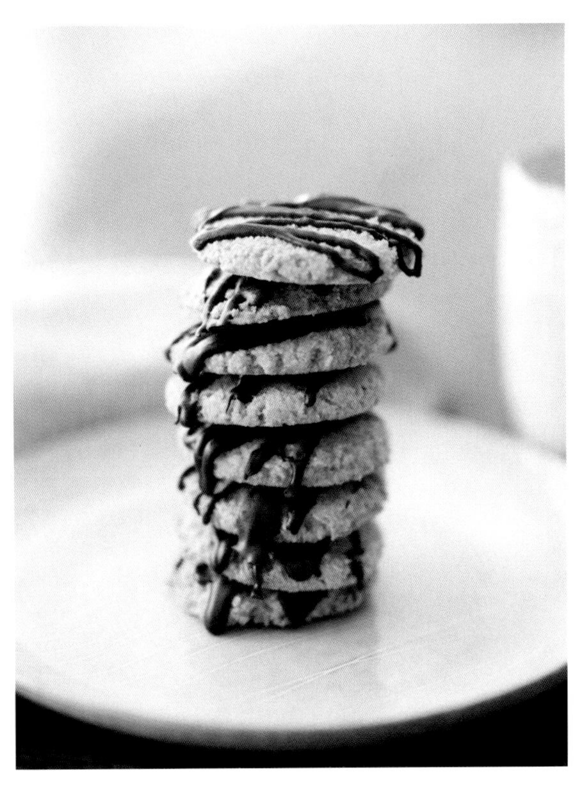

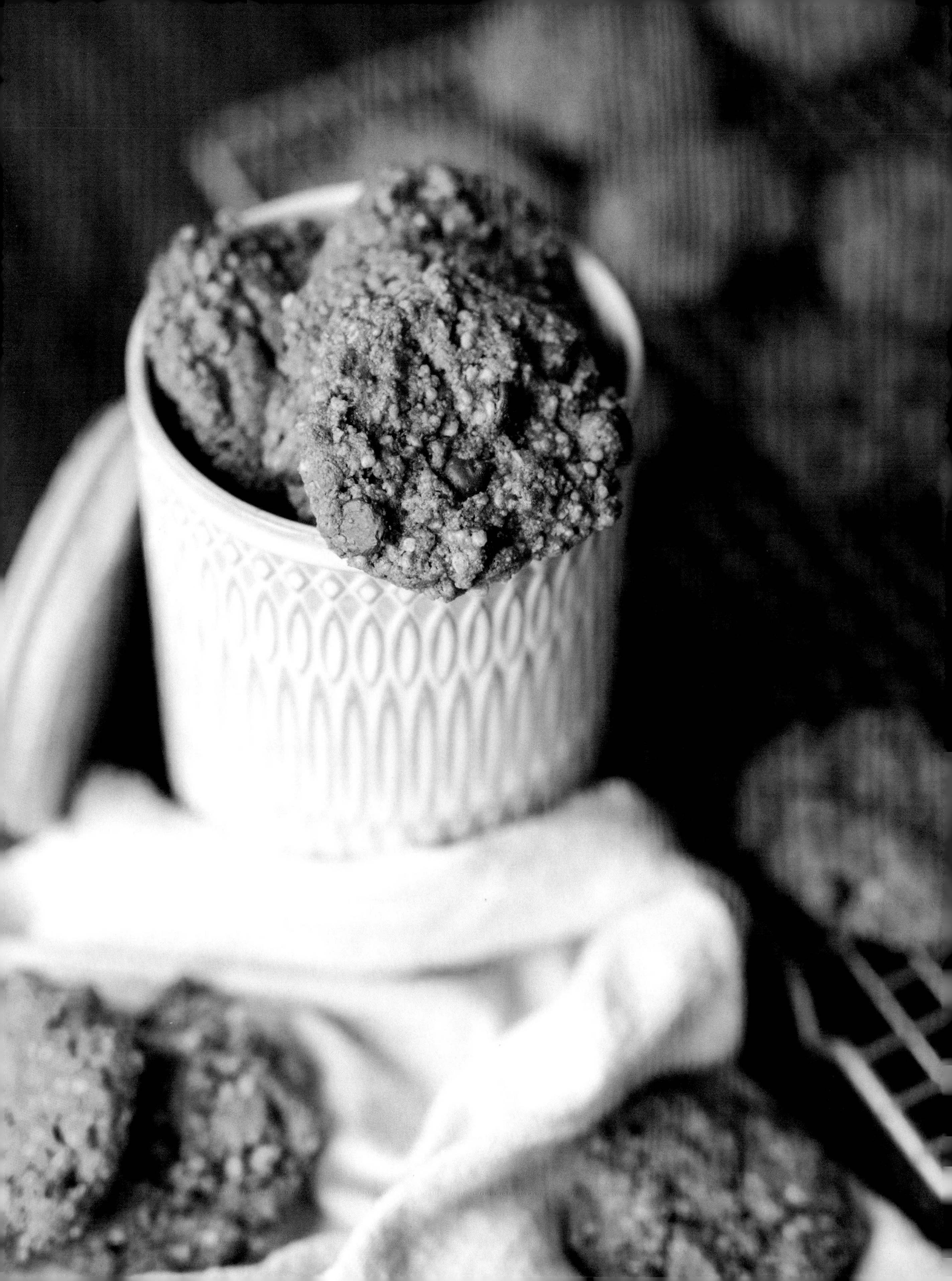

GLUTEN-FREE CRUNCH COOKIES

Dairy-Free, Gluten-Free

PREP 10 minutes | COOK 10 minutes | TOTAL 20 minutes | MAKES 2 dozen cookies

I love a chocolate chip cookie that is soft but has a little crunch to it. In this version, I use puffed quinoa to achieve the crunch. I order it from nuts.com. These cookies are gluten-free and dairy-free and sweetened with coconut sugar, but you would never know it. They have quickly become my family's favorite.

INGREDIENTS

1/2 cup palm shortening

3/4 cup coconut sugar

1 egg

2 teaspoons vanilla

1 1/2 cups almond flour

2 Tablespoons coconut flour

1/2 teaspoon baking soda

1/4 teaspoon salt

1 1/4 cups puffed quinoa

1 cup dairy-free chocolate chips

DIRECTIONS

1. Preheat the oven to 375 degrees.
2. In a large bowl in a stand-up mixer, mix together the palm shortening and coconut sugar until creamy.
3. Add the egg and vanilla and mix well.
4. Add the almond flour, coconut flour, baking soda and salt.
5. Mix well, stopping to scrape down the sides of the bowl and mix again.
6. Add the puffed quinoa and mix until just combined.
7. Stir in the chocolate chips by hand.
8. Scoop the dough onto parchment-lined baking sheets.
9. Lightly press the cookies and shape into rounds.
10. Bake for 10 minutes or until golden.
11. Cool on baking sheets for 2 minutes and then transfer the cookies to wire racks to cool completely.
12. Once cooled, store in an airtight container.

NO-BAKE PEANUT BUTTER CRUNCH BARS

Dairy-Free, Gluten-Free, Vegan

PREP 5 minutes | COOK 5 minutes | TOTAL 10 minutes* | MAKES 1 dozen bars

When my daughters came home from college to quarantine during the pandemic, I baked a lot of treats. I think it was my way of trying to make their newfound circumstances more fun. Each week I put together a batch of peanut butter bars, experimenting with different ingredients. I would keep a pan in the refrigerator and we would all slice off pieces to nibble on throughout the day. If you just take a little bite here and there and don't take a full bar at once, you are eating less, right? This recipe is the version we all liked best. I love that they are gluten-free and dairy-free and sweetened with pure maple syrup. They remind me of Special K bars but are made with healthier ingredients.

**Does not include setting time, which is noted in the directions.*

INGREDIENTS

1 3/4 cups natural peanut butter, divided

3/4 cup pure maple syrup

1 cup puffed quinoa (I like nuts.com brand)

1 cup salted peanuts, chopped

1 1/2 cups dairy-free chocolate chips or chopped dark chocolate

DIRECTIONS

1. Line a 9-by-9-inch square pan with parchment paper.
2. In a medium bowl, combine 1 1/2 cups peanut butter and the maple syrup.
3. Add the puffed quinoa and the chopped peanuts. Mix well.
4. Spread the peanut butter mixture into the parchment-lined pan and smooth.
5. Add the chocolate chips or dark chocolate and 1/4 cup peanut butter to a bowl and melt in the microwave or over a saucepan filled with simmering water.
6. Spread the melted chocolate mixture on top of the bars and smooth.
7. Place in the refrigerator for 2-3 hours until set.
8. Cut bars into squares and store in an airtight container in the refrigerator for up to 1 week.

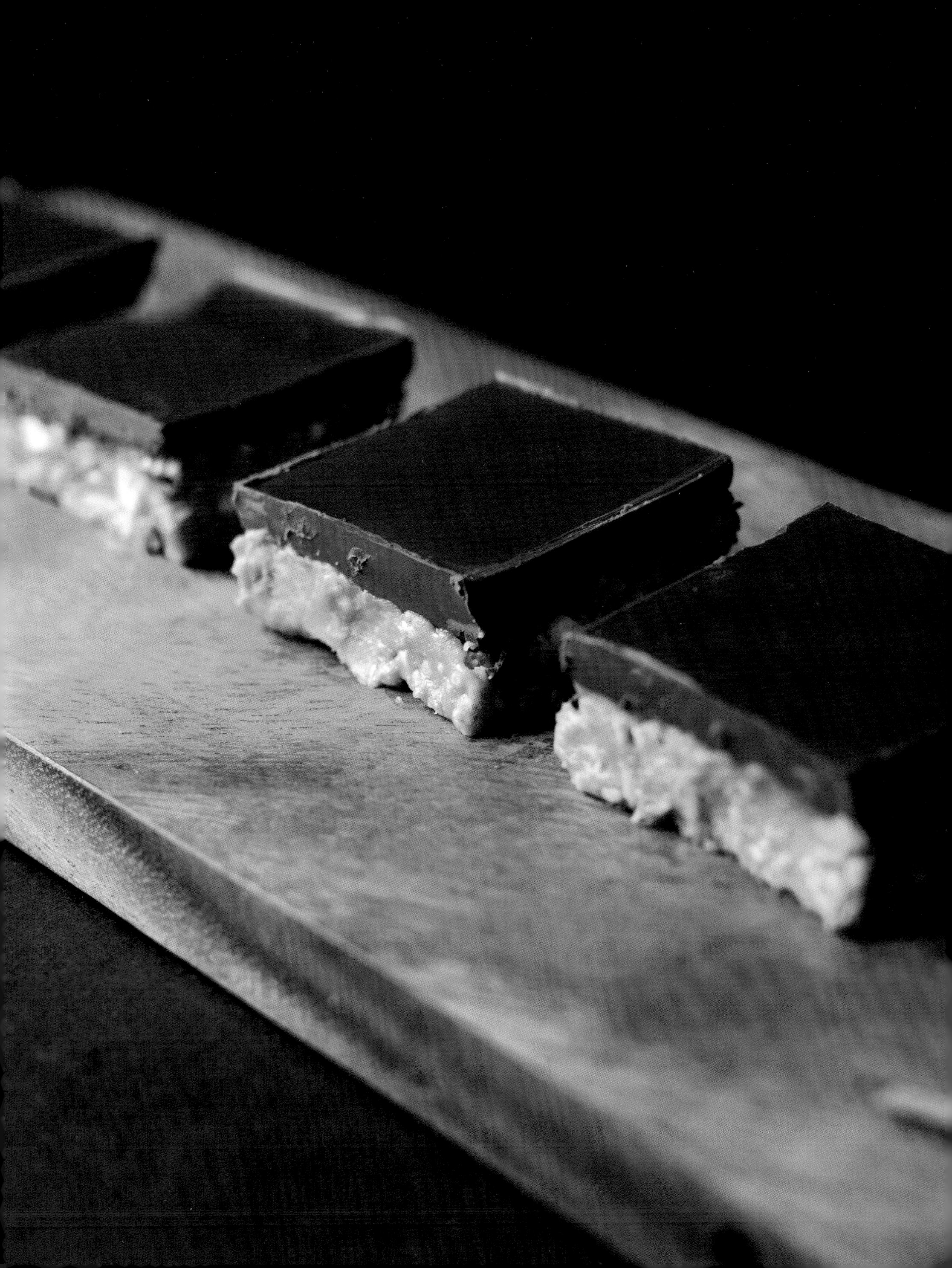

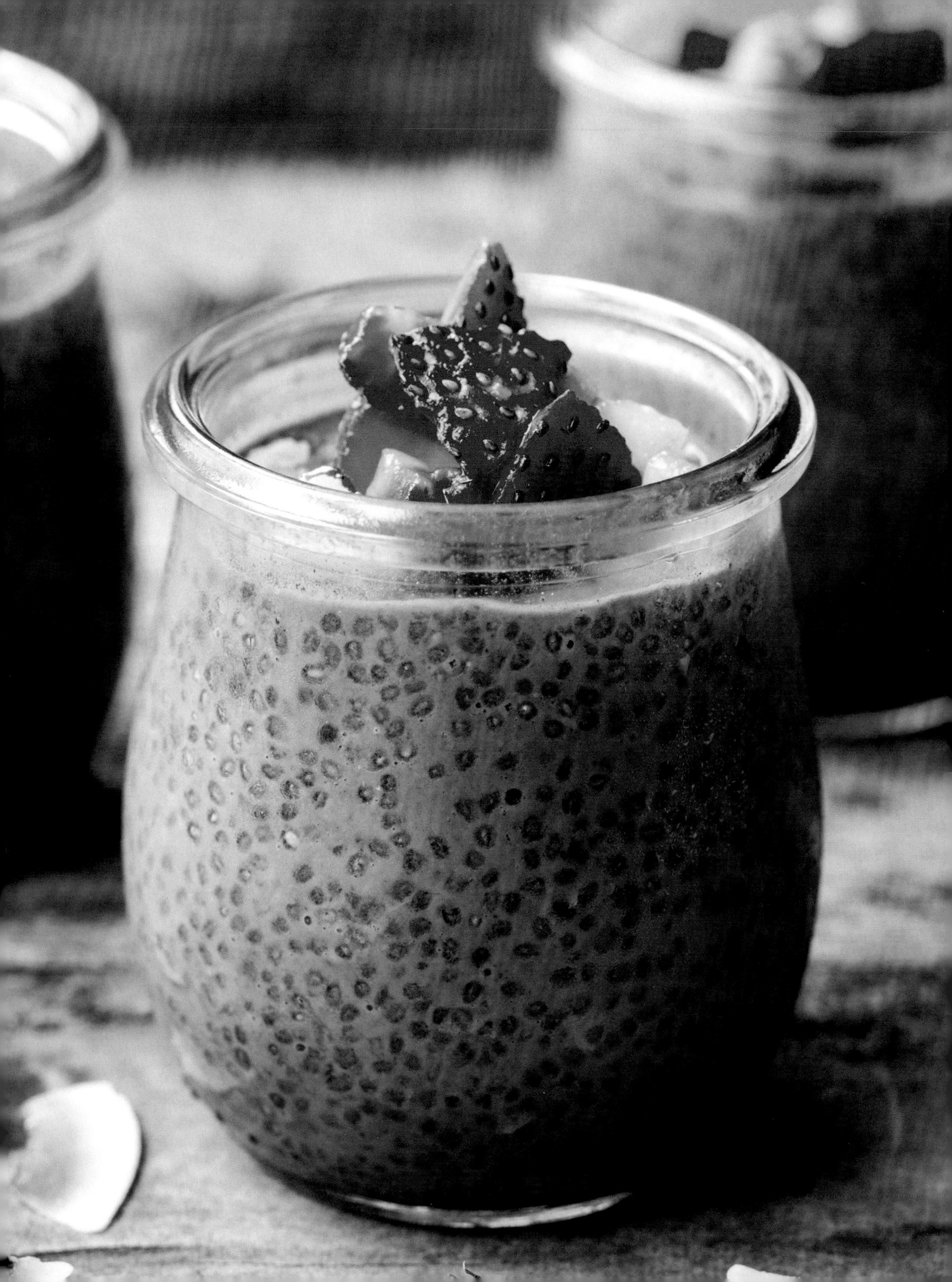

CHOCOLATE CHIA PUDDING

Dairy-Free, Gluten-Free, Grain-Free, Paleo, Vegan

PREP 10 minutes | COOK 0 minutes | TOTAL 10 minutes | SERVES 4

Chia seed pudding is easy to make and is great for a quick breakfast or snack. Chia seeds are full of fiber, omega-3 fatty acids and high-quality protein. Eating them in a pudding is a fun way to add them to your diet. In this recipe I add raw cacao powder, which gives the pudding a chocolate flavor and is loaded with antioxidants. I like to use pure maple syrup for the sweetener, but you can substitute the syrup with honey or the sweetener of your choice.

**Does not include setting time, which is noted in the directions.*

INGREDIENTS

8 Tablespoons chia seeds, divided

2 cups almond or other plant-based milk

1/4 cup pure maple syrup

2 Tablespoons raw cacao powder

Fresh berries, coconut or granola, for serving

DIRECTIONS

1. Take 4 glass jars and place 2 Tablespoons of chia seeds in each jar.
2. Blend the almond milk, maple syrup and raw cacao powder using an immersion or stand-up blender until well combined.
3. Pour a quarter of the milk mixture into each of the jars.
4. Using a fork, stir the chia seeds in each of the jars.
5. Let the puddings sit for 5 minutes and then stir them again with a fork, scraping the sides and breaking up any clumps of seeds.
6. Put the lids on the jars and refrigerate for at least 2 hours or overnight.
7. To serve: You can eat them as they are or top the puddings with fresh berries, coconut or granola.
8. Store in an airtight container in the refrigerator for up to 1 week.

GRAIN-FREE PUMPKIN BREAD

Dairy-Free, Gluten-Free, Grain-Free, Paleo (Adaptable for SCD)

PREP 10 minutes | COOK 65 minutes | TOTAL 1 hour 15 minutes | MAKES 1 loaf

It can be difficult to find good substitutes for baked goods when following a grain-free diet. I love pumpkin bread and was determined to create a grain-free and refined-sugar-free recipe that would satisfy my memories of fall treats. For this recipe, I baked many loaves before landing on the perfect combination of ingredients that produce a similar texture and taste to one with traditional ingredients. Even if you are not following a grain-free or gluten-free diet, you will love this healthier pumpkin bread. To adapt for SCD, use SCD-approved canned or homemade pumpkin purée and substitute honey for maple syrup.

INGREDIENTS

2 Tablespoons melted butter or coconut oil

2 1/2 cups almond flour

1/4 cup coconut flour

1 teaspoon baking soda

1/4 teaspoon sea salt

1 Tablespoon cinnamon

1/2 teaspoon ground ginger

1/2 teaspoon ground cloves

3 eggs

3/4 cup canned pumpkin

3/4 cup pure maple syrup

DIRECTIONS

1. Preheat oven to 350 degrees.
2. Lightly grease a 1-pound loaf pan with butter or coconut oil.
3. Sift together the almond flour, coconut flour, baking soda, sea salt, cinnamon, ginger and cloves. Set aside.
4. In a large bowl in a stand-up mixer, mix 3 eggs on high for 3 minutes until frothy.
5. Add the pumpkin and maple syrup and mix well.
6. Add the sifted dry ingredients and mix until combined.
7. Pour the batter into the prepared loaf pan.
8. Bake for 60-65 minutes or until done.
9. Let cool. Slice and serve.
10. Once cooled, store in an airtight container.

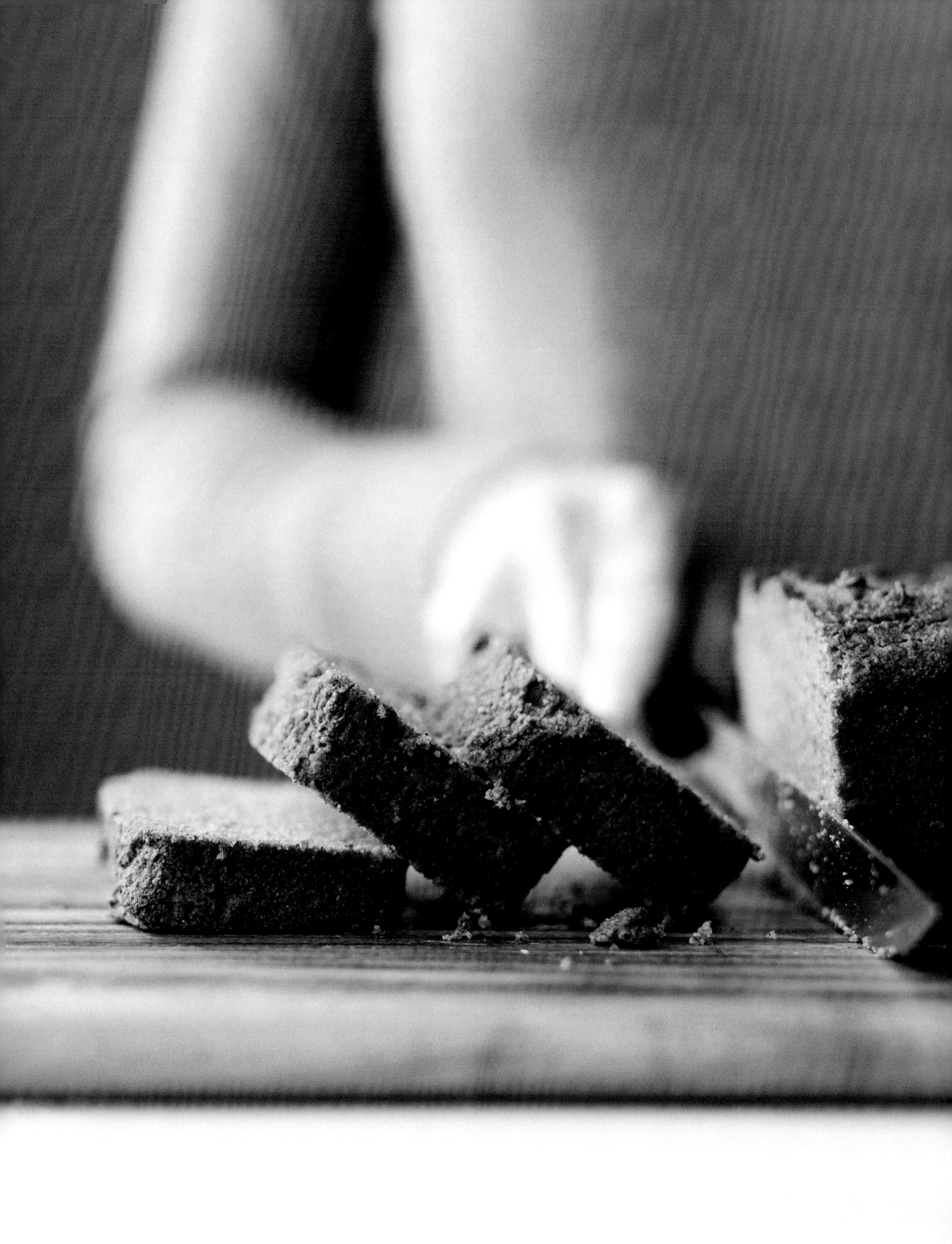

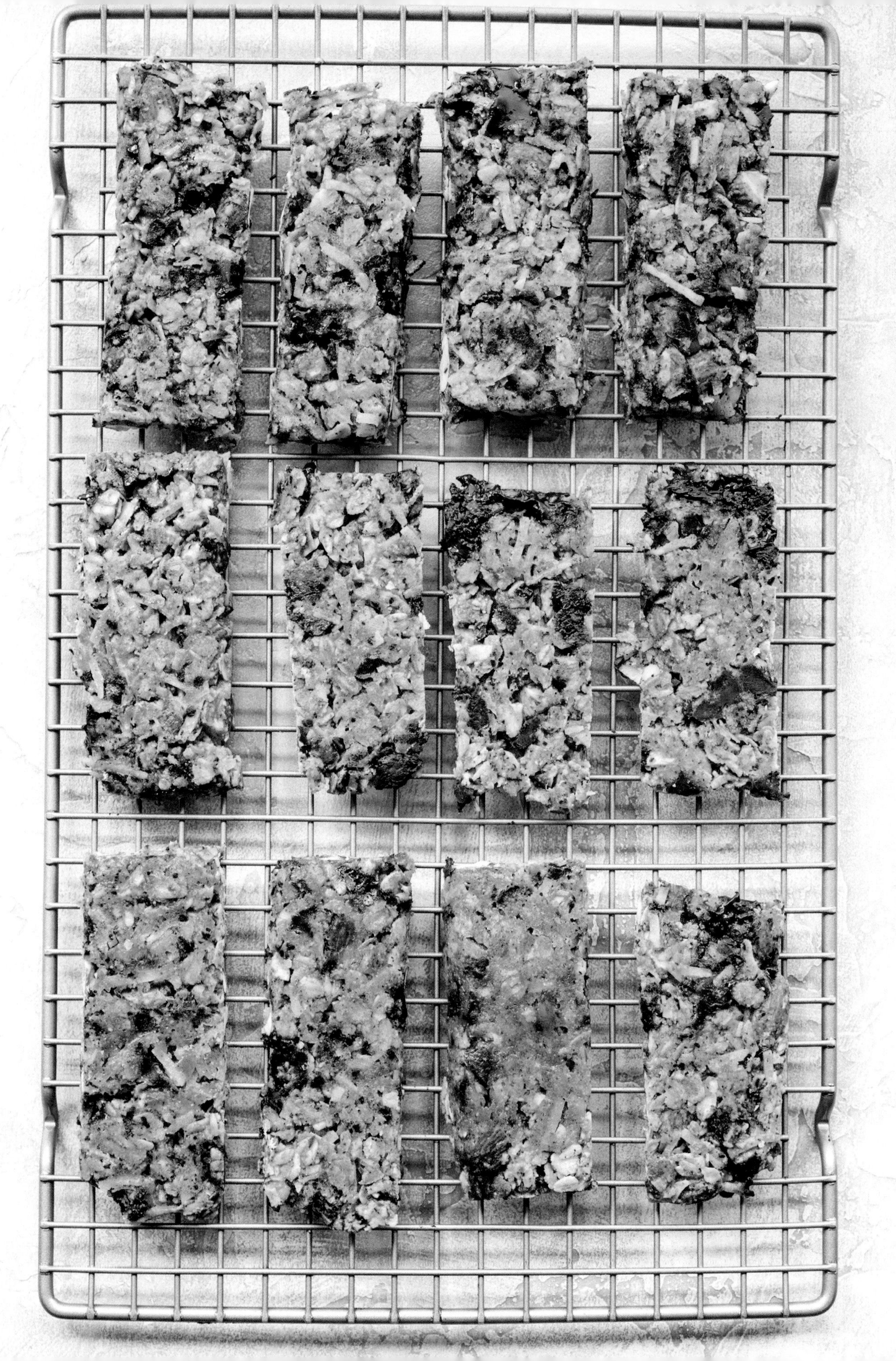

ALMOND JOY GRANOLA BARS

Dairy-Free, Gluten-Free, Vegan

PREP 20 minutes | COOK 30 minutes | TOTAL 50 minutes | MAKES about 1 dozen bars

I was that rare kid on Halloween who was excited when I got Mounds or Almond Joy candy bars while trick-or-treating. Everyone else hoped for Snickers or Reese's Peanut Butter Cups. Don't get me wrong, I liked those too, but I have always loved the combination of coconut, chocolate and almonds. These granola bars capture the flavor of an Almond Joy without all the refined sugar and overly processed ingredients.

DIRECTIONS

1. Preheat the oven to 300 degrees.
2. Line a 9-by-13-inch baking pan with parchment paper, allowing extra to hang over the long sides of the pan.
3. Place oats, almonds, coconut, chocolate and almond flour in a large bowl and mix well.
4. Place honey or maple syrup, almond butter, almond extract and salt in a medium bowl and stir until well combined.
5. Add the wet ingredients to the dry ingredients and mix well.
6. Spread the granola bar mixture into the prepared pan.
7. Place another sheet of parchment paper on top of the bars and press down with your hands until they are evenly distributed throughout the pan.
8. Remove the top sheet of paper and use a rubber spatula to smooth out any remaining uneven parts.
9. Bake for 25-30 minutes until golden.
10. Let cool for 5-10 minutes and then lift the granola bars out of the pan using the flaps of parchment as handles.
11. Place the bars with the parchment side up on a cutting board and remove the paper.
12. Cut into 12-15 bars depending on your desired size.
13. Transfer the bars to a wire rack and allow to cool.
14. Once cooled, store in an airtight container for up to 1 week.

INGREDIENTS

1 cup gluten-free oats

1 cup chopped almonds

1 cup unsweetened shredded coconut

3-ounce dairy-free dark chocolate bar, chopped

1/2 cup almond flour

1/2 cup honey or pure maple syrup

1/2 cup almond butter

1 teaspoon almond extract

1/2 teaspoon sea salt

PUFFED QUINOA AND PEANUT BUTTER PROTEIN BITES

Dairy-Free, Gluten-Free (Adaptable for Vegan)

PREP 10 minutes | COOK 0 minutes | TOTAL 10 minutes* | MAKES 2 dozen bites

It is nice to have a healthy snack on hand after a workout or to hold you over between meals. Quick and easy to make, these protein bites fit the bill. They have plenty of protein and good fat to keep you satisfied. The honey and chocolate chips add just the right amount of sweetness too. I also love the crunch of the puffed quinoa. I order it from nuts.com. To adapt for paleo, substitute peanut butter for other nut butter. To adapt for vegan, substitute pure maple syrup for honey.

**Does not include setting time, which is noted in the directions.*

INGREDIENTS

1/2 cup natural peanut butter or other nut butter

3/4 cup puffed quinoa

1 1/2 cups almond flour

1/3 cup honey or maple syrup

1/4 teaspoon sea salt

1/2 teaspoon vanilla

1/2 cup dairy-free mini chocolate chips or chopped dark chocolate

DIRECTIONS

1. In a medium bowl, combine all the ingredients except the chocolate chips.
2. Mix together well until it forms a soft dough.
3. Mix in the chocolate chips or chopped dark chocolate.
4. Roll the mixture into balls.
5. Place the protein bites in the freezer until set.
6. Store in an airtight container in the refrigerator for 5 days or in the freezer for 1 month.

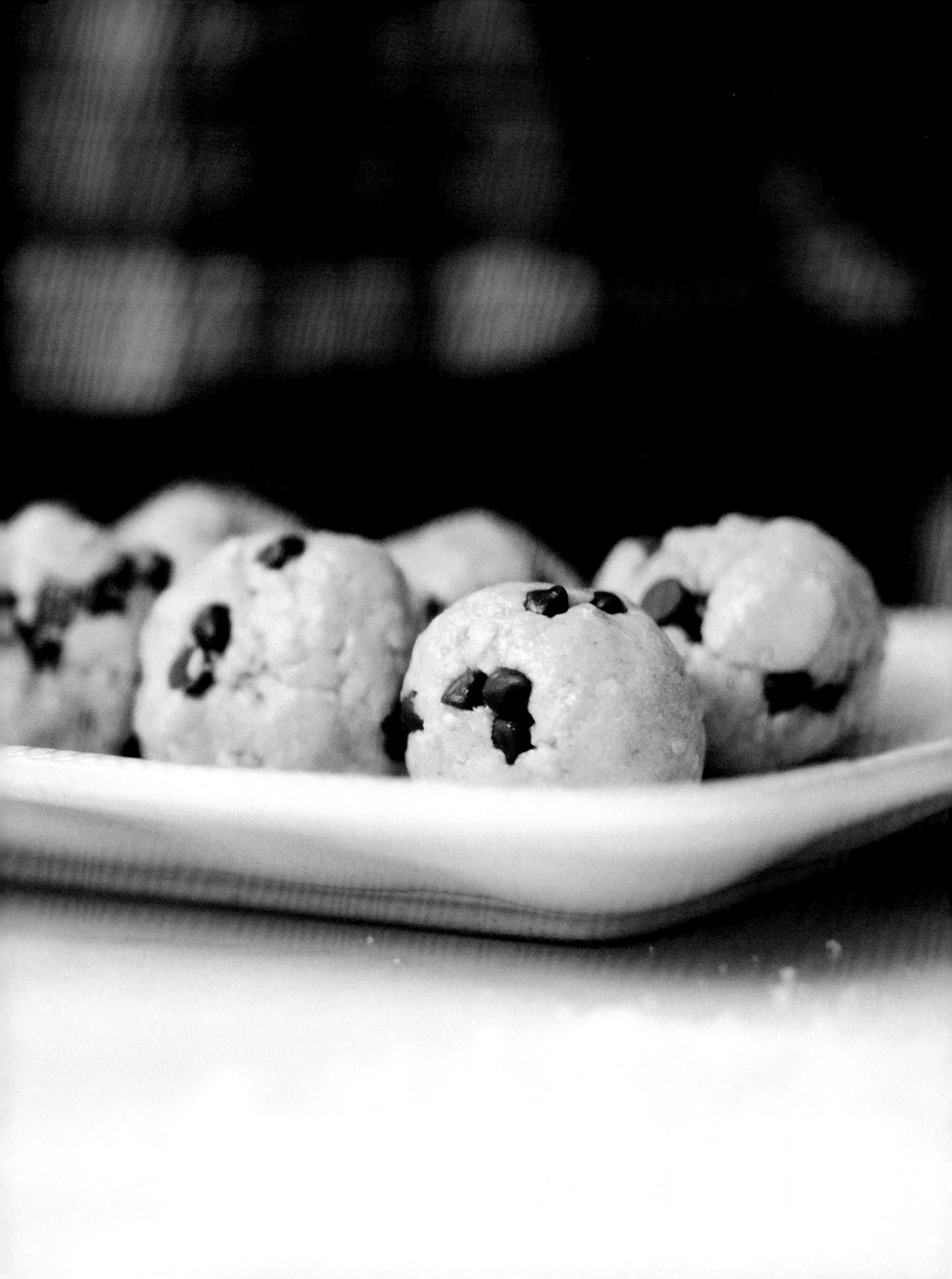

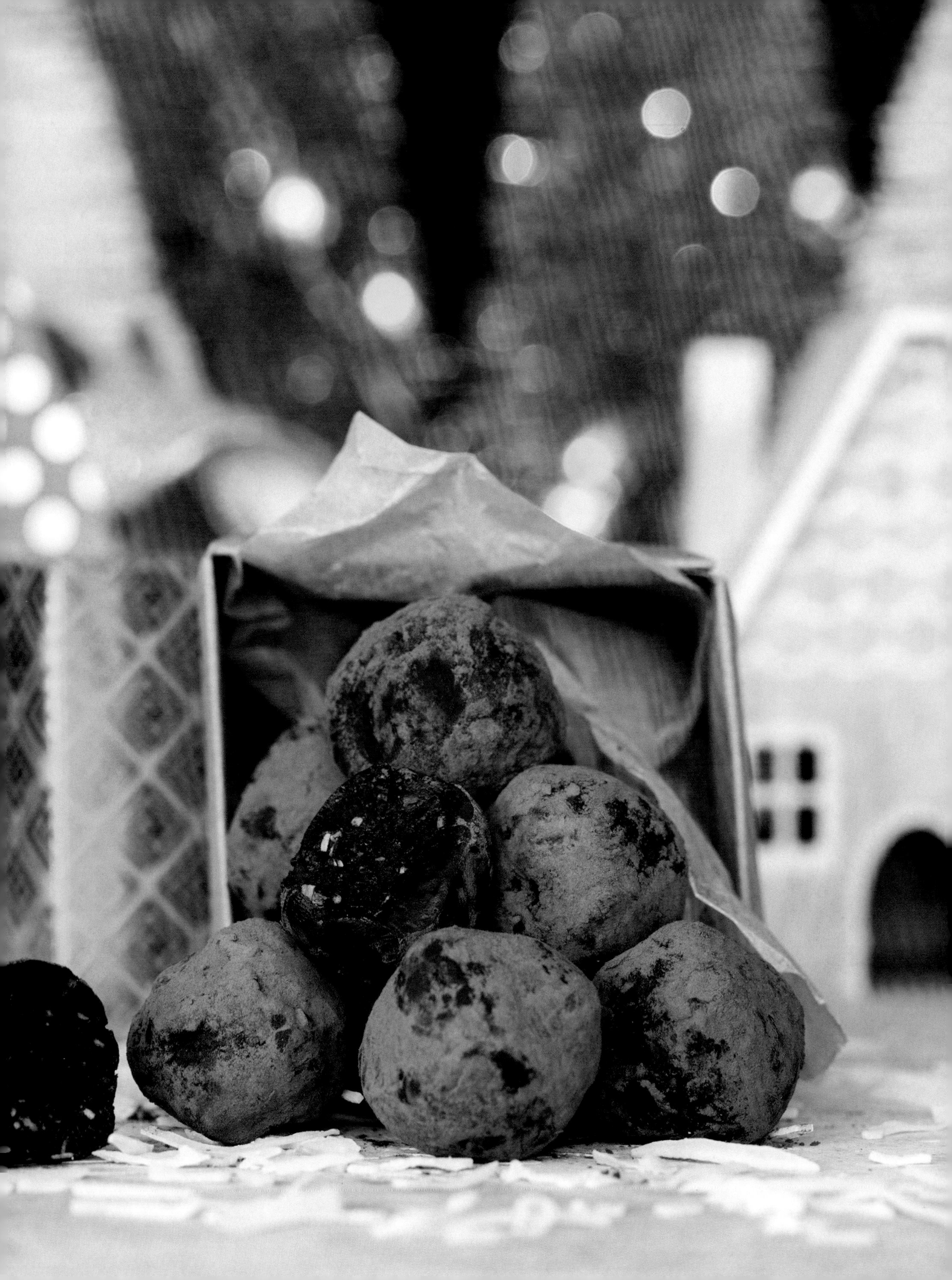

COCOA TRUFFLES

Dairy-Free, Gluten-Free, Grain-Free, Paleo (Adaptable for Vegan)

PREP 45 minutes | COOK 0 minutes | TOTAL 45 minutes | MAKES 5 dozen truffles

The recipe for these cocoa truffles was inspired by Honey Mama's chocolate bars. The Honey Mama's version is one of my favorite sweet treats made with whole healthy ingredients. If you haven't tried it, I highly recommend doing so soon. It is made without refined sugar, gluten, dairy or soy. You can find it in the refrigerated section of Fresh Thyme and some co-ops and natural grocery stores and at honeymamas.com.

I was working on a dairy-free and refined-sugar-free chocolate truffle recipe and thought I would try using the ingredients listed on the Honey Mama's bars. I created several batches using different ratios of the ingredients and finally landed on one I loved. This is a great homemade treat for gifting or enjoying yourself. To adapt for vegan, substitute pure maple syrup for honey.

INGREDIENTS

1 cup unsweetened shredded coconut

1/2 cup coconut oil

1 cup local raw honey

1/3 cup cashew or almond butter

2 teaspoons vanilla

3/4 teaspoon pink Himalayan sea salt

2 cups Dutch process cocoa powder

Extra cocoa powder, for coating the truffles

DIRECTIONS

1. Place the coconut in a small food processor or blender and blend until it is chopped fine. Set aside.
2. Using a hand or stand-up mixer, whip the coconut oil and honey until light and creamy.
3. Add the cashew or almond butter, vanilla and Himalayan sea salt and mix well.
4. Add the coconut and blend until well combined.
5. Using a spatula, fold in the cocoa powder before running the mixer again. This will help keep the cocoa powder from flying all over your kitchen.
6. Mix the ingredients well.
7. Chill the mixture in the refrigerator until firm.
8. Take a tablespoon-sized scoop of the chocolate mixture and roll into a ball.
9. Roll the ball in the extra cocoa powder and repeat until all of the chocolate is gone.
10. Store in an airtight container in the refrigerator for 1-2 weeks or in the freezer for 1 month.

HONEY ALMOND BRITTLE

Dairy-Free, Gluten-Free, Grain-Free, Paleo, SCD

PREP 5 minutes | COOK 18 minutes | TOTAL 23 minutes* | MAKES about 20 pieces

Growing up, peanut brittle was a treat we had during Christmastime. When I first learned to make it, I was amazed by how the addition of baking soda made the hot liquid sugar mixture puff up, causing the candy to be light and airy once it cooled. Science in the kitchen. As an adult, when I was following the Specific Carbohydrate Diet, the only sweetener I could have was honey. I experimented with creating treats using honey in place of sugar. Honey almond brittle is one of the recipes I came up with. This version has almond butter and almonds, which makes it paleo compliant, but you can substitute peanut butter and peanuts if you prefer. I also add a little cayenne pepper in the recipe to give it some kick. (Not too much!) You can omit it if you want a more traditional flavor.

**Does not include setting time, which is noted in the directions.*

INGREDIENTS

1 cup honey

1/4 cup almond butter

2 Tablespoons butter or ghee

1 cup toasted slivered almonds

1 teaspoon vanilla

1/2 teaspoon salt

1/4 teaspoon cayenne, optional

1 teaspoon baking soda

DIRECTIONS

1. Pour the honey into a medium-sized saucepan and place over low to medium-low heat.
2. Cook for 16-18 minutes or until it reaches 315 degrees on a candy thermometer.
3. Turn off the stove and add the almond butter, butter or ghee, almonds, vanilla, salt and cayenne.
4. Add the baking soda and stir.
5. Pour the bubbling mixture onto a parchment-lined baking sheet, spreading evenly.
6. Cool in the refrigerator or freezer until hardened.
7. Break into large pieces.
8. Store in an airtight container in the refrigerator.

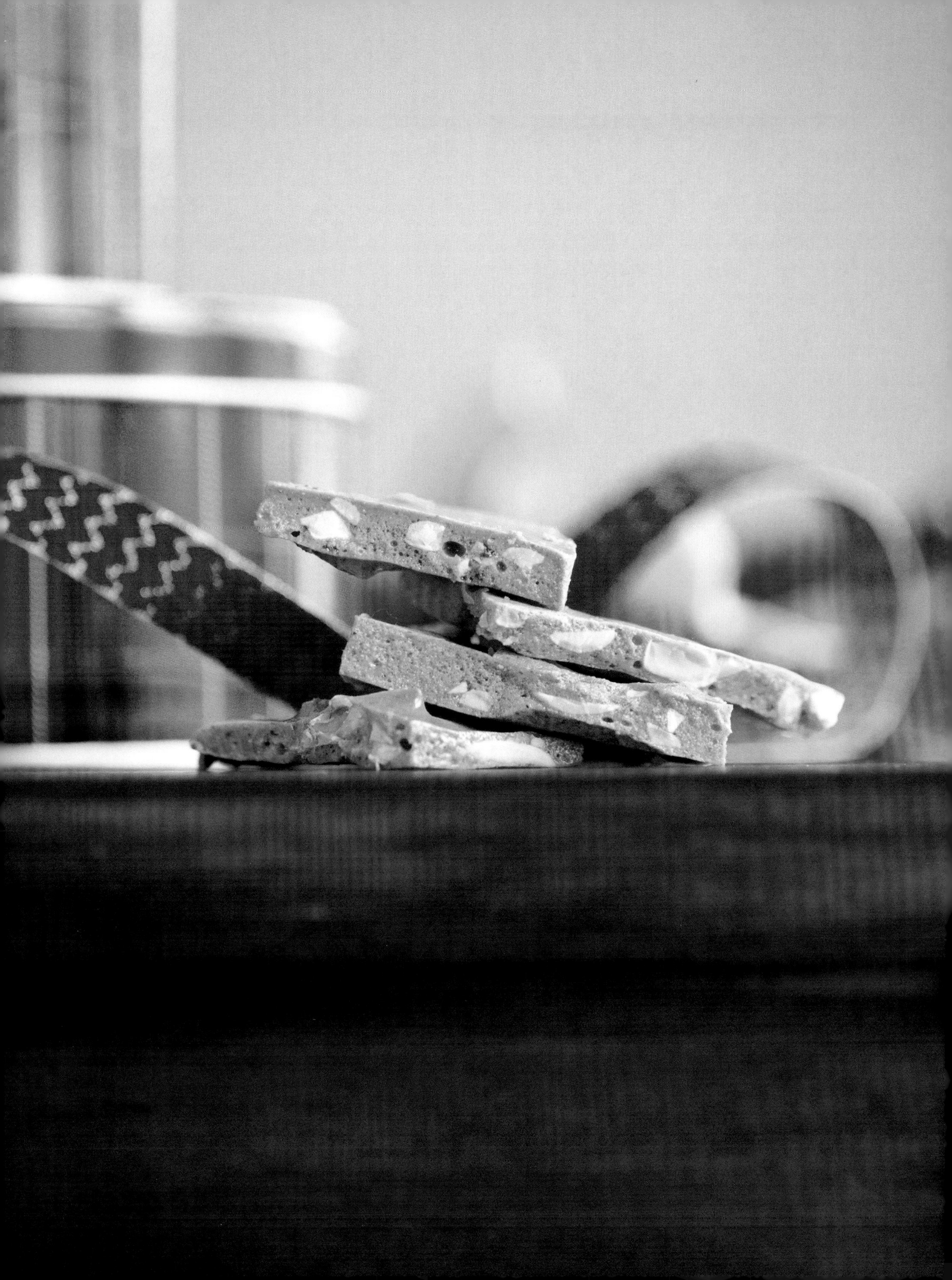

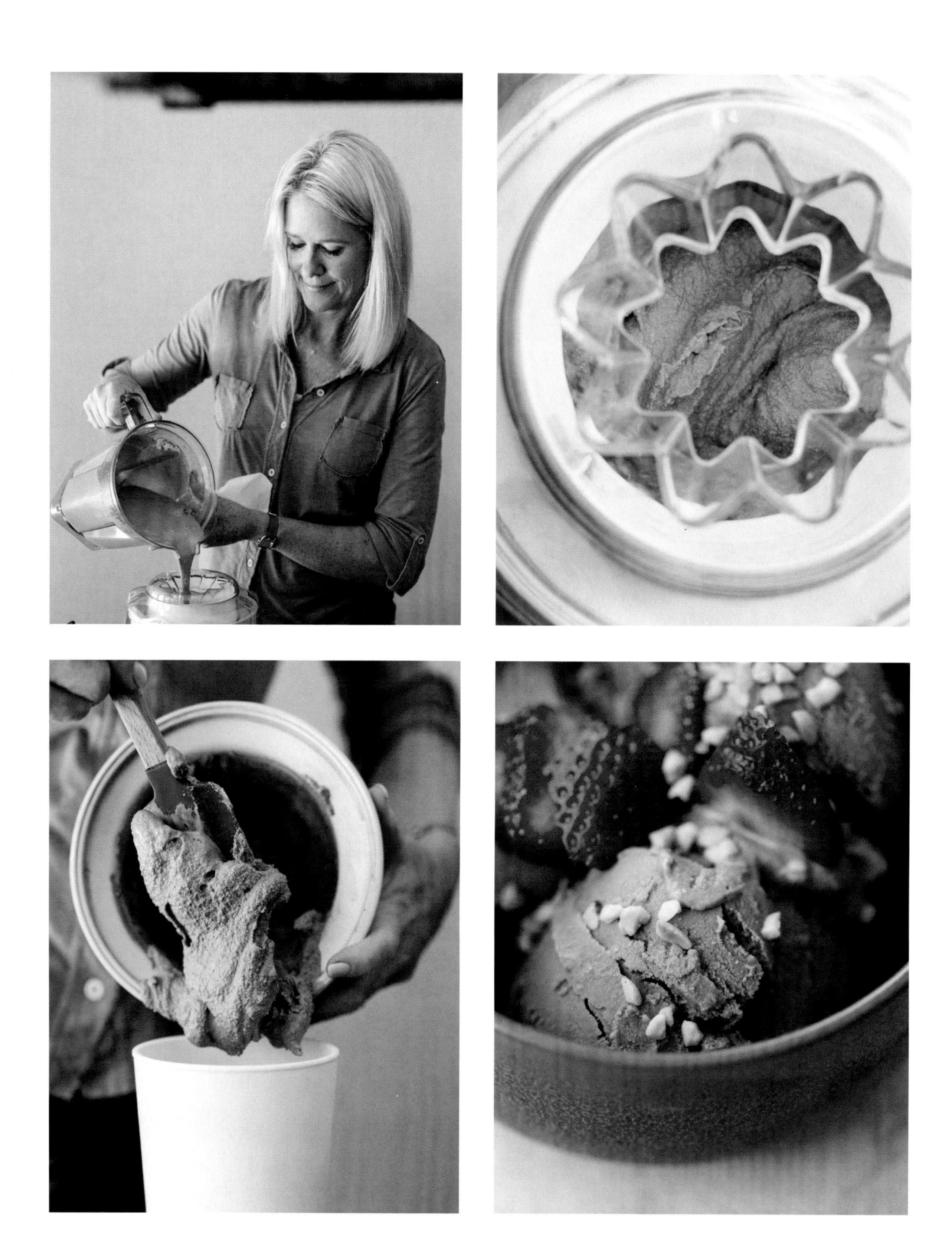

CASHEW CHOCOLATE ICE CREAM

Dairy-Free, Gluten-Free, Grain-Free, Paleo, Vegan

PREP 35 minutes | COOK 0 minutes | TOTAL 35 minutes* | MAKES 1 quart of ice cream

The cashews in this dairy-free ice cream give it an incredibly creamy texture, making it difficult to tell that it is dairy-free. It is hard to believe that a few simple ingredients can produce this delicious healthy treat! After you have finished freezing the ice cream in your ice cream maker, it's usually the texture of soft serve ice cream. You can eat it right away or store in the freezer for later. When stored in the freezer, it will harden a lot more than store-bought ice cream because it is not whipped and aerated the way commercially produced ice cream is. Set it out on the counter for 20-30 minutes before serving or zap it in the microwave to soften.

**Does not include soaking time, which is noted in the directions.*

DIRECTIONS

1. Place the cashews in a medium bowl and cover with filtered water.
2. Loosely cover and soak the cashews at room temperature for 6 hours or in the refrigerator overnight.
3. Fill a blender with 2 cups of chilled filtered water.
4. Drain the cashews and add them to the blender.
5. Add the maple syrup, cacao, sea salt and vanilla.
6. Blend on high until smooth and creamy.
7. Pour the mixture into an ice cream maker following the manufacturer's directions.
8. It should take about 20-30 minutes to reach the consistency of soft serve ice cream.
9. Serve immediately or store in an airtight container in the freezer.

INGREDIENTS

2 cups raw cashews

2 cups filtered water plus more for soaking cashews

3/4 cup pure maple syrup

1/2 cup raw cacao powder

1/4 teaspoon sea salt

1 Tablespoon real vanilla extract

PEANUT BUTTER MOLTEN CAKES

Dairy-Free, Gluten-Free, Grain-Free, SCD

PREP 5 minutes | COOK 25 minutes | TOTAL 30 minutes | SERVES 4

When I was following the Specific Carbohydrate Diet, it was difficult to find a sweet treat that met the diet's rigorous guidelines. While searching the internet for SCD-approved dessert recipes, I came across several flourless peanut butter brownie recipes made with eggs, honey and natural peanut butter. I tried a few versions and discovered that I enjoyed them the most when they were still warm.

I decided to tweak the same basic ingredients and make molten peanut butter cakes reminiscent of the molten chocolate cakes I would occasionally order for dessert at a restaurant before following the diet. They turned out great and satisfied my sweet tooth while still following the SCD guidelines. Today when I make them I add a little dark chocolate to the center of the cakes. Both versions make a delicious grain-free and dairy-free dessert.

INGREDIENTS

2 eggs

1 egg yolk

1 cup natural peanut butter

2/3 cup honey

1 teaspoon vanilla

1/2 teaspoon baking soda

1/4 teaspoon sea salt

4 Tablespoons chopped dairy-free dark chocolate, optional

DIRECTIONS

1. Preheat oven to 350 degrees.
2. Lightly grease 4 6-ounce ramekins and place on a sheet pan.
3. Using a hand or stand-up mixer, whip the 2 eggs and 1 egg yolk on high speed for 2 minutes.
4. Add the peanut butter, honey, vanilla, baking soda and sea salt. Mix until well combined.
5. Fill each ramekin 1/3 full with the peanut butter batter.
6. If using the chocolate, add 1 Tablespoon of chopped dark chocolate to each ramekin.
7. Fill to 2/3 full with remaining batter.
8. Bake for 25 minutes or until golden brown. The top and edges should be firm like a brownie and the inside warm and gooey.
9. Let cool for 5 minutes and serve.

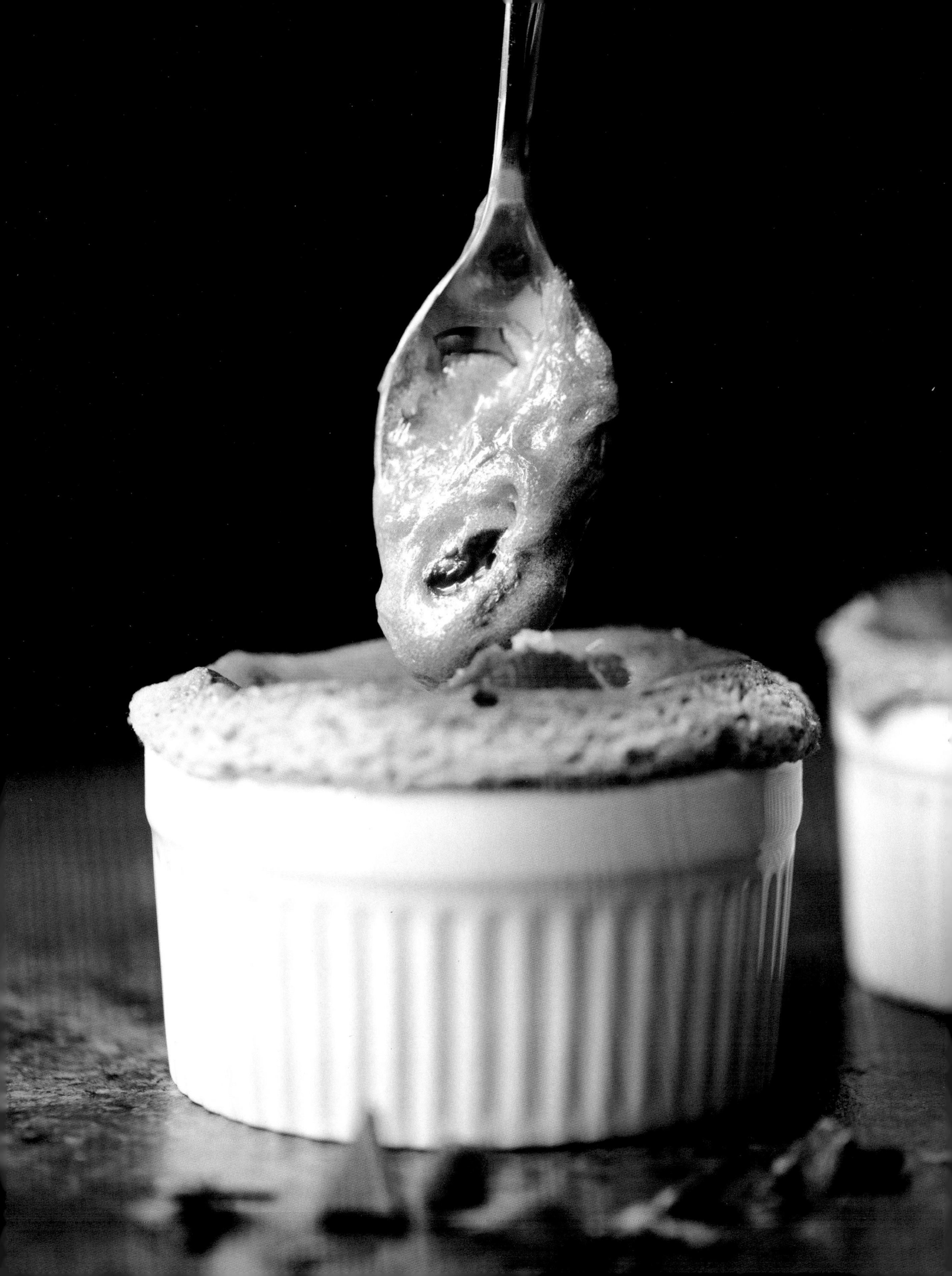

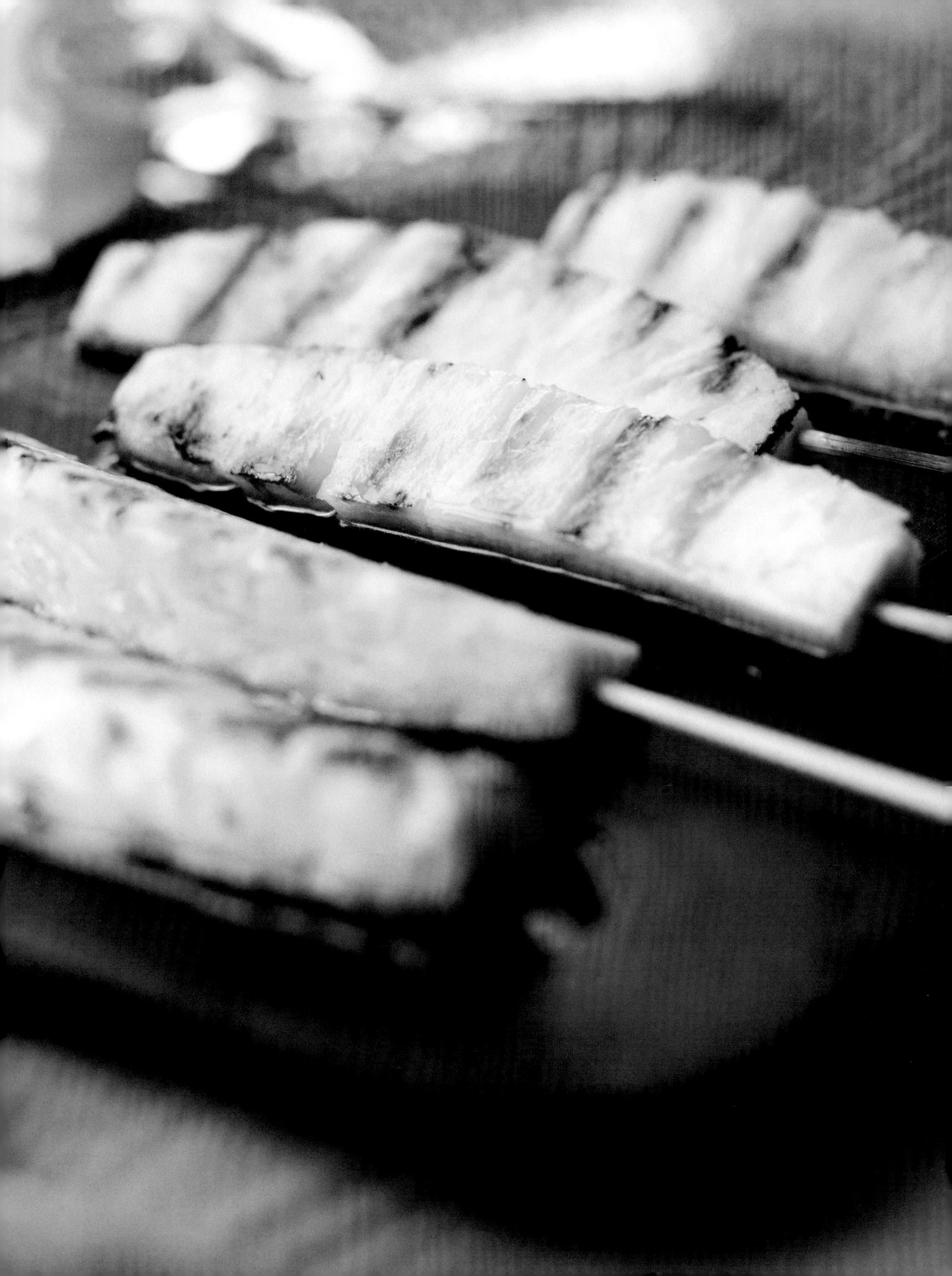

GRILLED PINEAPPLE

Gluten-Free, Grain-Free, SCD (Adaptable for Paleo)

PREP 10 minutes | COOK 10 minutes | TOTAL 20 minutes | MAKES 1 dozen skewers

Grilled pineapple is a simple, healthy dessert that is easy to prepare. Cooking pineapple on a hot grill makes the already sweet fruit warm, soft and extra juicy. The addition of honey and a little butter gives it a nice caramel flavor. If using bamboo skewers, soak them in warm water for 30 minutes or longer before using. This will keep them from catching fire and burning up on the grill. To adapt for paleo, substitute ghee for butter.

INGREDIENTS

1 whole ripe pineapple

12 bamboo or other skewers

1/2 cup honey

2 Tablespoons butter

DIRECTIONS

1. Slice off the top and bottom of the pineapple.
2. Turn the pineapple upright on the cutting board.
3. Using a serrated knife, cut off the rough skin following the shape of the pineapple.
4. Cut the pineapple lengthwise into quarters.
5. Cut the core off of each quarter.
6. Cut each quarter into 3 spears.
7. Skewer each pineapple spear lengthwise onto a skewer.
8. Preheat the grill to medium-high and lightly oil the grates.
9. Place the honey and butter in a saucepan and warm over medium heat until the butter has melted and they are well combined.
10. Brush the honey mixture onto all sides of each pineapple spear.
11. Grill the pineapple for 4-5 minutes per side until golden brown.

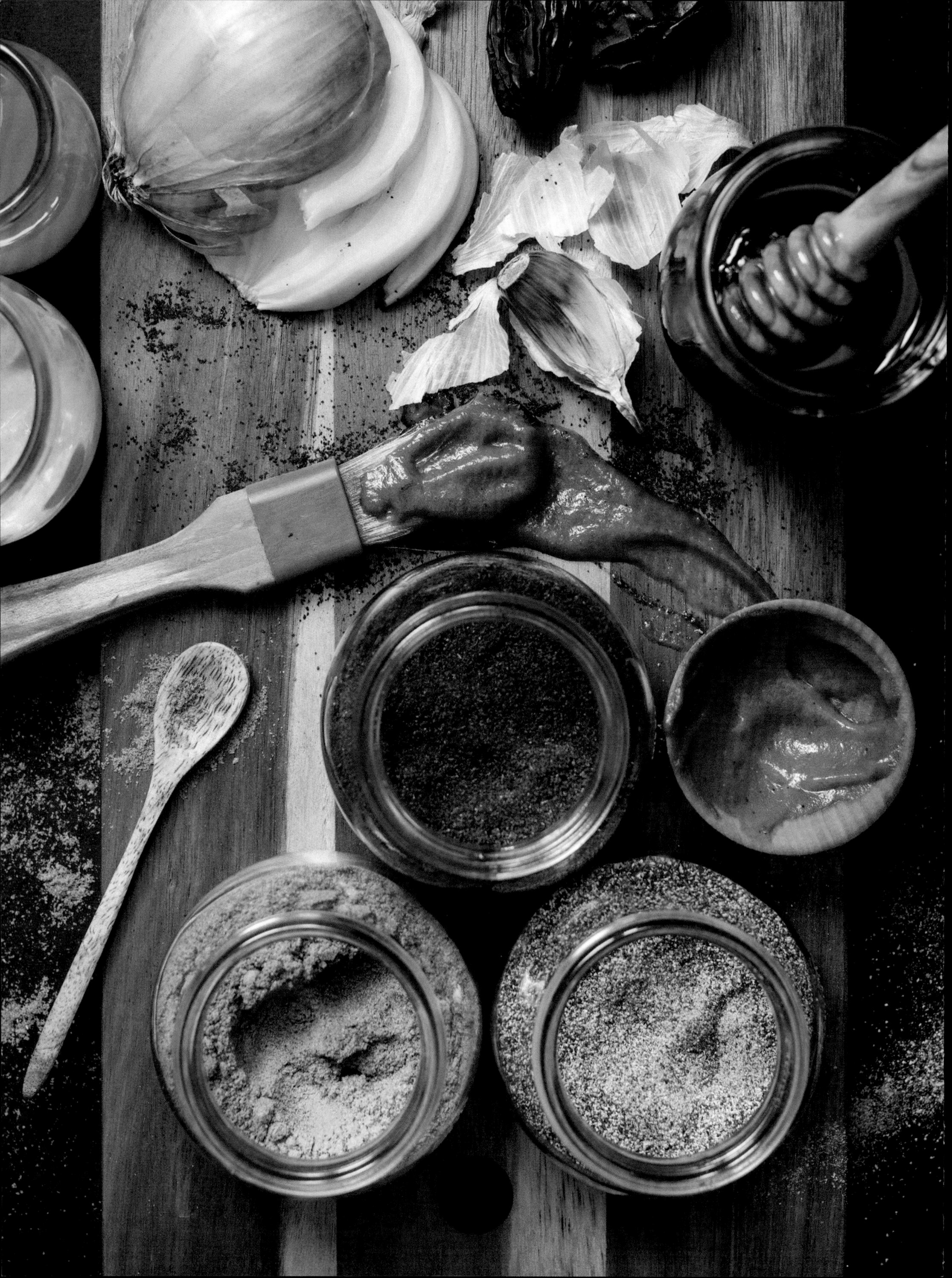

BASICS, CONDIMENTS, DRESSINGS AND SPICE BLENDS

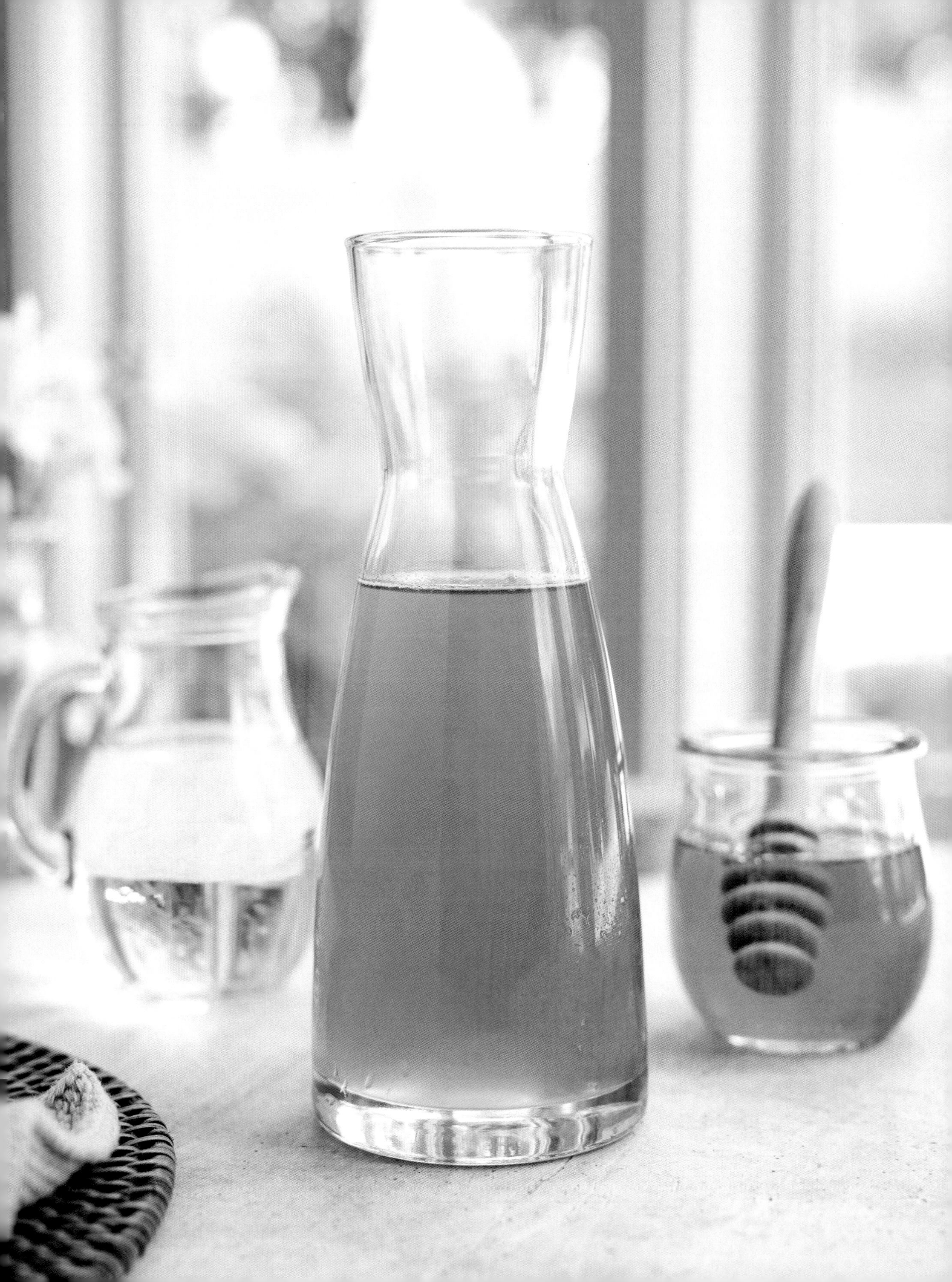

HONEY SIMPLE SYRUP

Dairy-Free, Gluten-Free, Grain-Free, Paleo, SCD

PREP 0 minutes | COOK 5 minutes | TOTAL 5 minutes | MAKES about 2 cups

When I was following the Specific Carbohydrate Diet, honey was the only sweetener allowed. Honey is a monosaccharide, which is easily absorbed during digestion and fits in the strict guidelines of the diet. It continues to be my sweetener of choice. As another benefit, raw honey contains antioxidants and anti-inflammatory properties. Research has also shown that local raw honey helps with seasonal allergies, too. I like to have this simple syrup on hand for sweetening cold liquids and drinks where honey on its own doesn't dissolve well.

INGREDIENTS

2 cups local raw honey

1 cup water

DIRECTIONS

1. Combine honey and water in a saucepan over medium heat.
2. Bring to a simmer and then remove from heat and let cool.
3. Store in an airtight container in the refrigerator for up to 2 weeks.

GHEE

Gluten-Free, Grain-Free, Paleo, SCD

PREP 5 minutes | COOK 20 minutes | TOTAL 25 minutes | MAKES 1 1/2 cups

Ghee (also known as clarified butter) is a great lactose-free and casein-free cooking fat. Ghee is made by cooking butter to separate and remove the milk solids. It's a nice option for people who are sensitive to dairy but still want the flavor of butter in their cooking. Ghee has wonderful flavor and a high smoke point, making it the perfect choice for high-heat cooking.

INGREDIENTS

1 pound unsalted grass-fed butter

DIRECTIONS

1. Melt the butter over medium-low heat and simmer gently.
2. Bubbles will start to form and a foam will emerge on top. Skim off the foam as it forms.
3. At about 10-15 minutes after it starts bubbling, the milk solids will brown and fall to the bottom of the pan.
4. Remove the pan from the heat.
5. Line a strainer with a few layers of cheesecloth or a clean fine dishcloth.
6. Strain the butter through and discard the browned milk solids.
7. Store in an airtight container at room temperature for 1 month or in the refrigerator for up to 1 year.

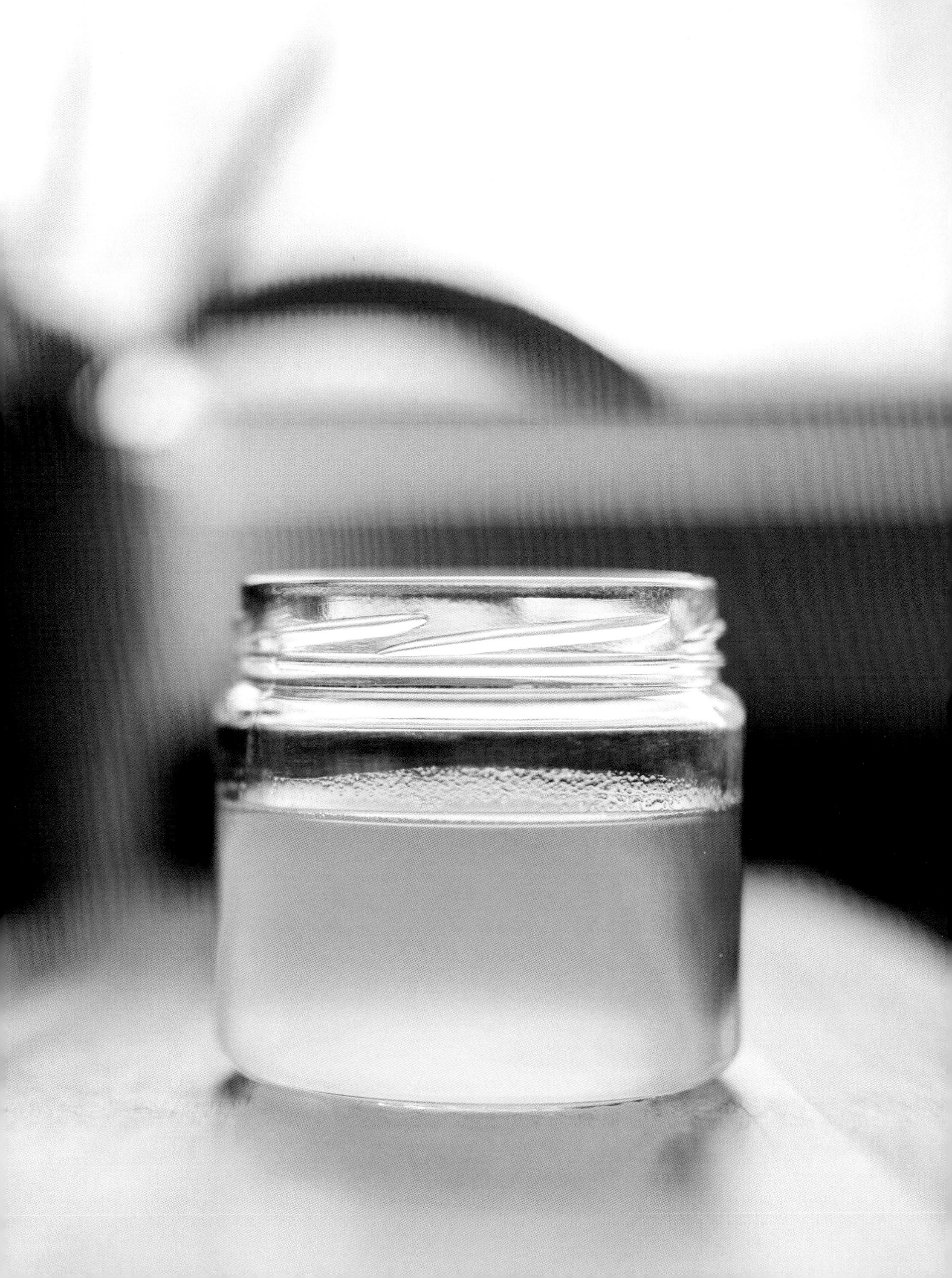

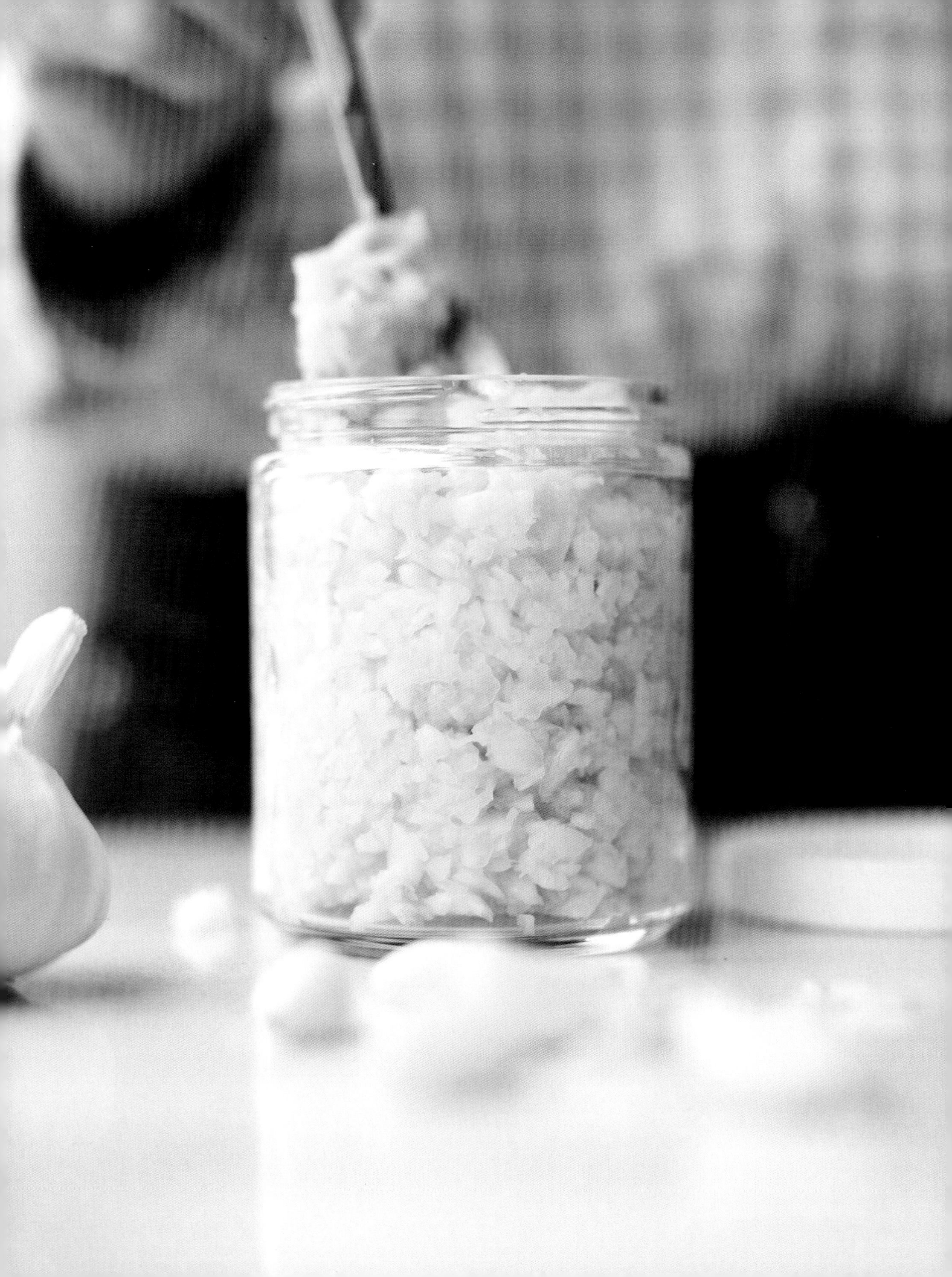

MINCED GARLIC

Dairy-Free, Gluten-Free, Grain-Free, Paleo, SCD, Vegan

PREP 5 minutes | COOK 0 minutes | TOTAL 5 minutes | MAKES 1/2 cup

I love garlic and use it often in my cooking. To save time, I like to prep it ahead and store it in the refrigerator. To store longer than a week, you can scoop the minced garlic into an ice cube tray and place the tray in the freezer until set. Then transfer the frozen cubes of garlic to a freezer bag or container and return it to the freezer.

INGREDIENTS

3/4 cup garlic cloves
1/2 teaspoon sea salt
Olive oil

DIRECTIONS

1. Place peeled garlic cloves and salt in a mini food processor.
2. Add enough olive oil to lightly cover the cloves.
3. Pulse the food processor until the garlic is minced.
4. Transfer the minced garlic to a glass jar and top with olive oil.
5. Store in an airtight container in the refrigerator for up to 1 week. Minced garlic cubes will last in the freezer for 3 months.

CHIMICHURRI

Dairy-Free, Gluten-Free, Grain-Free, Paleo, SCD, Vegan

PREP 5 minutes | COOK 0 minutes | TOTAL 5 minutes | MAKES 1 1/2 cups

Chimichurri is an uncooked sauce that originated in Argentina. It is made with fresh parsley, garlic and red pepper flakes. In my version I like to include cilantro. This recipe is easy to make and goes well with grilled meats, fish and vegetables.

INGREDIENTS

1 cup of fresh cilantro

1 cup of fresh flat-leaf parsley

5 cloves garlic, minced

1 Tablespoon cumin

1 teaspoon salt

1 teaspoon crushed red pepper flakes

3 Tablespoons fresh lemon juice

3/4 cup olive oil

DIRECTIONS

1. Place all the ingredients in a food processor and blend for 30 seconds.
2. Scrape down the sides of the food processor bowl.
3. Blend again for another 30 seconds.
4. Serve immediately or refrigerate.
5. If refrigerated, bring to room temperature before serving.
6. Store in an airtight container in the refrigerator for up to 3 days.

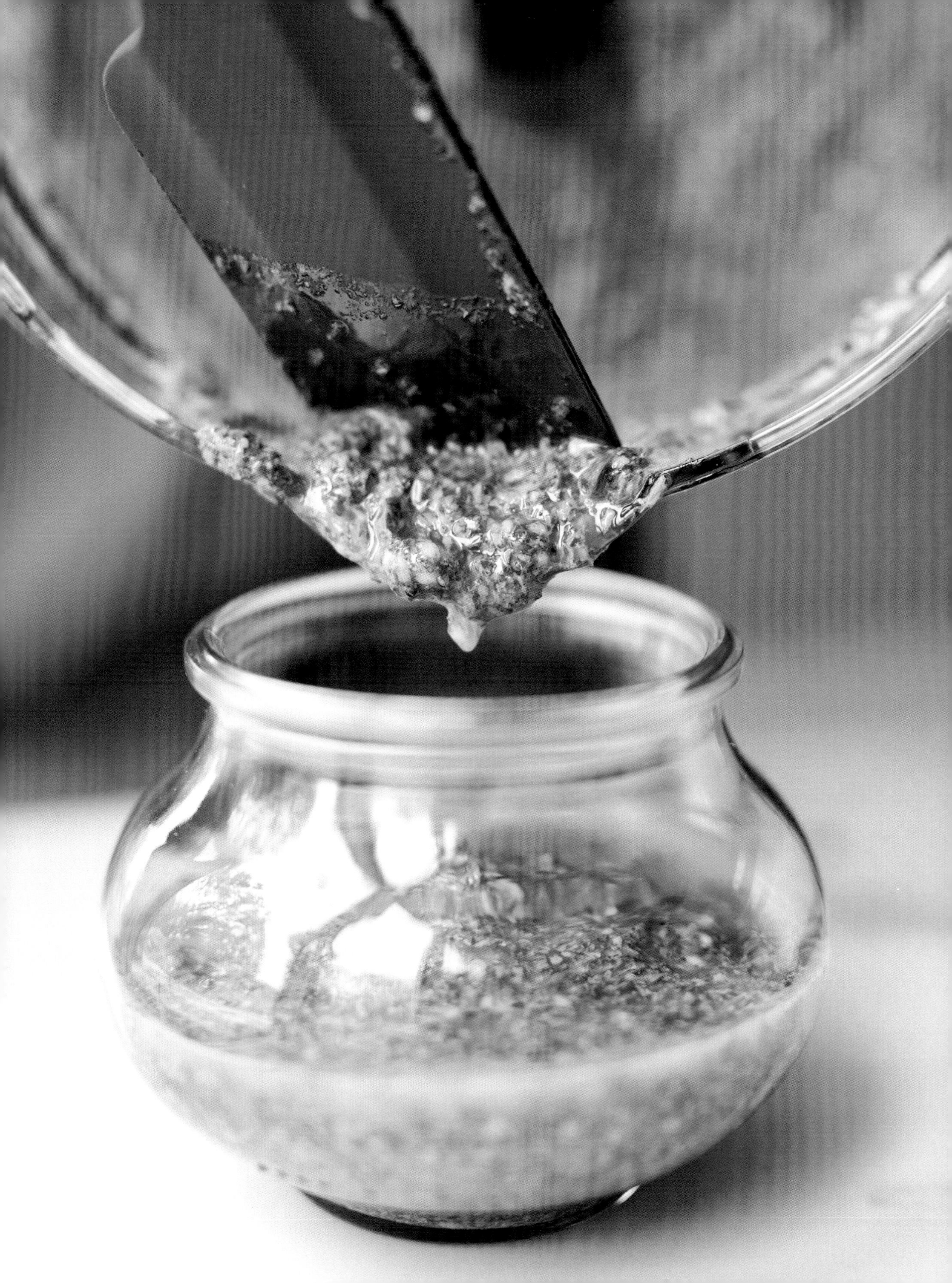

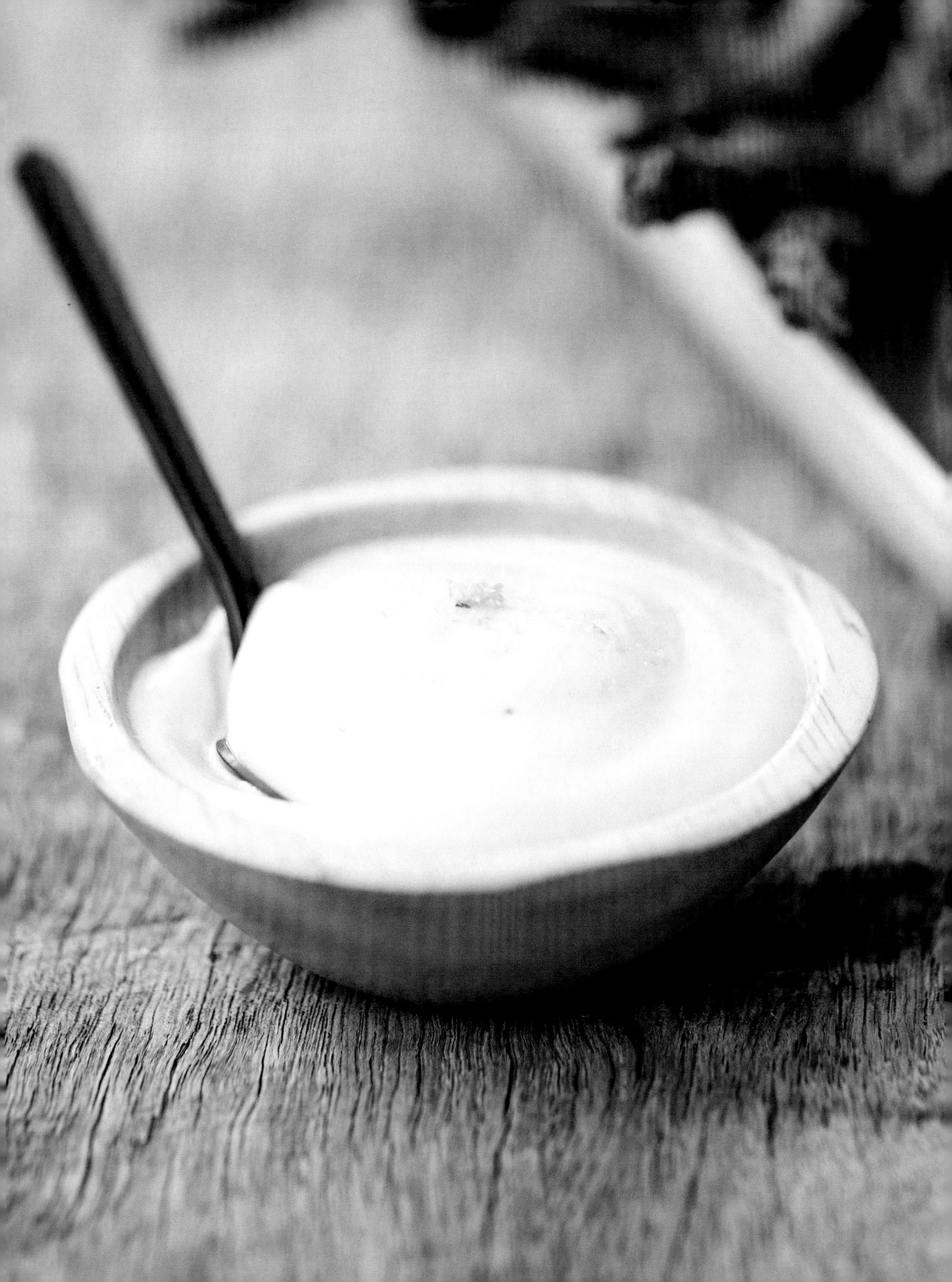

LEMONY AQUAFABA

Dairy-Free, Gluten-Free, Grain-Free, Vegan

PREP 5 minutes | COOK 0 minutes | TOTAL 5 minutes | MAKES 1 cup

Aquafaba is the liquid left over from cooked chickpeas. It has the consistency of egg whites and is often used as an egg substitute in vegan cooking. I use it to make a lemony sauce that reminds me of hollandaise. Serve it with grilled vegetables or any dish that could benefit from a lemony plant-based condiment.

INGREDIENTS

1/4 cup aquafaba from a can of chickpeas

1 Tablespoon fresh lemon juice

1/2 teaspoon sea salt

1/8 teaspoon cayenne pepper

3/4 cup olive oil

DIRECTIONS

1. Drain can of chickpeas, reserving 1/4 cup of aquafaba.
2. Place aquafaba, lemon juice, sea salt and cayenne pepper in a mini food processor.
3. With food processor running, slowly add olive oil until combined.
4. Store in an airtight container in the refrigerator for 1 week.

BARBECUE SAUCE

Dairy-Free, Gluten-Free, Grain-Free, Paleo, SCD (Adaptable for Vegan)

PREP 5 minutes | COOK 2 hours 10 minutes | TOTAL 2 hours 15 minutes
MAKES about 6 cups

When I was following the Specific Carbohydrate Diet, I couldn't use bottled condiments and sauces because of the added sugars and other additives, which motivated me to create a barbecue sauce I could use with some of my favorite recipes. I sweeten the sauce with dates and honey and use tomatoes without any added sugars. I still prefer this sauce over bottled sauce. To adapt for vegan, substitute pure maple syrup for honey.

INGREDIENTS

1/4 cup olive oil

2 cups chopped onions

4 teaspoons chopped garlic

1 date, pitted and chopped

1 1/2 teaspoons sea salt

1 teaspoon cumin

1 teaspoon chili powder

1/2 teaspoon black pepper

2 1/2 teaspoons Dijon mustard

1/2 cup honey

1/2 cup apple cider vinegar

1 28-ounce can crushed tomatoes, no added sugar

1 cup water

DIRECTIONS

1. In a saucepan over medium-high heat, sauté the onions in olive oil for 4-5 minutes.
2. Add the garlic and date and sauté for 3 minutes.
3. Add the salt, cumin, chili powder and pepper and mix well.
4. Add Dijon mustard, honey, vinegar, tomatoes and water.
5. Bring to a boil and then simmer over low heat for 2-3 hours.
6. Store in an airtight container in the refrigerator for up to 5 days.

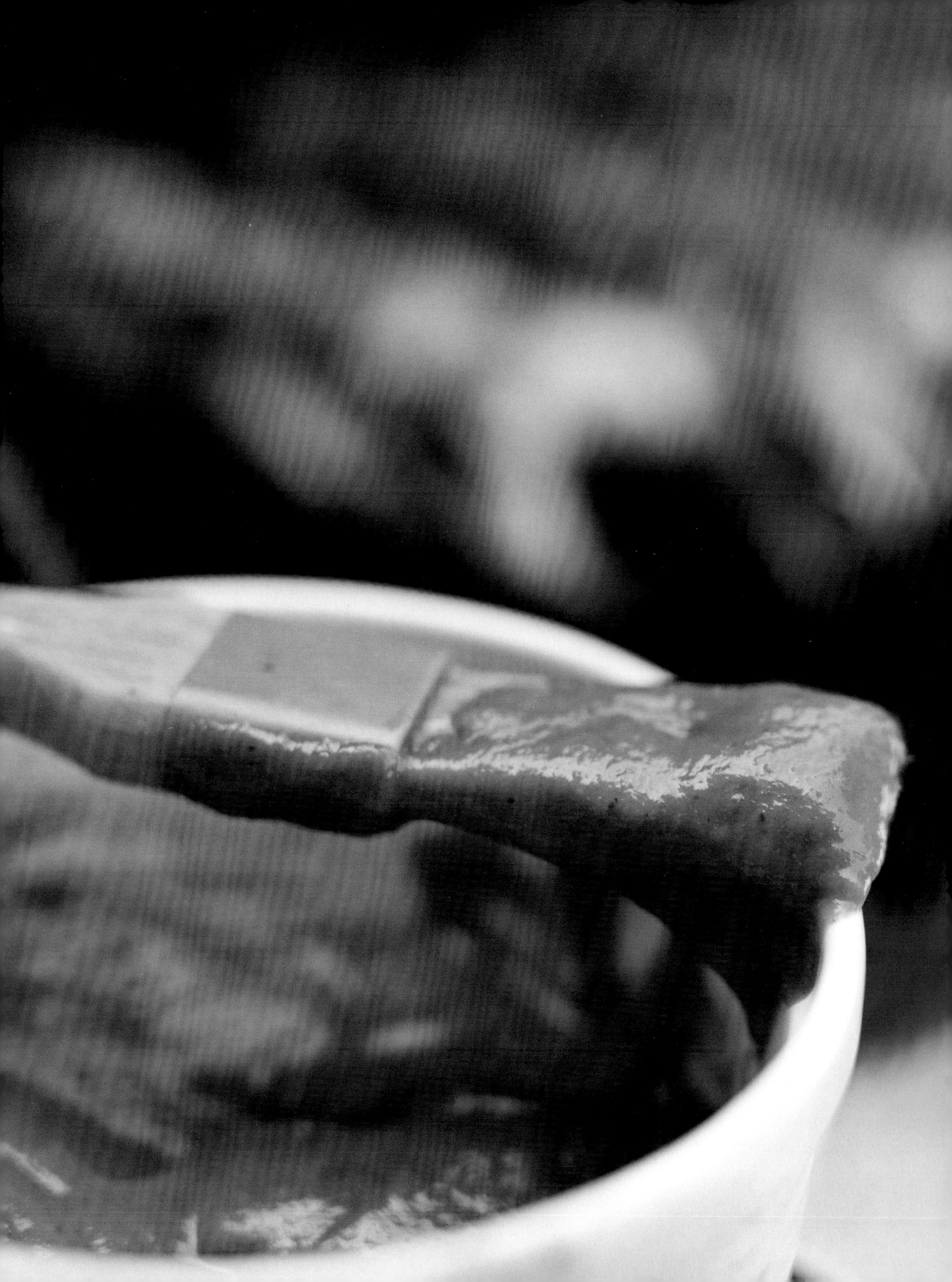

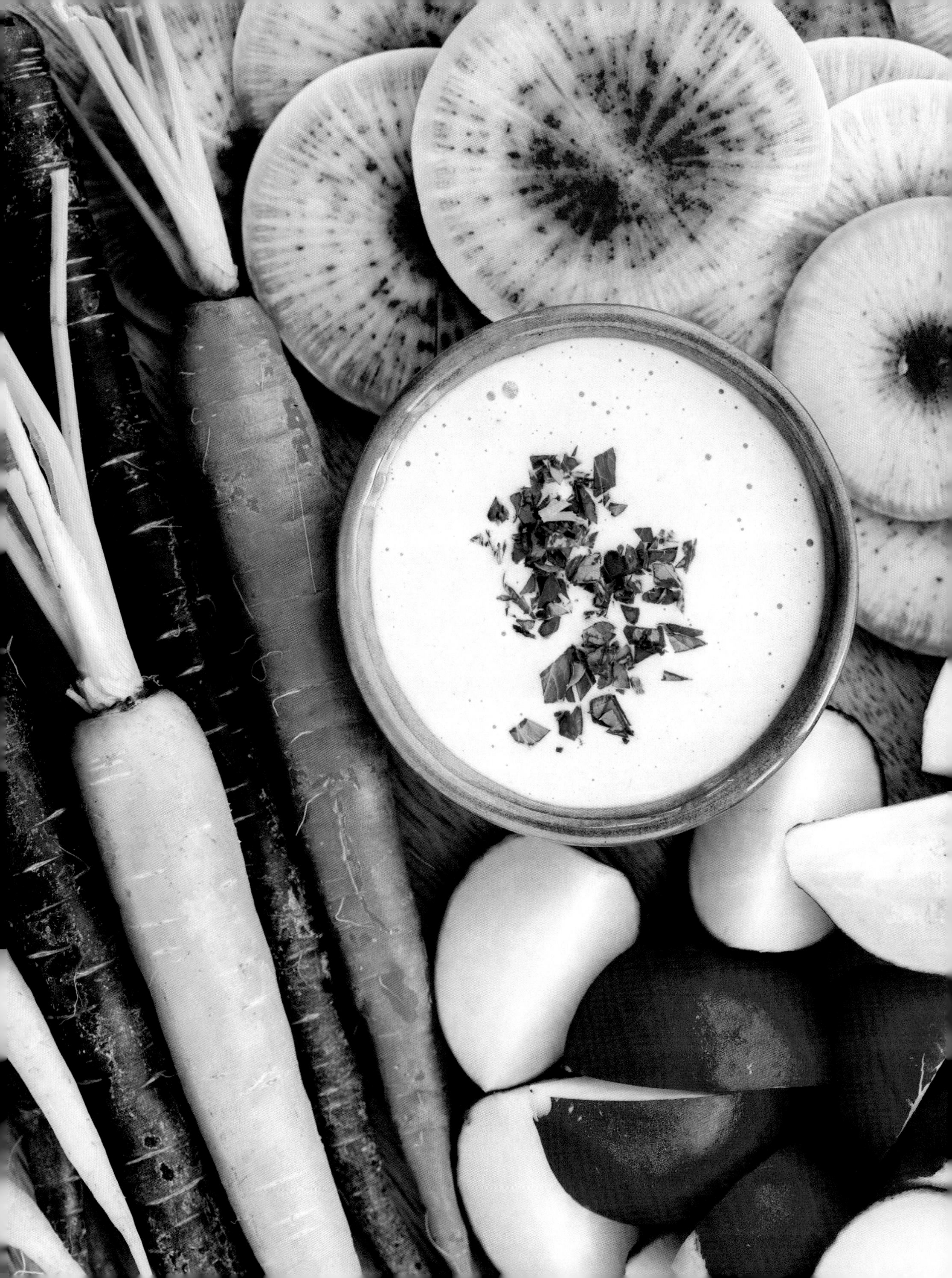

LEMON GARLIC TAHINI

Dairy-Free, Gluten-Free, Grain-Free, Paleo, SCD, Vegan

PREP 5 minutes | COOK 0 minutes | TOTAL 5 minutes | MAKES 1 cup

Tahini is a traditional Middle Eastern sauce made from ground toasted sesame seeds. Adding a few flavorful ingredients to it creates a delicious and versatile condiment. This version is tasty as a salad dressing or dip. It is also lovely drizzled over grilled meats, roasted vegetables and grain bowls. This creamy sauce is simple to make, takes very little time and will elevate any dish.

INGREDIENTS

1/2 cup tahini
1/4-1/2 cup water
1/4 cup fresh lemon juice
2 cloves garlic, minced
3/4 teaspoon sea salt
1/2 teaspoon cumin

DIRECTIONS

1. Place all ingredients in a small food processor or blender.
2. Blend until smooth.
3. Adjust the amount of water to achieve desired consistency.
4. Store in an airtight container in the refrigerator for up to 1 week.

TARTAR SAUCE

Dairy-Free, Gluten-Free, Grain-Free, Paleo, SCD (Adaptable for Vegan)

PREP 5 minutes | COOK 0 minutes | TOTAL 5 minutes | MAKES 1 3/4 cups

Homemade tartar sauce is easy to make and tastes much better than the store-bought versions. The dill and lemon juice make it fresh and bright. It is the perfect accompaniment for fish and seafood dishes. To adapt for vegan, use vegan mayonnaise.

INGREDIENTS

1 cup homemade or good-quality mayonnaise

2/3 cup chopped dill pickles (I like Grillo's brand)

1 Tablespoon fresh chopped dill

1 Tablespoon fresh lemon juice

1/4 teaspoon sea salt

1/4 teaspoon black pepper

DIRECTIONS

1. Place all the ingredients in a small bowl and combine.
2. Adjust seasoning to taste.
3. Store in an airtight container in the refrigerator for up to 1 week.

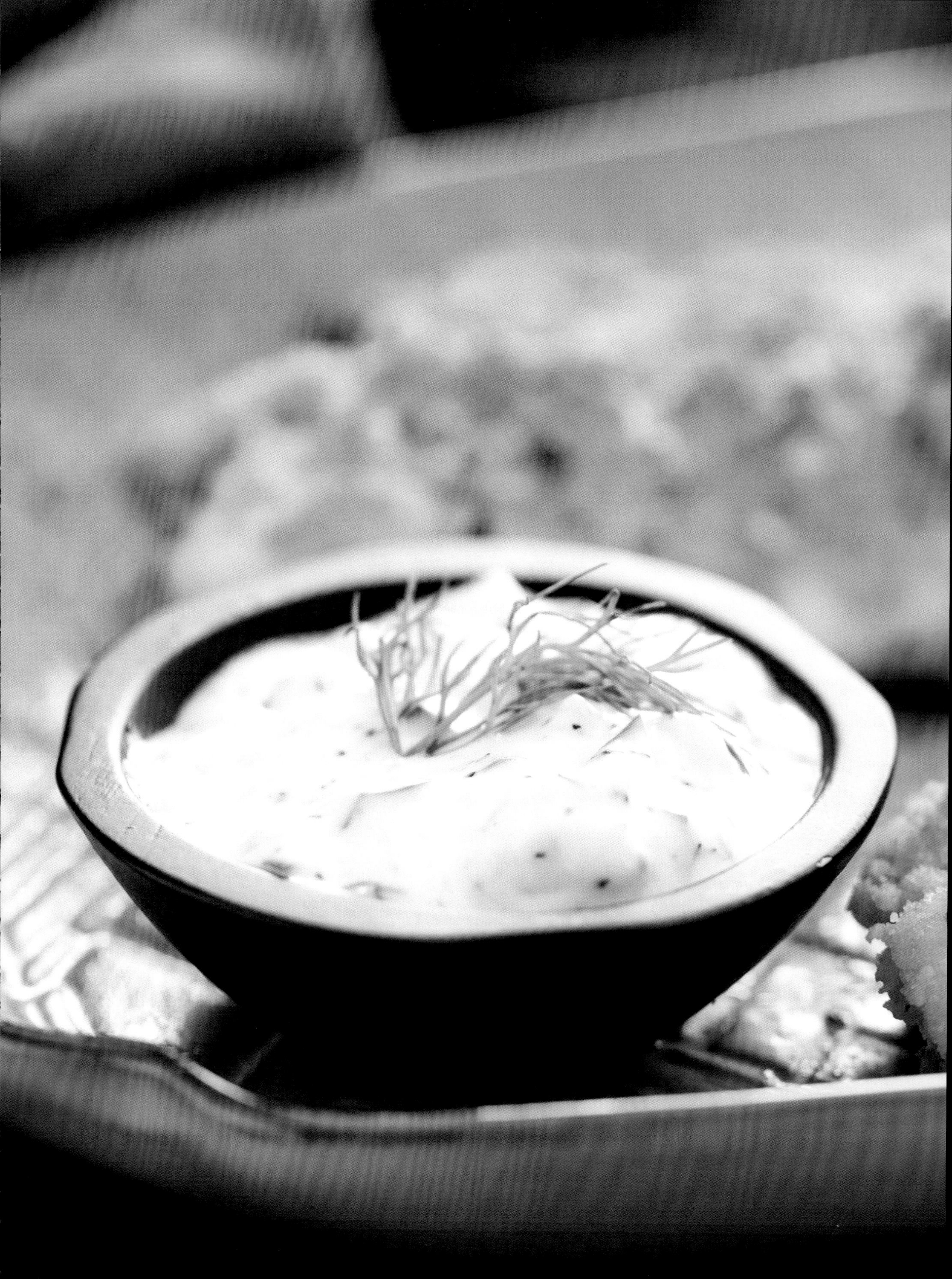

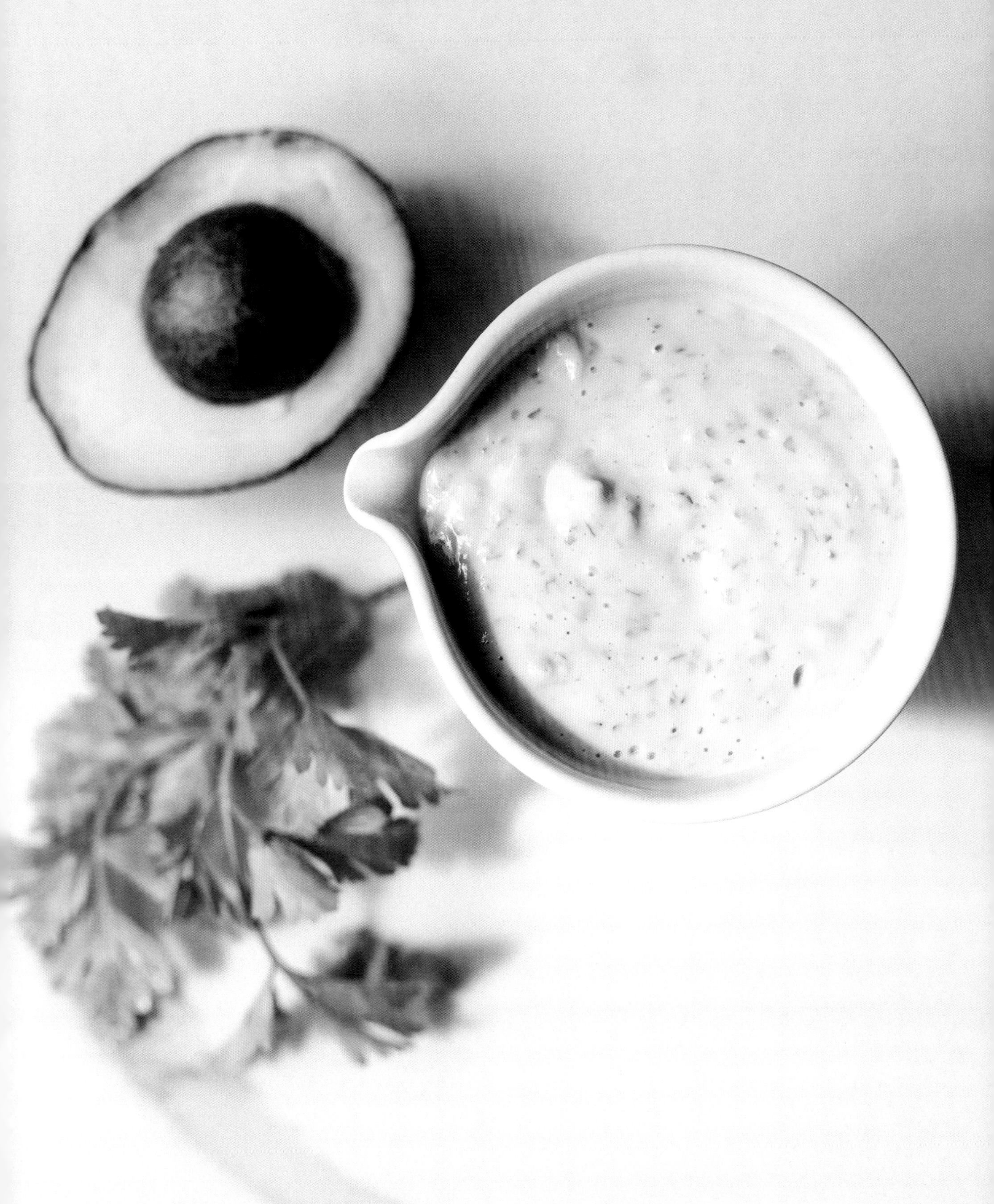

AVOCADO HERB DRESSING

Dairy-Free, Gluten-Free, Grain-Free, Paleo, SCD (Adaptable for Vegan)

PREP 5 minutes | COOK 0 minutes | TOTAL 5 minutes | MAKES about 2 cups

I love that this dressing is creamy, flavorful and very versatile. It works well with leafy green salads and as a dip for vegetables. You can also use it as a spread for wraps and sandwiches. In this recipe, I use parsley, basil and chives, but you can use any combination of fresh herbs you'd like. To adapt for vegan, use vegan mayonnaise.

INGREDIENTS

1 avocado, diced

1/2 cup of homemade or good-quality mayonnaise

1/2 cup fresh parsley leaves

1/4 cup fresh basil leaves

1/4 cup fresh chives

2 garlic cloves, minced

3 Tablespoons lemon juice

1 teaspoon sea salt

1/4 teaspoon white pepper

1/2-3/4 cup water

DIRECTIONS

1. Place all of the ingredients except for the water in a mini food processor and blend well.
2. Gradually add water until you achieve the desired consistency.
3. Store in an airtight container in the refrigerator for up to 5 days.

DAIRY-FREE CILANTRO RANCH

Dairy-Free, Gluten-Free, Grain-Free, Paleo, SCD (Adaptable for Vegan)

PREP 10 minutes | COOK 0 minutes | TOTAL 10 minutes | MAKES 1 1/4 cups

Ranch dressing is an American staple for kids and adults alike. Unfortunately, the bottles lining the shelves in grocery stores are full of processed ingredients and chemical preservatives. Making it from scratch is easy though. This version is dairy-free and seasoned with fresh cilantro, cumin, cayenne and lime juice to give it a Southwestern twist. I like to use it as a dip for vegetables or dressing on Buffalo chicken and taco salads. To adapt for vegan, use vegan mayonnaise.

INGREDIENTS

1/3 cup canned full-fat coconut milk, preferably without guar gum

1/2 cup homemade or good-quality mayonnaise

1/3 cup chopped fresh cilantro

1 Tablespoon minced fresh onion

2 garlic cloves, minced

1 Tablespoon fresh lime juice

1/2 teaspoon cumin

1/8 teaspoon cayenne

1/2 teaspoon sea salt

DIRECTIONS

1. Shake the can of coconut milk vigorously before opening, as the milk can separate.
2. In a small bowl, whisk together the mayonnaise and coconut milk until smooth.
3. Add the remaining ingredients and combine well.
4. Store in an airtight container in the refrigerator for up to 1 week.

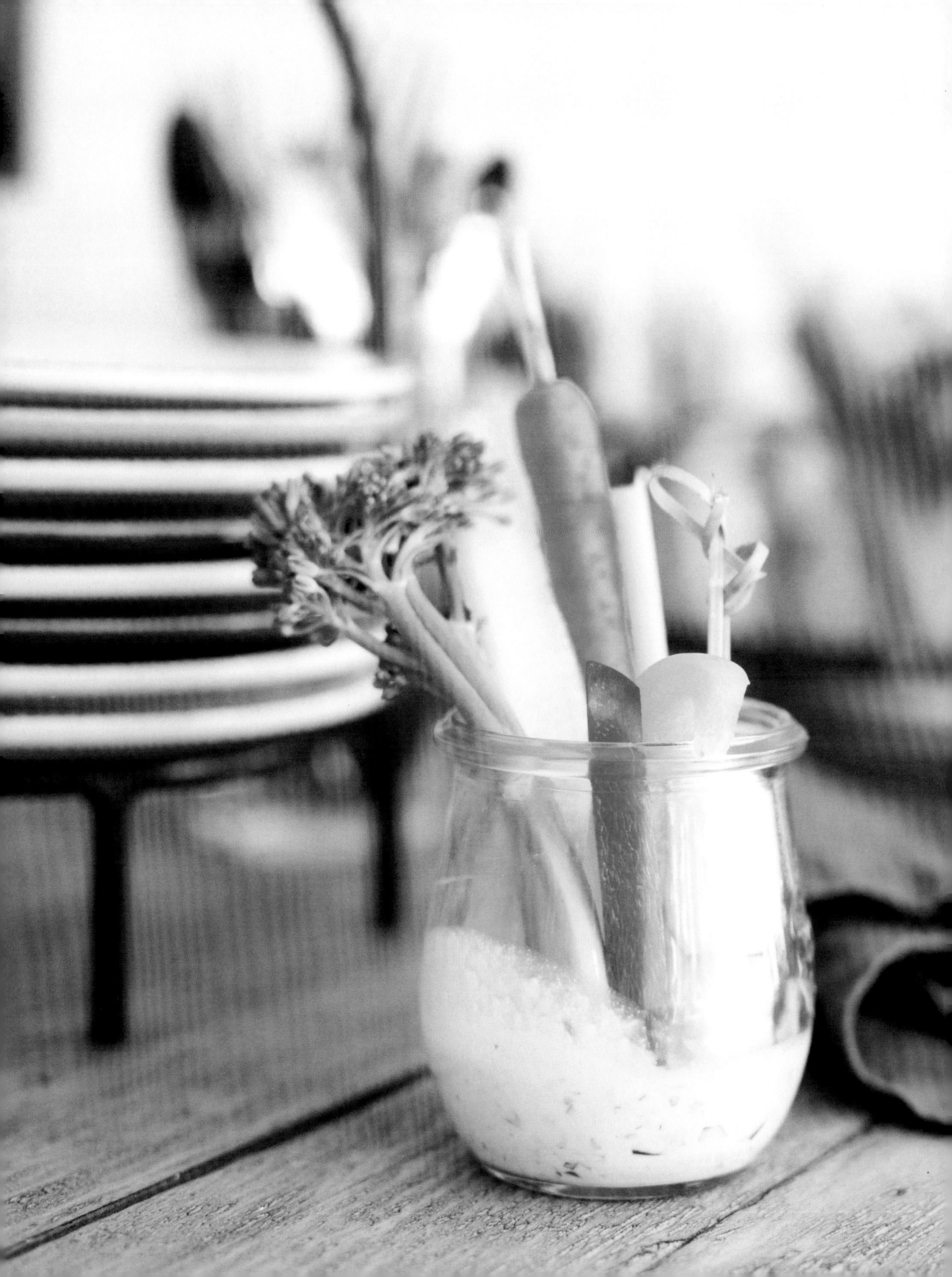

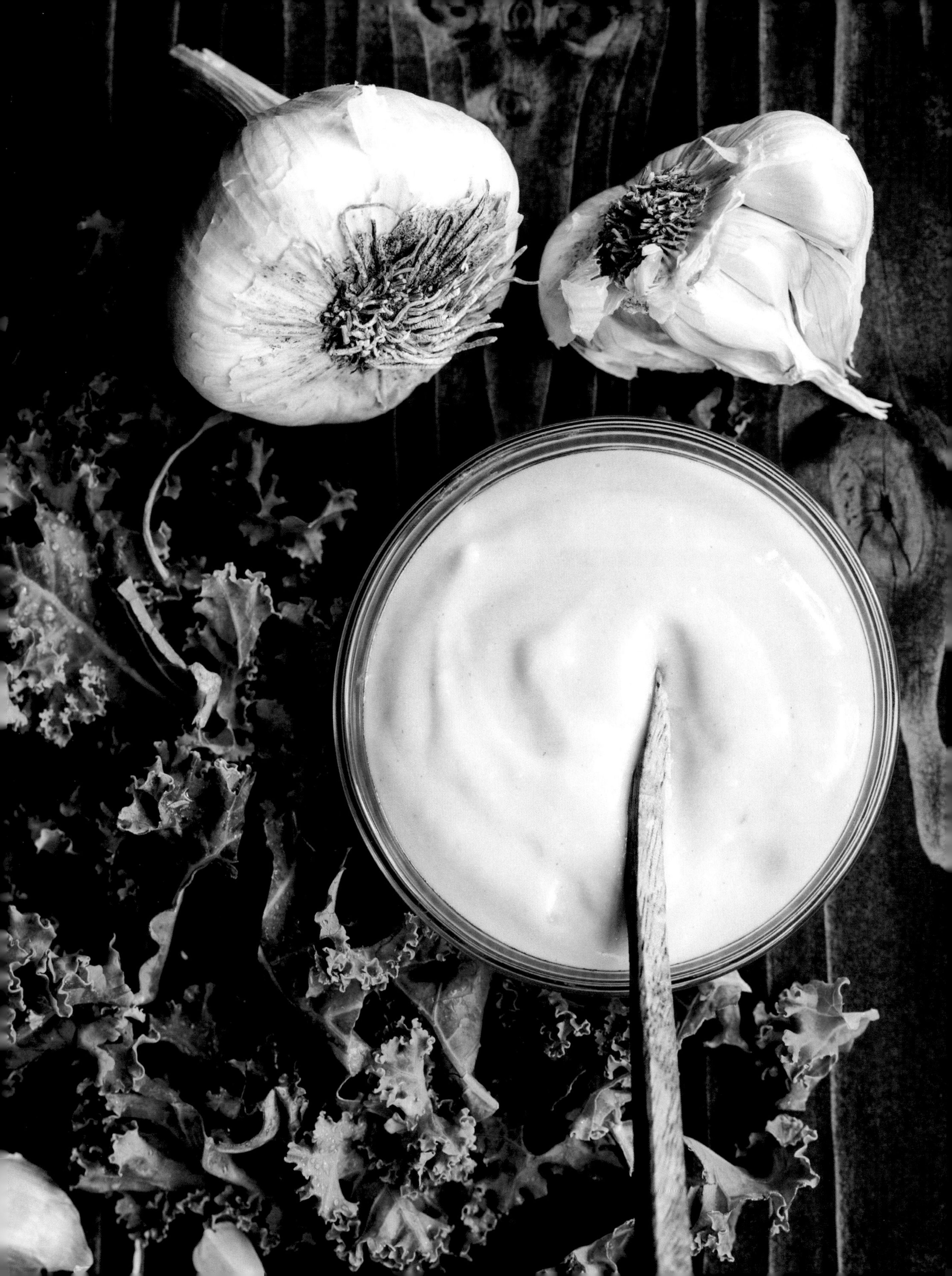

GARLIC DRESSING

Dairy-Free, Gluten-Free, Grain-Free, Paleo, SCD, Vegan

PREP 5 minutes | COOK 0 minutes | TOTAL 5 minutes | MAKES about 3/4 cup

I created a garlic dressing that is thick and full of flavor. Toss it with a simple green salad or serve it as a condiment for grilled or roasted meats and vegetables. I like to make it in my mini food processor since it's a small recipe. You can also make it in a blender.

INGREDIENTS

3 cloves garlic, minced
2 Tablespoons Dijon mustard
Juice from 1 lemon
1/4 teaspoon salt
1/2 cup olive oil

DIRECTIONS

1. Place garlic, Dijon mustard, lemon juice and salt in a mini food processor and blend well.
2. With food processor running, slowly add olive oil until combined.
3. Store in an airtight container in the refrigerator for up to 5 days.

SHALLOT VINAIGRETTE

Dairy-Free, Gluten-Free, Grain-Free, Paleo, SCD (Adaptable for Vegan)

PREP 5 minutes | COOK 0 minutes | TOTAL 5 minutes | MAKES about 3/4 cup

When I was following the Specific Carbohydrate Diet, I started reading the labels on everything to look for ingredients I wasn't allowed to eat. I was surprised to see so many sweeteners, stabilizers and additives in salad dressings and other condiments. Out of necessity, I started making my own dressings and found that I actually liked them better. This shallot vinaigrette is one of my favorite simple dressings to make, and it keeps well in the refrigerator. To adapt for vegan, substitute pure maple syrup for honey.

INGREDIENTS

1/2 cup olive oil

3 Tablespoons white balsamic vinegar or lemon juice

2 teaspoons Dijon mustard

1 teaspoon honey

1/4 teaspoon salt

1 Tablespoon minced shallots

DIRECTIONS

1. Add all ingredients to a small jar and seal.
2. Shake the dressing until well combined.
3. Store in an airtight container in the refrigerator for up to 1 week.
4. Shake well to re-emulsify before serving.

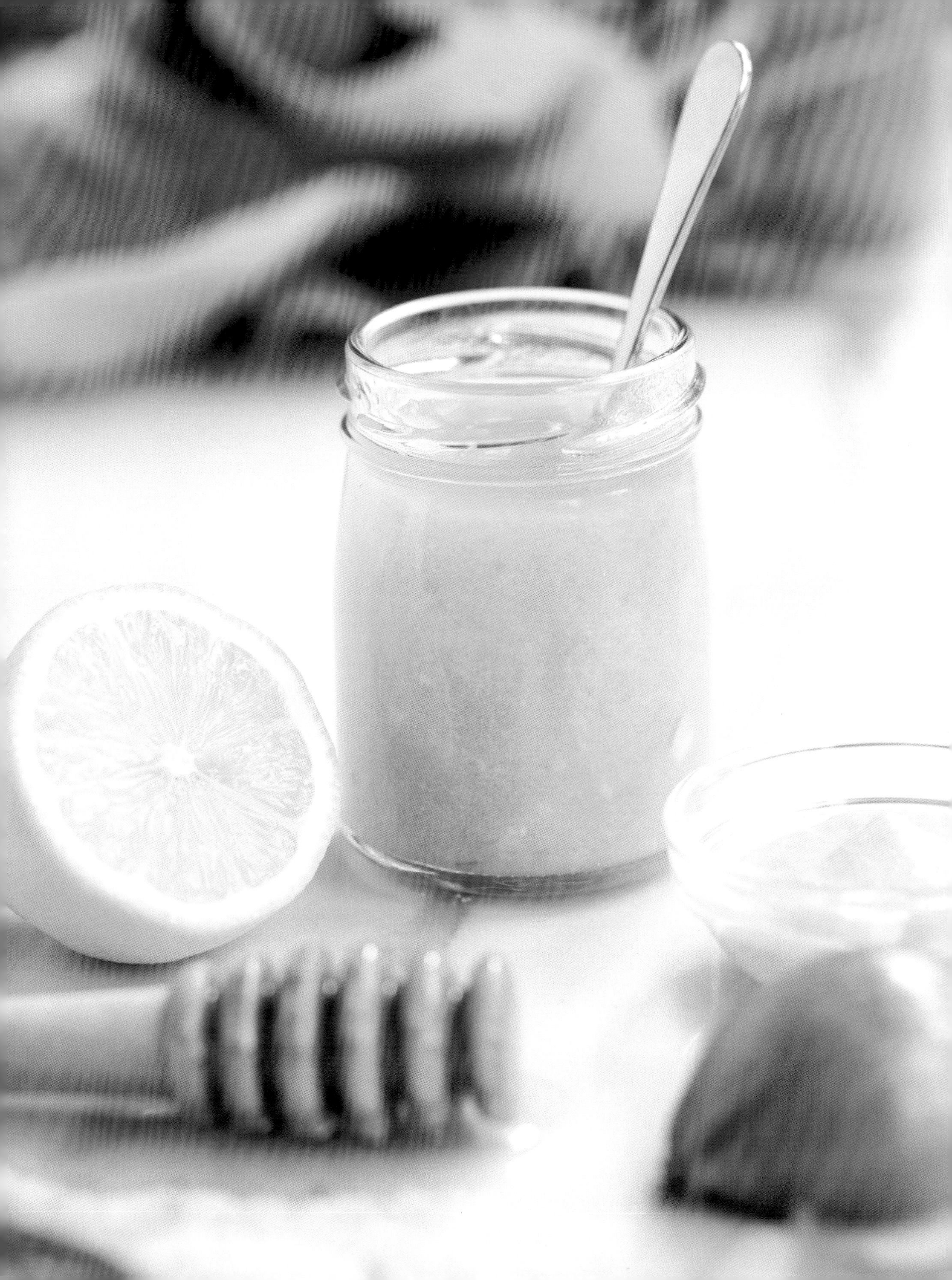

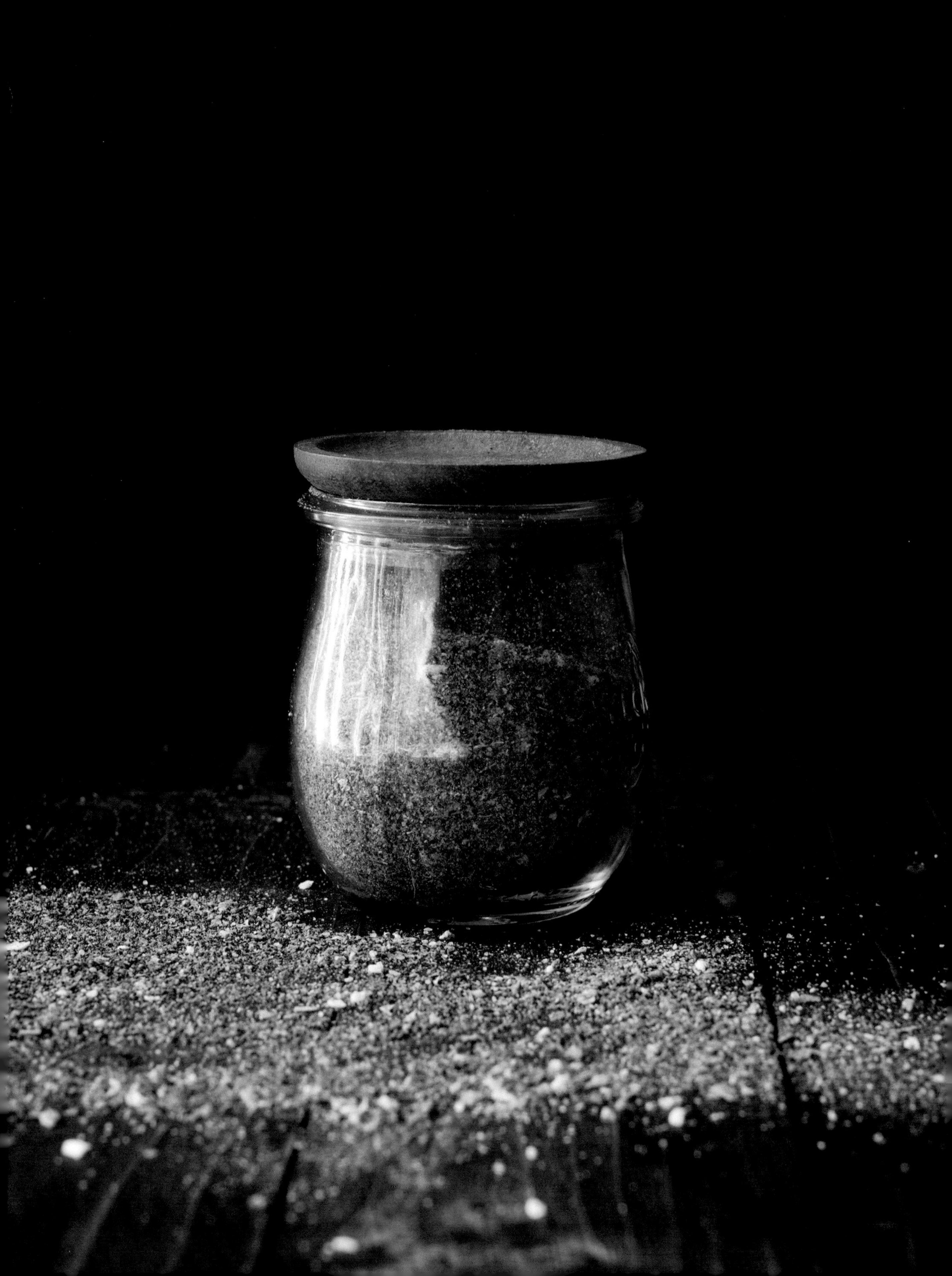

TACO SEASONING

Dairy-Free, Gluten-Free, Grain-Free, Paleo, SCD, Vegan

PREP 5 minutes | COOK 0 minutes | TOTAL 5 minutes | MAKES 6 Tablespoons

I like to make my own taco seasoning to keep on hand in my spice cabinet. The store-bought packets are convenient, but they also contain additives, starches and fillers. This recipe is easy and makes a perfectly balanced taco seasoning mix. It is smoky with a mild kick of heat. If you like more heat, you can increase the amount of crushed pepper flakes or add some cayenne pepper. This recipe makes a little over six tablespoons—the equivalent of three packets of taco seasoning. You can use this with beef, poultry, seafood and vegetables for Mexican flavor.

INGREDIENTS

2 teaspoons salt

1 Tablespoon cumin

3 Tablespoons chili powder

1 teaspoon smoked paprika

2 teaspoons oregano

1 teaspoon garlic powder

1/4 teaspoon crushed pepper flakes

1 teaspoon dried minced onion

DIRECTIONS

1. Add all ingredients to a bowl and mix thoroughly.
2. Store in an airtight container for up to 6 months.

DRY SPICE RUB

Dairy-Free, Gluten-Free, Grain-Free, Paleo, SCD, Vegan

PREP 5 minutes | COOK 0 minutes | TOTAL 5 minutes | MAKES about 3/8 cup

Mixing spices to create a dry rub is a great way to add plenty of flavor to grilled or roasted meats without taking the time necessary for a marinade. This combination pairs well with pork, chicken and turkey. You can add the rub to the meat you are preparing right on the spot or up to an hour before cooking. If you don't have a mortar and pestle, you can use a small food processor or coffee grinder to crush the peppercorns and fennel seeds. I recommend running bread through the grinder afterward to absorb the excess oils from the spices before using for something else later. You can also place the whole spices in a sealed bag and roll them with a rolling pin to crush.

INGREDIENTS

2 teaspoons black peppercorns

2 teaspoons fennel seeds

2 Tablespoons dried oregano

1 Tablespoon dried minced onion

2 teaspoons granulated garlic

1 teaspoon crushed red pepper flakes

1 Tablespoon sea salt

DIRECTIONS

1. Using a mortar and pestle, crush the peppercorns and fennel seeds.
2. Add the oregano, onion, garlic, red pepper and sea salt. Combine well.
3. Rub the spice mixture on pork, chicken or turkey before grilling or roasting.

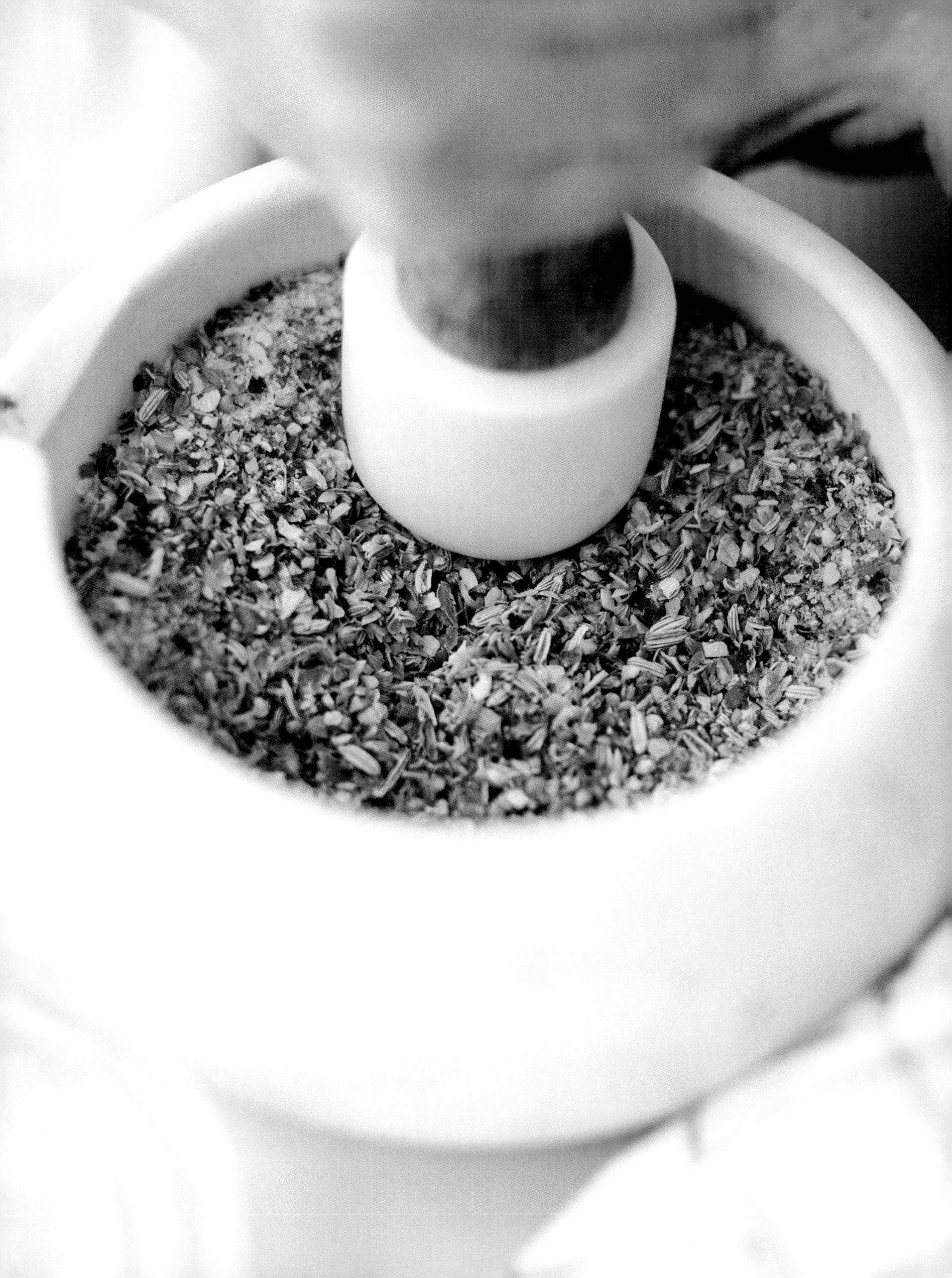

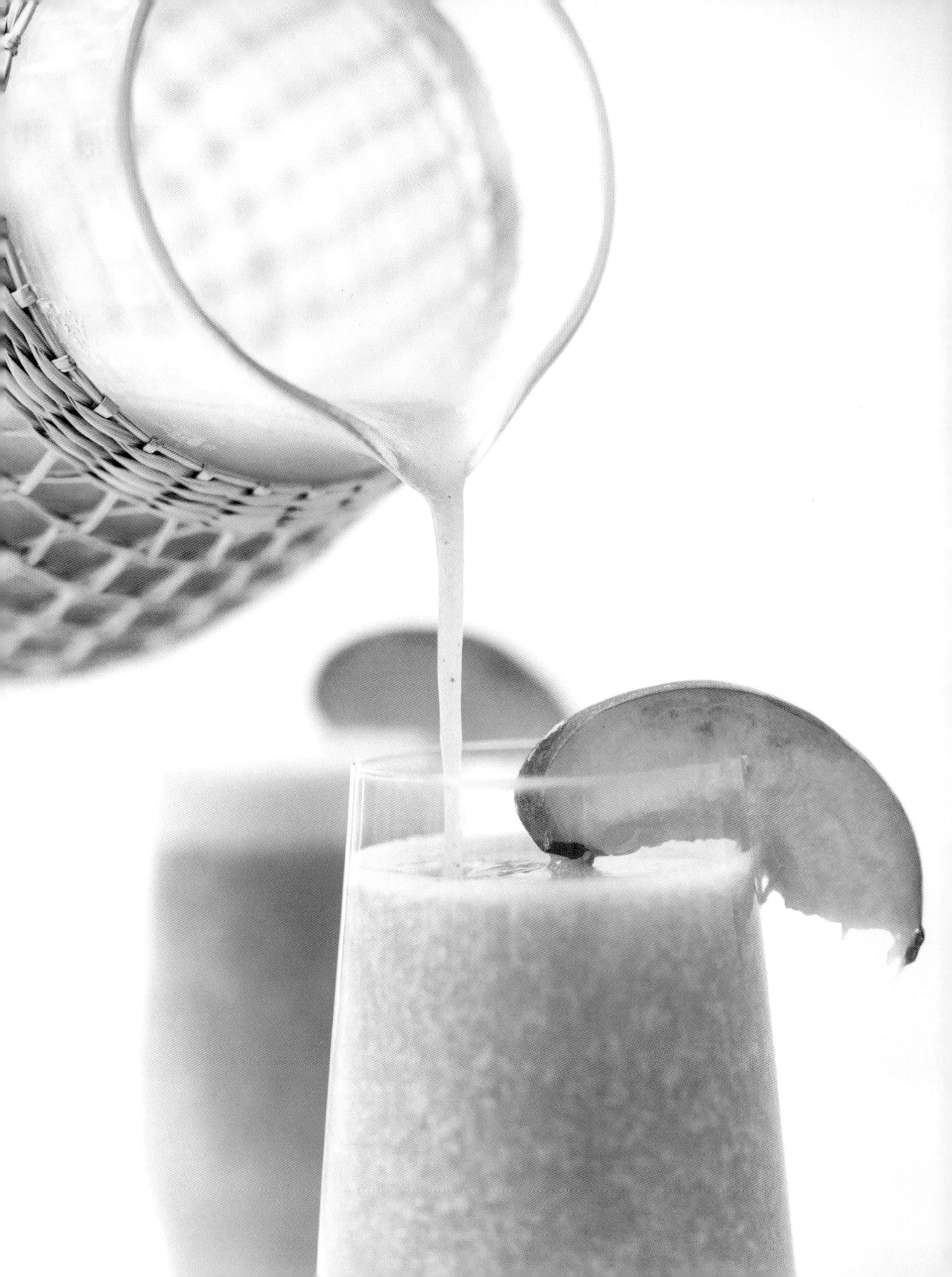

DRINKS AND COCKTAILS

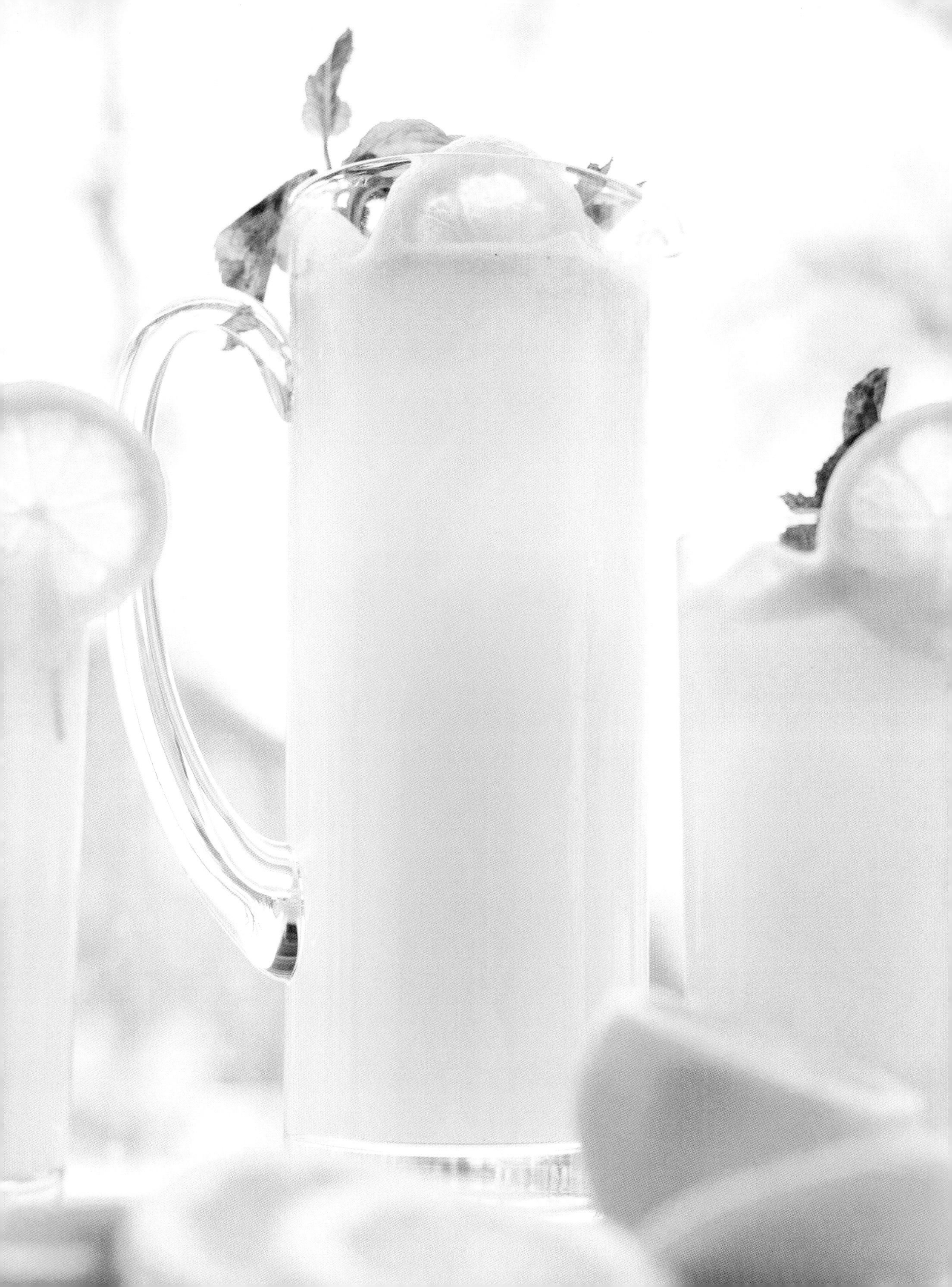

EASY FRESH LEMONADE WITH MINT

Dairy-Free, Gluten-Free, Grain-Free, Paleo, SCD (Adaptable for Vegan)

PREP 5 minutes | COOK 0 minutes | TOTAL 5 minutes | MAKES about 5 cups

This lemonade is so simple to make. The recipe uses the whole lemon, peel included, so no juicing is required. The essential oils in the peel not only add great flavor, but they also help to boost immunity, aid digestion and neutralize free radicals. The lemonade is sweetened with a honey simple syrup, so no refined sugars, artificial colorings or flavorings. It is wonderful on its own or you can add vodka for a refreshing summer cocktail. To adapt for vegan, substitute sugar-based simple syrup for honey simple syrup.

INGREDIENTS

3 lemons, cut into 8 pieces each

1 ounce fresh mint

4 1/2 cups water

1 cup EFK Honey Simple Syrup (page 209)

Pinch of sea salt

Lemon slices and fresh mint, for serving

DIRECTIONS

1. Place all ingredients in a blender and blend on medium for 7-8 seconds. Do not blend longer or the lemonade may turn bitter.
2. Pour through a mesh strainer into a pitcher with ice.
3. Pour into glasses garnished with lemon slices and fresh mint.

CHERRY LIMEADE

Dairy-Free, Gluten-Free, Grain-Free, Paleo, SCD (Adaptable for Vegan)

PREP 15 minutes | COOK 0 minutes | TOTAL 15 minutes | MAKES about 6 cups

This is a refreshing drink enjoyed by people of all ages. This recipe is easy to make and much healthier than the version from a soda tap. Using fresh cherries adds some extra work with the pitting, but I think it's worth it. I found a great cherry pitting tool on Amazon that pits six cherries at a time. It speeds up the process and works great. I highly recommend the minimal investment if you like to use fresh cherries in recipes. To adapt for vegan, substitute sugar-based simple syrup for honey simple syrup.

INGREDIENTS

3 cups fresh or previously frozen cherries, pitted

2/3 cup EFK Honey Simple Syrup (page 209)

4 cups water

2 limes, quartered

Sparkling water

DIRECTIONS

1. Place the pitted cherries, EFK Honey Simple Syrup and water in a blender and blend on high for 8-10 seconds.
2. Add the quartered limes and blend for an additional 5 seconds.
3. Pour through a mesh strainer into a pitcher.
4. Pour 6-8 ounces into a glass with ice and add 2 ounces of sparkling water.
5. Stir and enjoy.

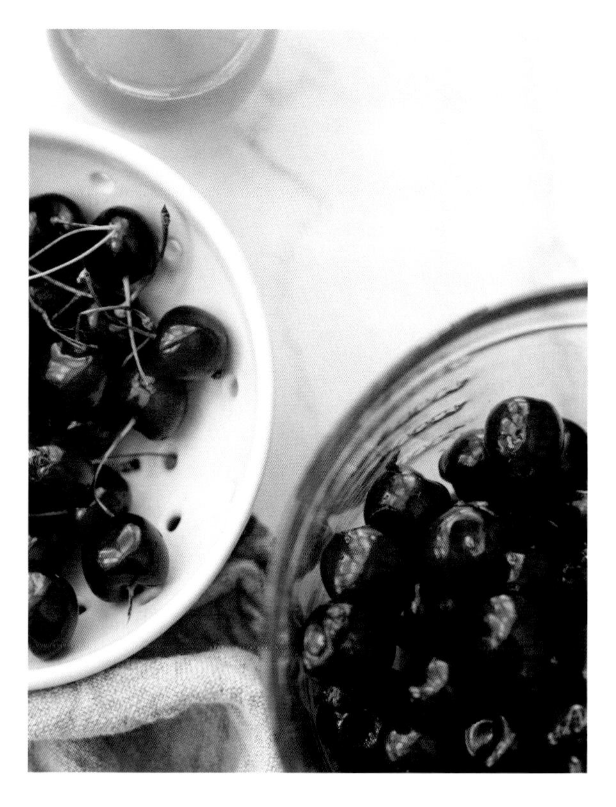

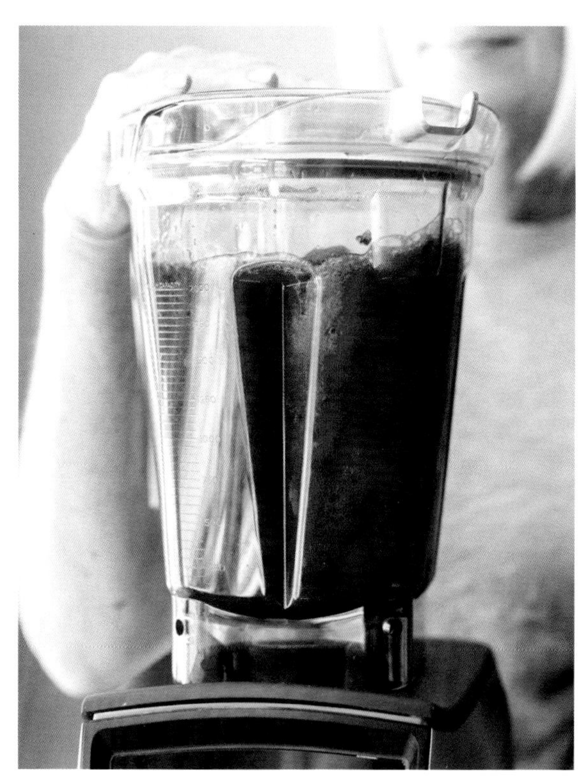

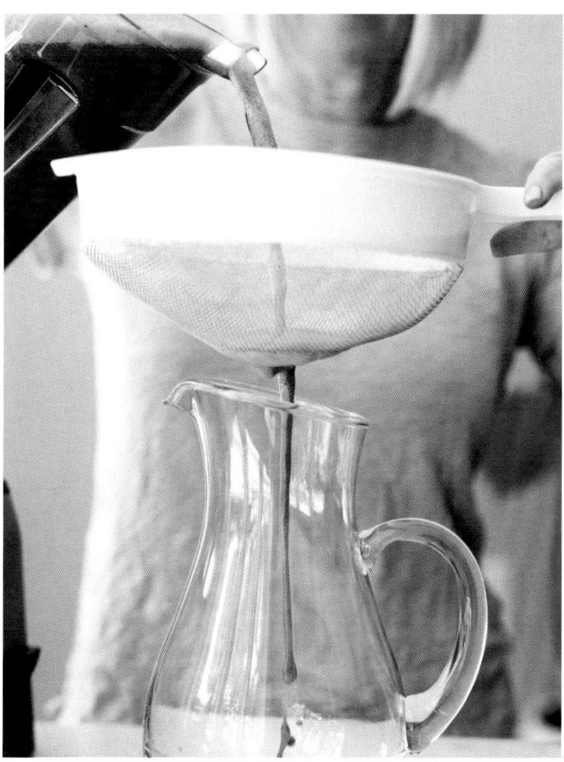

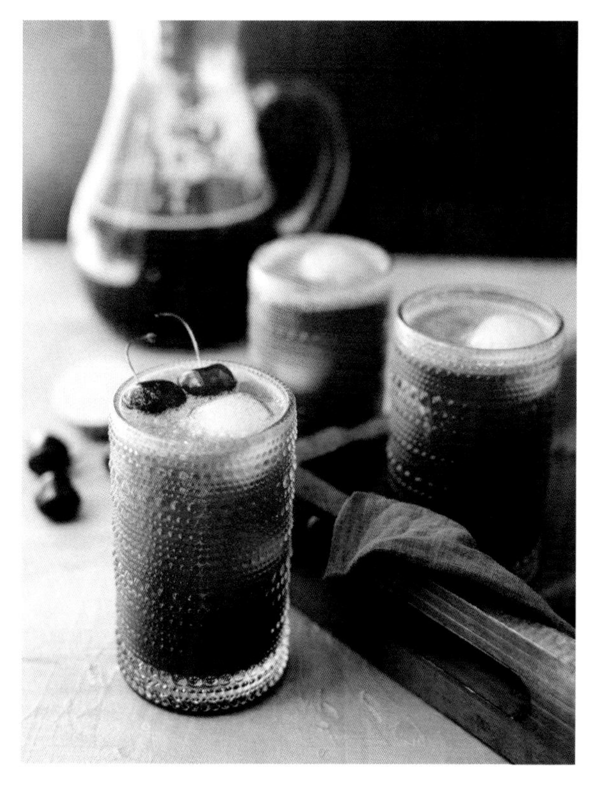

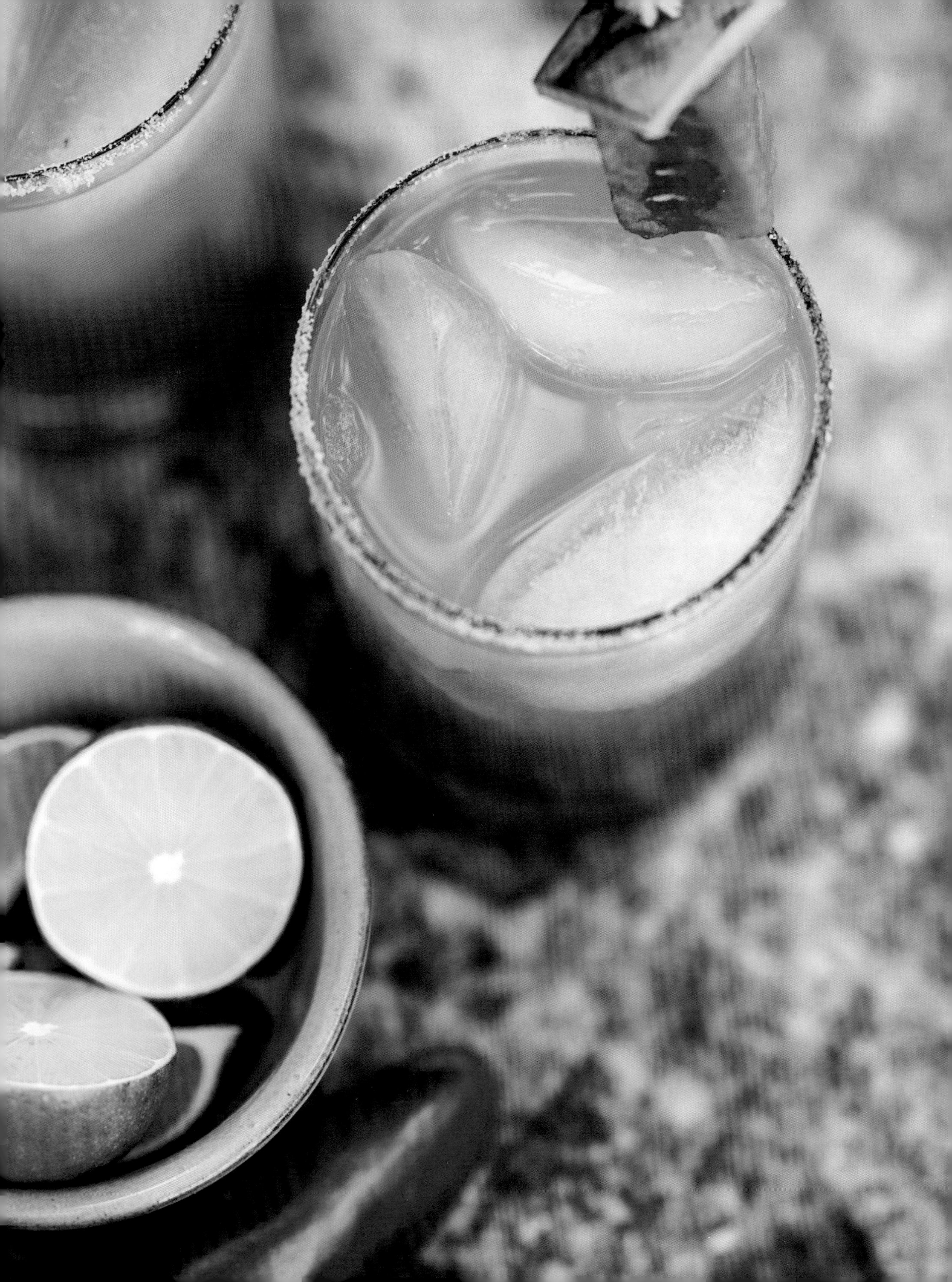

SPICY WATERMELON MARGARITA

Dairy-Free, Gluten-Free, Grain-Free, Paleo, SCD (Adaptable for Vegan)

PREP 20 minutes | COOK 10 minutes | TOTAL 30 minutes | MAKES about 8 cocktails

I really enjoy a good margarita. Drinking one transports me to a beach and puts me in vacation mode. In the summer, it is nice to take advantage of the seasonal options and use fresh watermelon for a twist on this classic cocktail. Plus the color is gorgeous. A spicy simple syrup made with honey and jalapeños adds the right amount of heat to balance the sweetness of the watermelon. To adapt for vegan, substitute sugar for honey.

INGREDIENTS

2 jalapeños

1 cup honey

Water

2 cups diced watermelon

20 limes

Pink Himalayan sea salt

16 ounces tequila blanco

Watermelon cubes, watermelon rind and limes or jalapeño slices, for serving

DIRECTIONS

1. Roughly chop the jalapeños.
2. In a small saucepan, combine the honey, jalapeños and 1/2 cup water.
3. Bring to a simmer and cook for 3 minutes if you prefer a less spicy drink and up to 5 minutes for a spicier drink.
4. Strain the spicy honey syrup into a jar or glass container and cool.
5. Place watermelon and 1/4 cup water in a blender and blend 1-2 minutes.
6. Strain watermelon juice through a fine sieve.
7. Juice limes to make 8 ounces juice.
8. Run a lime wedge around the rim of a cocktail glass and dip in pink salt.
9. Add ice to glass.
10. In a cocktail shaker, add 2 ounces watermelon juice, 1 ounce lime juice, 1 ounce honey syrup, 2 ounces tequila and a few ice cubes. You can double this to make 2 drinks at a time.
11. Shake well.
12. Strain into cocktail glass.
13. Garnish with watermelon cubes and rind, limes or jalapeño slices.

PEACH FLIP

Dairy-Free, Gluten-Free, Grain-Free, Paleo, SCD (Adaptable for Vegan)

PREP 5 minutes | COOK 0 minutes | TOTAL 5 minutes | MAKES 4 cocktails

Growing up, we took summer vacations at a lake in the Midwest with my mother's extended family. One of the relatives would make different batches of special cocktails in the evenings for the adults in the group. They also made nonalcoholic versions for the kids. One of my favorites was the Peach Flip made with fresh, ripe peaches and lemonade concentrate. In this version I omit the sugary lemonade concentrate and substitute fresh lemon and honey. To make this recipe nonalcoholic, omit the vodka and add club soda after blending. This drink looks and tastes like a summer sunset. To adapt for vegan, substitute sugar for honey.

INGREDIENTS

2 medium peaches

1 large or 2 small lemons, rind removed

1/3 cup honey

1 cup vodka

4 cups ice

DIRECTIONS

1. Place all ingredients in a blender.
2. Blend well.

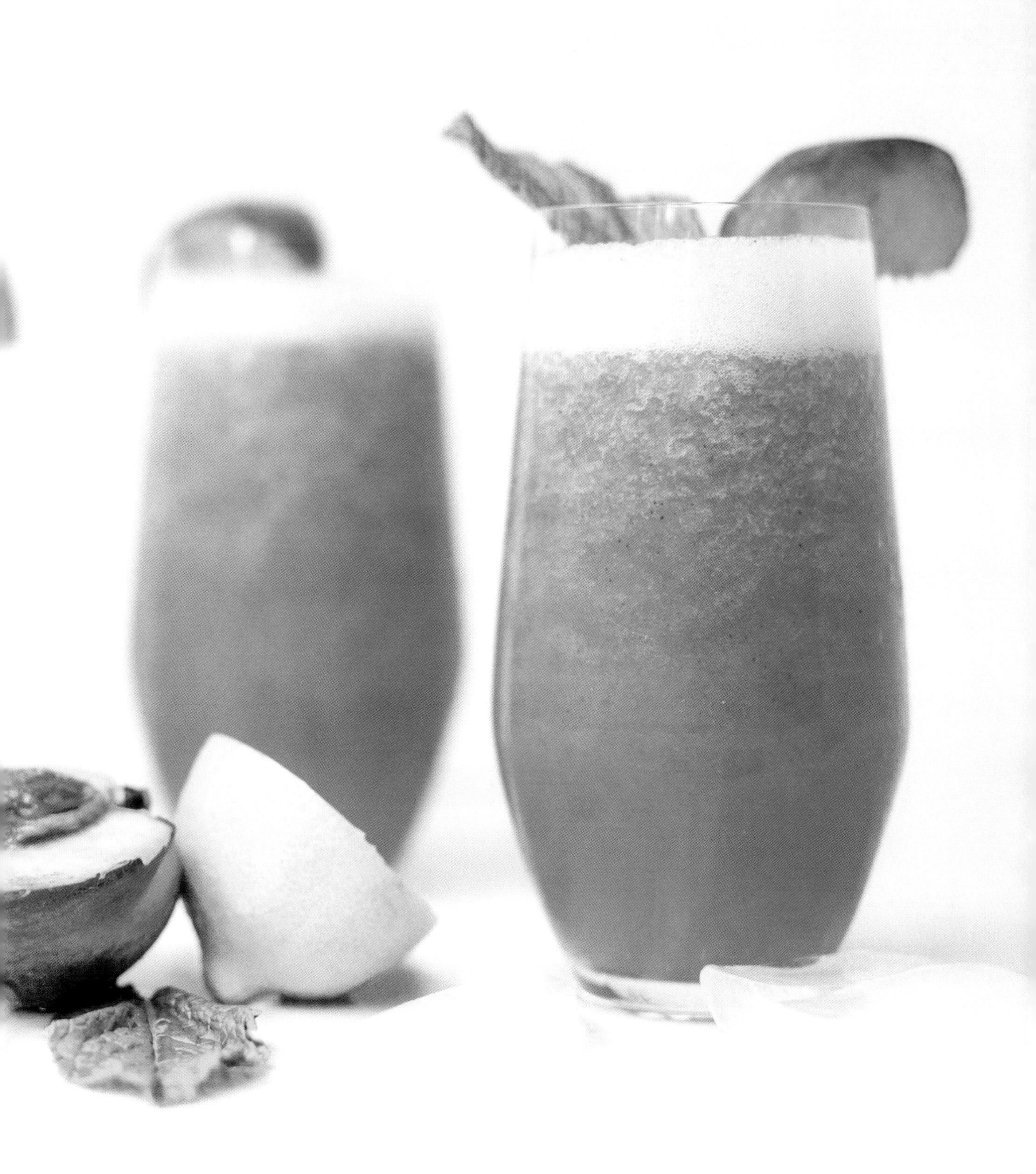

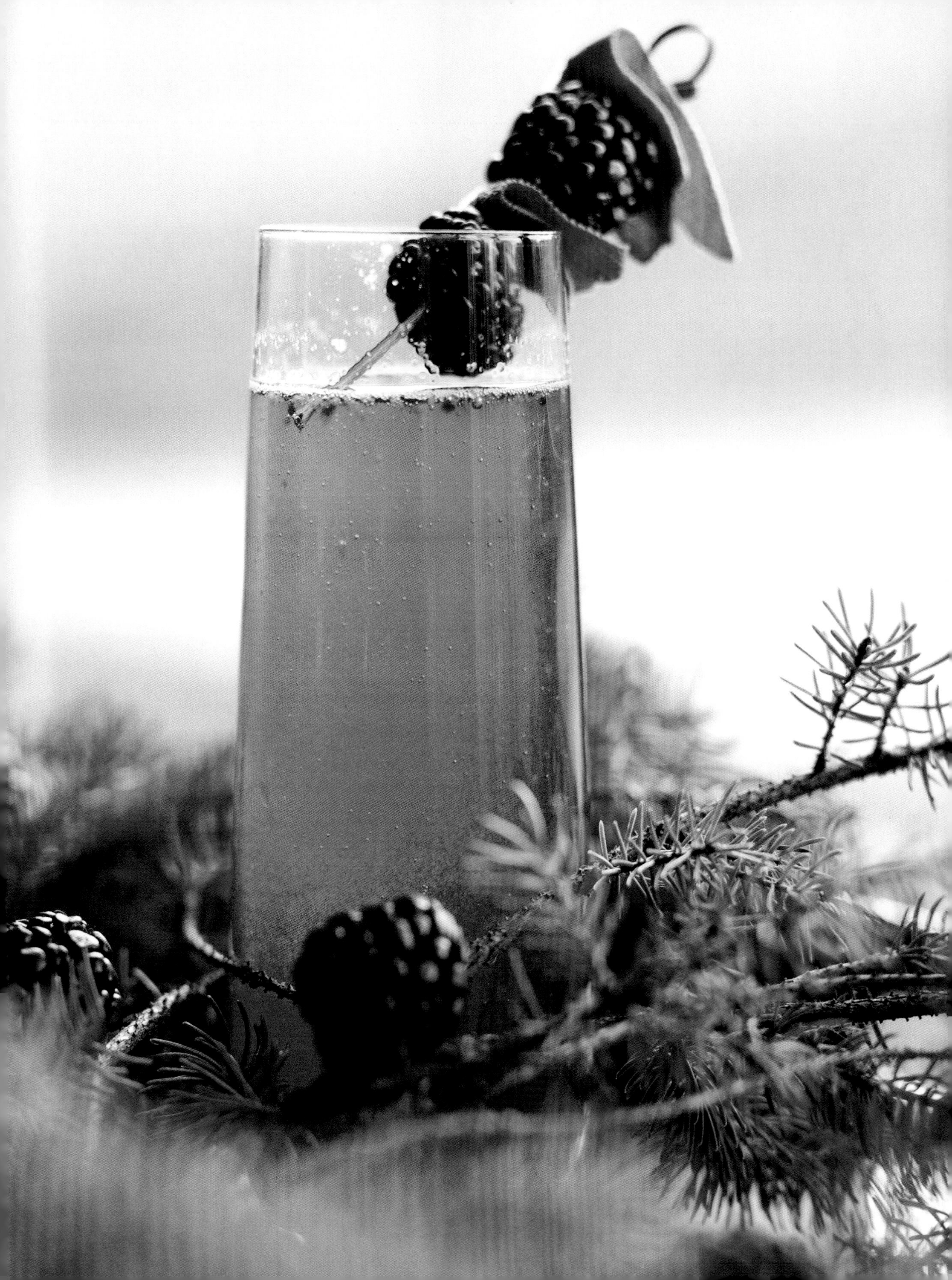

BLACKBERRY SAGE PROSECCO

Dairy-Free, Gluten-Free, Grain-Free, Paleo, SCD (Adaptable for Vegan)

PREP 5 minutes | COOK 55 minutes | TOTAL 60 minutes | MAKES about 12 cocktails

Adding a fruit syrup or liqueur is a fun way to dress up a glass of prosecco or other sparkling wine. In this recipe I make a blackberry and sage syrup and sweeten it with honey. The combination adds a delicious fruity and earthy flavor as well as a beautiful color to the sparkling wine. It is a festive and perfect drink to serve before or after a meal. To adapt for vegan, substitute sugar for honey.

INGREDIENTS

4 cups fresh or frozen blackberries

1 cup honey

1/2 cup vodka

1/2 cup water

1/2 cup fresh sage, chopped

Prosecco or other sparkling wine, chilled

DIRECTIONS

1. In a medium saucepan combine the blackberries, honey, vodka and water.
2. Bring to a boil and then reduce to a simmer.
3. Simmer for 30 minutes and then add the sage.
4. Simmer for an additional 15 minutes.
5. Strain the blackberry mixture through a fine sieve.
6. Allow the hot syrup to cool.
7. Pour 1-2 Tablespoons of the blackberry sage syrup into a glass.
8. Fill the rest of the glass with chilled prosecco and enjoy.
9. Store remaining syrup in an airtight container in the refrigerator for 1-2 months.

OAK ISLAND PRESS

Dairy-Free, Gluten-Free, Grain-Free, Paleo, SCD (Adaptable for Vegan)

PREP 15 minutes | COOK 0 minutes | TOTAL 15 minutes | MAKES about 12 cocktails

This refreshing citrus cocktail was created while we were on vacation with friends on Oak Island in Lake of the Woods. This remote island is accessed by boat from a small town in northern Minnesota. Before we crossed the lake to our friends' cabin, we gathered supplies at the neighborhood grocery store, grabbing an assortment of citrus fruits to use with a small citrus juicer. We hoped we could make fresh juice to create fun cocktails to enjoy before dinner. The end result was a big hit and we named it the Oak Island Press. It has since become a regular in my cocktail repertoire.

In this recipe, I list specific amounts and types of citrus fruits to get you started, but feel free to use any varieties and amounts you wish. I have used pomelos, blood oranges and clementines in the past. Get creative! This drink can also be served as a delicious mocktail without any spirits. To adapt for vegan, substitute sugar-based simple syrup for honey simple syrup.

INGREDIENTS

4 ruby red grapefruit

8 oranges

3 lemons

3 limes

EFK Honey Simple Syrup (page 209)

Club soda

Vodka or tequila

DIRECTIONS

1. Using a citrus juicer, juice all of the fruit and combine in a pitcher.
2. For each cocktail, fill a glass with ice.
3. Add 3 ounces of the fresh juice, 1 ounce of EFK Honey Simple Syrup, 2 ounces of club soda, and 2 ounces of vodka or tequila.
4. Stir well and serve.
5. Repeat as necessary.
6. Store remaining juice in the refrigerator for 2-3 days.

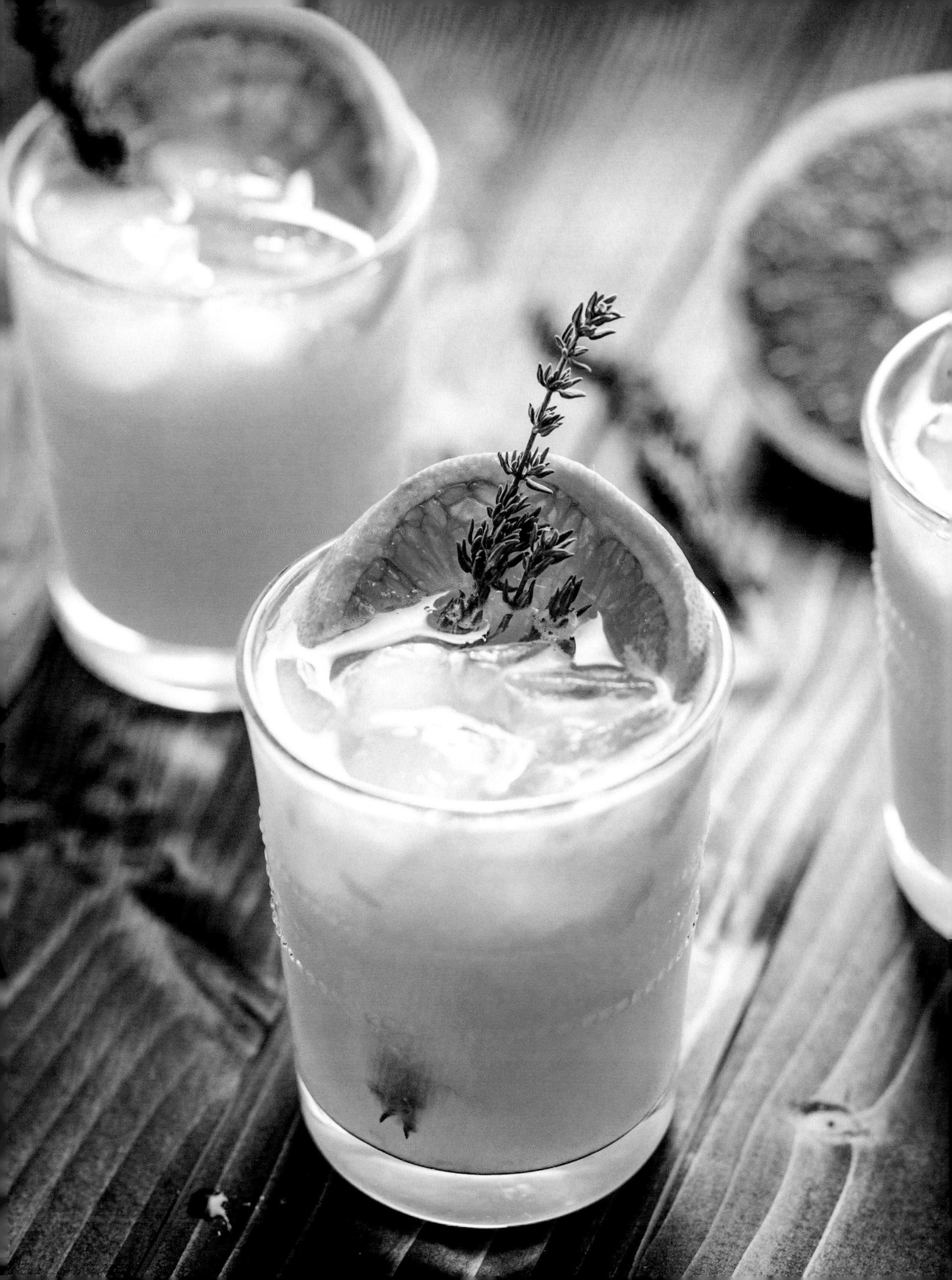

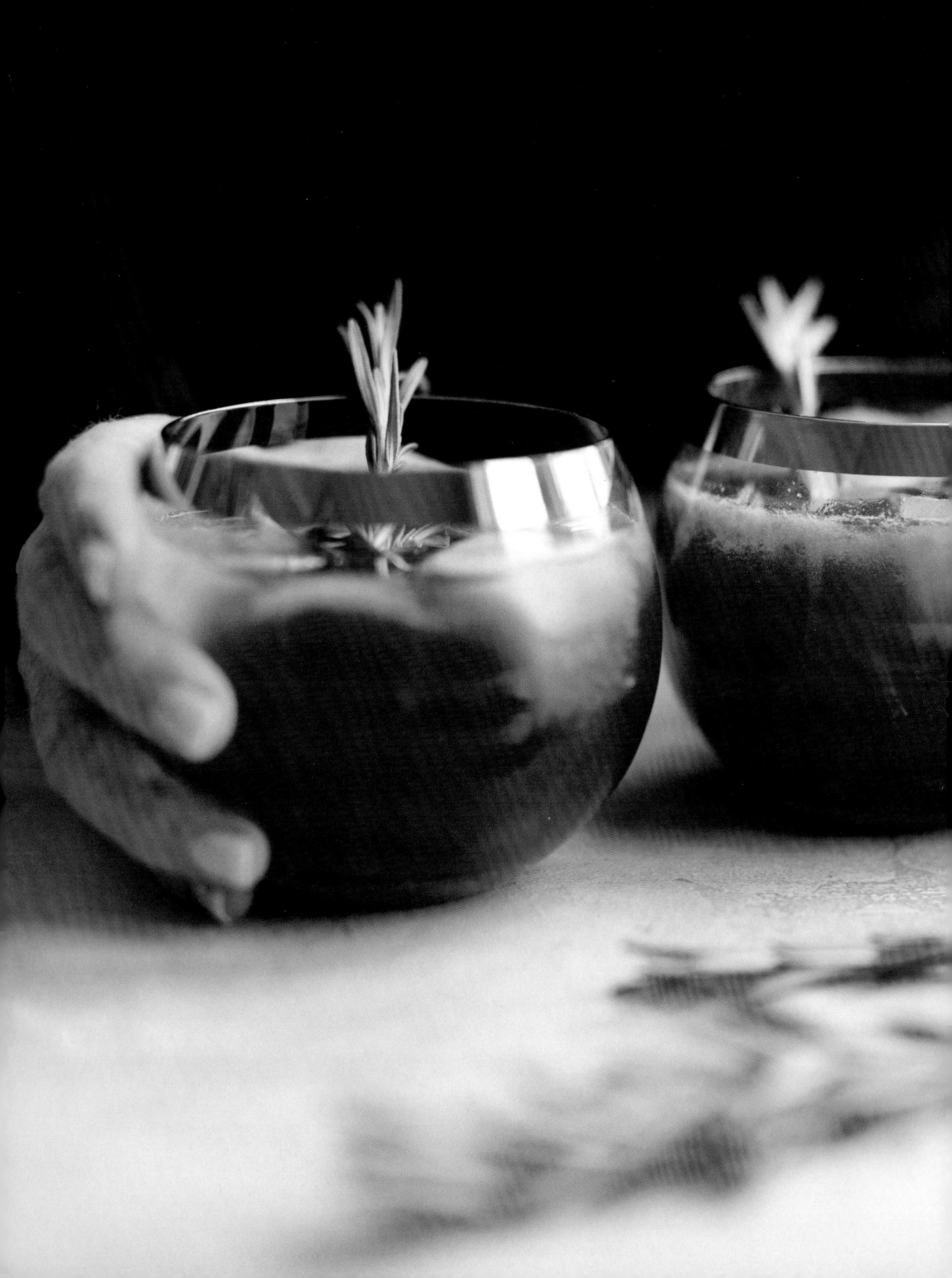

POMEGRANATE GINGER FIZZ

Dairy-Free, Gluten-Free, Grain-Free, Paleo, SCD (Adaptable for Vegan)

PREP 5 minutes | COOK 20 minutes | TOTAL 25 minutes | MAKES 2 cocktails

This is a festive cocktail that's fun to serve during the holidays. The pomegranate juice gives it a pretty color and adds a nice dose of antioxidants, too. The honey ginger syrup provides just the right amount of sweetness with a mild ginger flavor. For a nonalcoholic version, omit the vodka. To adapt for vegan, substitute sugar for honey.

INGREDIENTS (SYRUP)

4 Tablespoons freshly grated ginger

1 Tablespoon lemon zest

1 cup honey

1/2 cup water

INGREDIENTS (COCKTAIL)

4 ounces vodka

4 ounces 100% pomegranate juice

2 ounces honey ginger syrup

1 ounce freshly squeezed lemon juice

8 ounces club soda

Pomegranate seeds and rosemary sprigs, for serving

DIRECTIONS

1. For the honey ginger syrup, place all the syrup ingredients in a small saucepan.
2. Simmer over low heat for 15 minutes.
3. Strain the syrup into a jar or glass container and cool.
4. For the cocktail, combine the vodka, pomegranate juice, honey ginger syrup and lemon juice in a shaker or small pitcher and shake or mix well.
5. Pour the mixture into 2 glasses with ice.
6. Add 4 ounces club soda to each glass and stir.
7. Garnish with pomegranate seeds and a sprig of fresh rosemary.
8. Store remaining syrup in an airtight container in the refrigerator for up to 2 weeks.

GRAPEFRUIT AND MINT MEZCAL COCKTAIL

Dairy-Free, Gluten-Free, Grain-Free, Paleo (Adaptable for Vegan)

PREP 5 minutes | COOK 10 minutes | TOTAL 15 minutes | MAKES 3-4 cocktails

Mezcal is a unique spirit that is made only in Mexico. It's created by roasting the heart of the agave plant in the ground before it is distilled, which creates the wonderful smoky flavor that mezcal is known for. Pairing it with grapefruit and mint makes a refreshing cocktail. This recipe has a nice balance of citrus, herb, sweet and smoky flavors. The combination is delightful and perfect for an experienced or first-time mezcal drinker. To adapt for vegan, substitute sugar for honey.

INGREDIENTS (SYRUP)

1 cup honey

1/2 cup water

1 bunch of fresh mint

INGREDIENTS (COCKTAIL)

6 ounces mezcal

2 ounces St. Germain elderflower liqueur

4 ounces fresh grapefruit juice

4 ounces mint honey syrup

2 ounces fresh lime juice

12 ounces club soda

Grapefruit, sliced and quartered, and fresh mint, for serving

DIRECTIONS

1. For the mint honey syrup, combine honey and water in a saucepan over medium heat.
2. Bring to a simmer and then add the fresh mint.
3. Simmer for 2 minutes.
4. Strain the honey mixture to remove the mint.
5. Allow the syrup to cool.
6. For the cocktail, combine the mezcal, St. Germain, grapefruit juice, mint honey syrup, lime juice and club soda in a small pitcher.
7. Fill 3-4 glasses with ice and pour in the cocktail mix.
8. Add a slice of grapefruit and a sprig of mint.
9. Makes 3-4 cocktails.
10. Store remaining syrup in an airtight container in the refrigerator for up to 2 weeks.

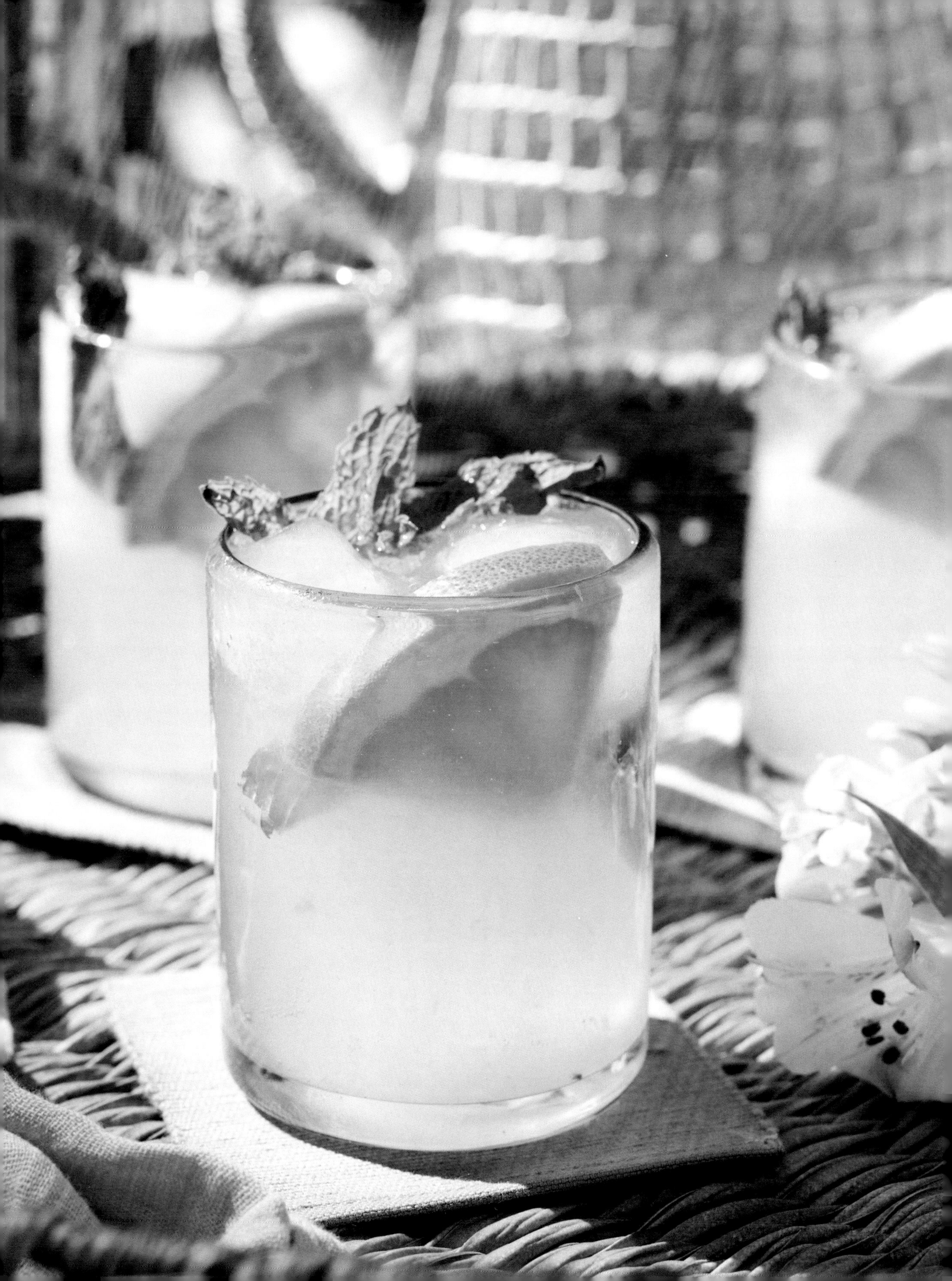

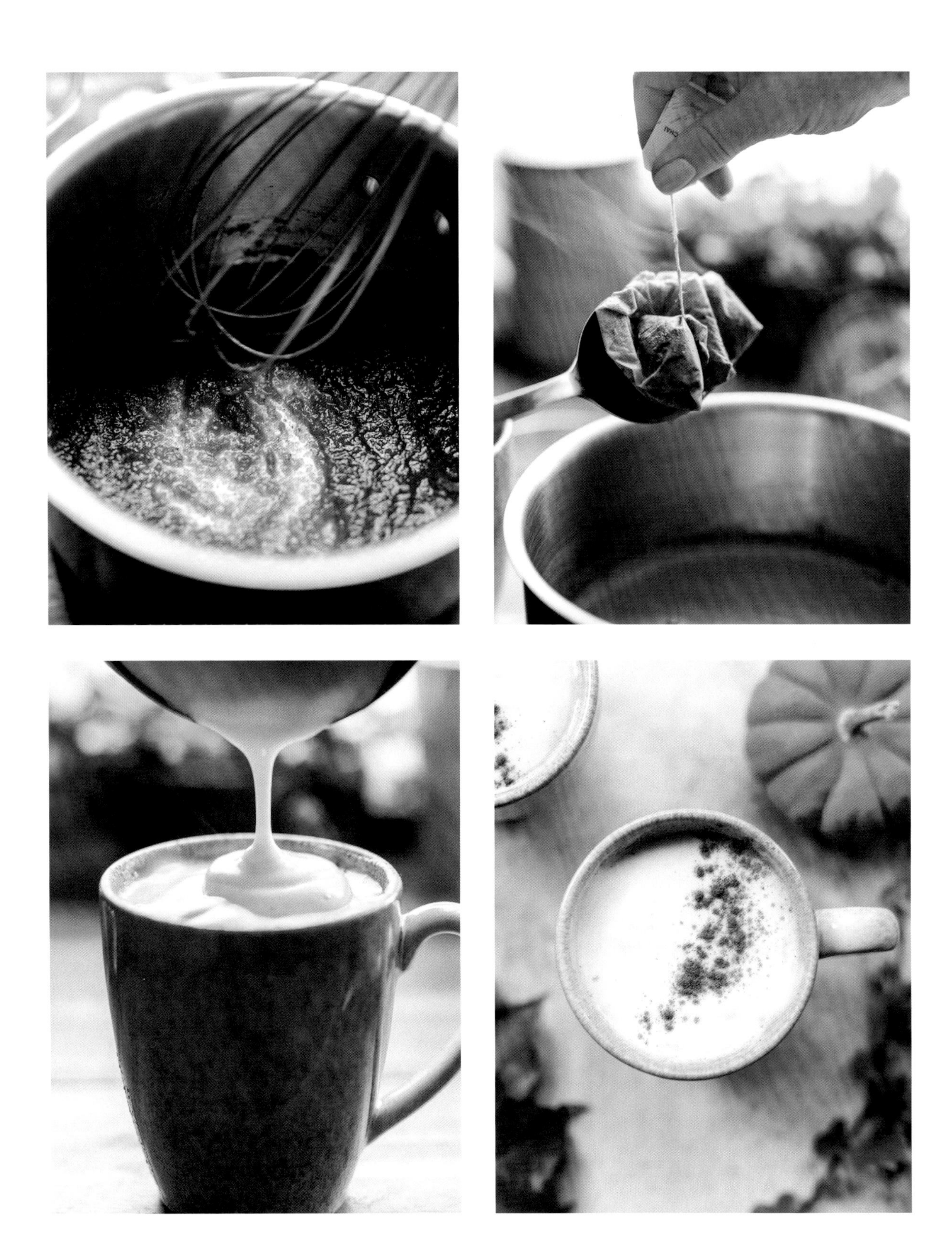

PUMPKIN SPICE CHAI LATTE

Dairy-Free, Gluten-Free, Grain-Free, Paleo, SCD, Vegan

PREP 2 minutes | COOK 15 minutes | TOTAL 17 minutes | MAKES 2 drinks

Nothing says fall like pumpkin spice, and enjoying these flavors in a warm drink is a great way to embrace the cooler temperatures of the season. This pumpkin spice chai latte is easy to make and has healthier ingredients than one you would buy at most coffee shops. It is made with real pumpkin and sweetened with pure maple syrup. I use a combination of almond and coconut milk so that this version is also dairy-free. Enjoy the latte served hot or poured over ice for a cold drink.

INGREDIENTS

3 Tablespoons canned pumpkin

2 Tablespoons pure maple syrup

1/2 teaspoon cinnamon

1/8 teaspoon ground cloves

1/8 teaspoon ground ginger

1/8 teaspoon ground nutmeg

1 3/4 cups almond milk

1/2 cup coconut milk

1/2 teaspoon vanilla

3 chai tea bags

Frothed almond milk or whipped coconut cream, for serving

DIRECTIONS

1. In a small saucepan combine the pumpkin, maple syrup and spices over medium heat, blending well.
2. Add the almond milk and coconut milk and whisk well to combine.
3. Bring the flavored milk to a boil.
4. Remove from heat and add the vanilla and 3 chai tea bags.
5. Steep the tea for 5 minutes.
6. Remove the tea bags and pour into 2 mugs.
7. Top with frothed almond milk or whipped coconut cream.

CHICKEN BONE BROTH

Dairy-Free, Gluten-Free, Grain-Free, Paleo, SCD

PREP 10 minutes | COOK 25 hours | TOTAL 25 hours 10 minutes | MAKES about 2 quarts

Bone broth is simple to make and can do amazing things for your body. It is helpful in healing and restoring gut health, protecting joints, supporting the immune system and boosting detoxification. It has also been shown to assist with sleep and improve skin and hair health. What makes bone broth different from stock is that it cooks for a longer period of time, at least 24 hours. The longer cooking time allows for more minerals and nutrients to be extracted from the bones into the broth. I drink bone broth in a mug with a little salt or use it when cooking in place of stock.

INGREDIENTS

1 whole free-range chicken

1 large onion, chopped

2 large carrots, chopped

3 celery sticks, chopped

4 cloves garlic, smashed

2 Tablespoons apple cider vinegar

Filtered water

1 bunch parsley

Sea salt

DIRECTIONS

1. Place the chicken, onion, carrots, celery, garlic and vinegar in a large slow cooker.
2. Fill with filtered water to cover.
3. Let the ingredients sit for 30-60 minutes to allow the vinegar to start pulling the minerals from the bones.
4. Turn the slow cooker on high and bring to a boil.
5. After one hour, remove the scum that rises to the top.
6. Turn the slow cooker to low and cook for 24 or more hours.
7. Add the parsley for the final 10 minutes of cooking.
8. Use a slotted spoon to remove the chicken carcass. The overcooked meat is mushy and flavorless but can be saved and fed to pets.
9. Strain the broth through a fine sieve.
10. Season to taste with sea salt.
11. Store in an airtight container in the refrigerator for up to 1 week or in the freezer for up to 1 month.

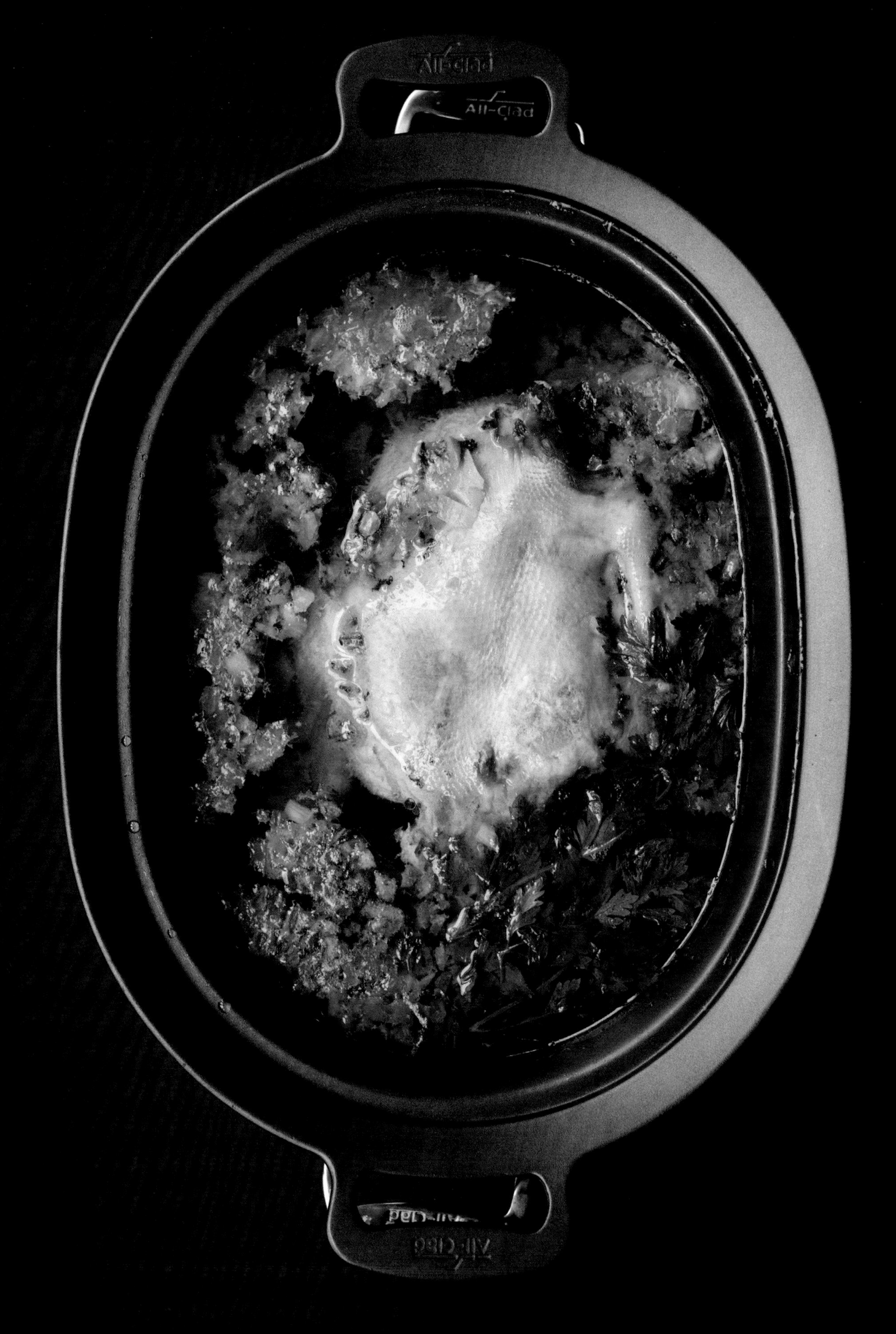
All-Clad

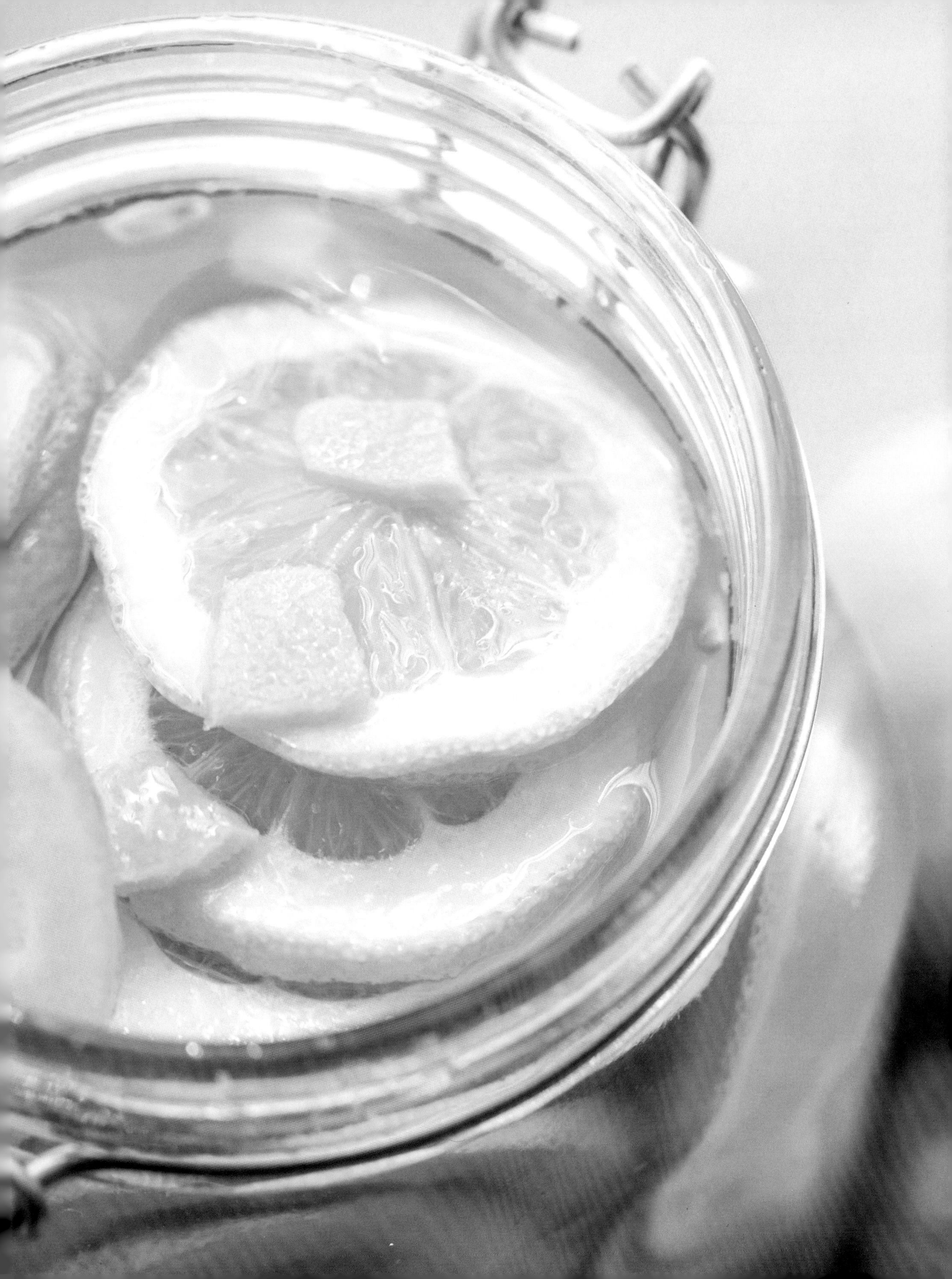

HONEY GINGER LEMON TEA

Dairy-Free, Gluten-Free, Grain-Free, Paleo, SCD

PREP 10 minutes | COOK 0 minutes | TOTAL 10 minutes

Colder weather means an increase in colds and sore throats. I like to keep a mixture of honey, lemon and ginger in my refrigerator to use in tea when someone in the house feels sniffles or a sore throat coming on. It is a soothing natural remedy.

INGREDIENTS

Local raw honey

Lemons

Ginger root

DIRECTIONS

1. Wash and slice the lemons.
2. Peel the ginger root and slice into small pieces.
3. Layer the slices of lemon and ginger pieces in a large jar or glass container.
4. Fill the jar with the honey and seal the lid.
5. To drink, add a scoop of honey with some lemon and ginger into a mug and fill with hot water.
6. Store in an airtight container in the refrigerator for up to 8 weeks.
7. The mixture will separate over time, so just give it a good stir to reblend, keeping the lemons and ginger covered with honey.

ACKNOWLEDGMENTS

First of all, I want to thank God for seeing me through a struggle in my life and inspiring me to use it for something good. Thank you for putting this book in my heart and helping me find a way to make it happen. You are faithful and good and I am grateful.

To my husband, Chris, there wouldn't be a book without you. Your constant encouragement and belief in me have been incredible. Thank you for being my number one taste tester, patiently sampling multiple recipe variations and listening to me talk about the slight differences between each one. Thank you for pushing me to not give up on this dream. I am beyond blessed to have you as my partner in life.

To my daughters, Lydia and Abby, thank you for always cheering me on. It is amazing to have the two women I admire the most be my biggest fans. I love you both so much.

To my mom, thank you for teaching me the gift of hospitality and passing down a love of cooking. And for spending all those nights in the hospital by my side. I couldn't have made it through the two weeks after surgery without you.

To my dad, thank you for introducing me to fine dining at a young age and ordering things like escargots and caviar for us to try. And for driving me to the Mayo Clinic every eight weeks for treatments when I was so sick.

To my sisters, Liz and Erin, I hit the jackpot in the sibling category. Your support of me is invaluable.

To my mother-in-law, Christine, thank you for always thinking I should be on TV doing a cooking demonstration instead of said TV chef. Your belief in my culinary abilities is unmatched.

To my Bible study girls, prayer group and Cabos Chicas, we are not meant to go through this world alone and I am grateful that the Lord placed each one of you in my life. Thank you for your prayers, friendship and support.

To Belén Fleming, my wildly talented photographer, working with you on this project has been the most enjoyable experience. You always find a way to capture my recipes and make them look drool worthy. You are incredibly gifted, and I appreciate your attention to detail. You have stretched me creatively and professionally. Collaborating with you on food shoot days is one of my favorite things.

To Julie Burton, thank you for creating ModernWell, the beautiful coworking space where I found the amazing women who helped me with this project. Your sincere support and encouragement of each member there is what makes it so special. The ModernWell magic is real. You are an incredible human being.

To Chris Olsen, Julie Burton and the rest of the team at Publish Her, thank you for your vision and enthusiasm in making my dream of publishing a cookbook a reality. Your belief in my mission has been validating. The experience and knowledge you have shared has been extraordinary. Thank you for creating a unique publishing company that gives authors more of a voice in the process.

To Nina Badzin, thank you for editing all of my recipes and helping me find the right words to share the stories behind them. I have learned so much about writing from you. You are a delight to work with.

To the followers of the Emily's Fresh Kitchen website and social media, thank you for making my recipes and being so kind. We are on this journey to cooking our way to better health together!

Emily Maxson, Author
Emily's Fresh Kitchen Cookbook

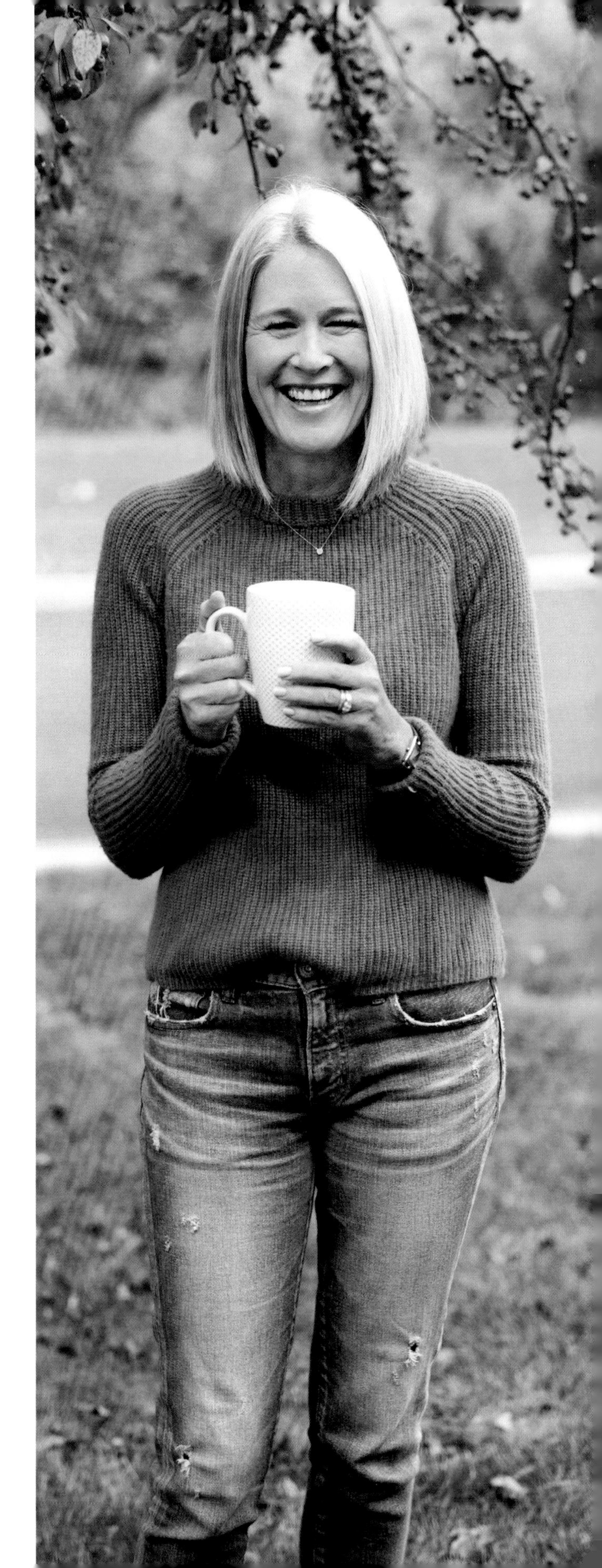

INDEX

C

H

I

J

K

P

Q

R

S

T

V

W

Y

Z

ISBN: 979-8-9850242-2-7
Printed in the United States of America
First Printing: 2022

Published by Publish Her, LLC
2909 South Wayzata Boulevard
Minneapolis, MN 55405
www.publishherpress.com

Photographs by Belén Fleming

Book design by Chris Olsen

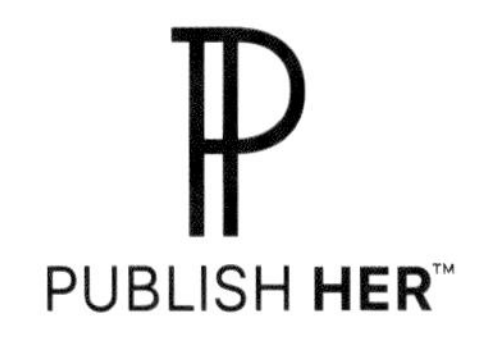